Quick Look Nursing:

Maternal and Newborn Health

JANET ARENSON, MS, RN
Clinical Practitioner of Nursing
Delaware State University
Dover, Delaware

PATRICIA DRAKE, MS, RNC
Instructor
School of Nursing
University of Delaware
Newark, Delaware

World Headquarters
Jones and Bartlett Publishers
40 Tall Pine Drive
Sudbury, MA 01776
978-443-5000
info@jbpub.com
www.jbpub.com

Jones and Bartlett Publishers Canada
6339 Ormindale Way
Mississauga, Ontario L5V 1J2
CANADA

Jones and Bartlett Publishers
International
Barb House, Barb Mews
London W6 7PA
UK

Jones and Bartlett's books and products are available through most bookstores and online booksellers. To contact Jones and Bartlett Publishers directly, call 800-832-0034, fax 978-443-8000, or visit our website, www.jbpub.com.

Substantial discounts on bulk quantities of Jones and Bartlett's publications are available to corporations, professional associations, and other qualified organizations. For details and specific discount information, contact the special sales department at Jones and Bartlett via the above contact information or send an email to specialsales@jbpub.com.

Library of Congress Cataloging-in-Publication Data
Arenson, Janet.
    Maternal and newborn health / Janet Arenson, Patricia Drake.
      p. ; cm. -- (Quick look nursing)
    Includes bibliographical references and index.
    ISBN-13: 978-0-7637-3887-7
    ISBN-10: 0-7637-3887-5
    1. Maternity nursing.   I. Drake, Patricia. II. Title. III. Series.
    [DNLM: 1. Maternal-Child Nursing. 2. Pregnancy Complications.
    WY 157.3 A681m 2007]
    RG951.A74 2007
    618.2--dc22
                                    2006010563
6048

Production Credits
Acquisitions Editor: Kevin Sullivan
Associate Editor: Amy Sibley
Production Director: Amy Rose
Associate Production Editor: Kate Hennessy
Senior Marketing and Project Manager: Emily Ekle
Text Design: Shawn Girsberger
Composition: Shawn Girsberger
Manufacturing and Inventory Coordinator: Amy Bacus
Cover Illustrator: Cara Judd
Cover Layout Design: Timothy Dziewit
Printing and Binding: Malloy, Inc.
Cover Printing: Malloy, Inc

Printed in the United States of America
10 09 08 07 06   10 9 8 7 6 5 4 3 2 1

CONTENTS

PART IX. SIGNIFICANT MEDICAL COMPLICATIONS OF PREGNANCY

PART X. COMPLICATIONS OF LABOR, DELIVERY, AND POSTPARTUM

PART XI. COMPLEX PSYCHOSOCIAL SITUATIONS

PART XII. SELECTED COMPLICATIONS IN THE NEWBORN

PREFACE

During our many years of experience in nursing education and practice, students and staff nurses have asked for guidance in identifying essential content for maternity nursing practice. This book is intended as a quick reference for nursing students, new graduates preparing for licensing examinations, and nurses in perinatal clinical practice. It identifies the most important facts and summarizes current information relevant to maternal and newborn nursing. This resource is not intended to replace more comprehensive maternity textbooks. Readers are also directed to online resources for professional and patient education.

ACKNOWLEDGMENTS

Many people have been supportive of our efforts as we prepared this manuscript. Colleagues in our schools have given encouragement and validated our choices for essential content. We gratefully acknowledge the following individuals. Karen Morin, DSN, RN, encouraged us to undertake the project, reviewed chapters as we completed them, and gave advice whenever requested. Greg Barkley, technical illustrator, prepared figures used in several chapters. Patricia Arenson served as a model for some of the drawings and sketched some additional figures. Michael Arenson assisted with the computer technology needed to submit the materials electronically. Special thanks to our husbands and children for their patience and understanding of the time commitment needed for this project: Michael Arenson, Peter Drake, Mary Jane Drake, Kathryn Drake, Patricia Arenson, and Rebecca Arenson.

I

Reproduction

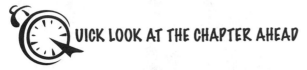

QUICK LOOK AT THE CHAPTER AHEAD

External reproductive organs of the female, called the vulva, are the mons pubis, labia majora, labia minora, clitoris, urethral meatus, paraurethral and vulvovaginal glands, and the perineal body.

Internal reproductive organs of the female are the vagina, uterus, fallopian tubes, ovaries, and the bony pelvis.

These organs aid sexual intercourse and serve as the birth passage.

The size and shape of the true pelvis (the inlet, the midpelvis, and the outlet) are the indicators that a fetus can travel through the birth canal.

A female whose true pelvis is too small for vaginal birth must deliver by cesarean section.

1

Female Anatomy

Nurses need to know the external and internal female anatomical structures and their functions to understand
- how pregnancy occurs
- the resultant changes in a woman's body during pregnancy
- the birth process
- the return to the nonpregnant state.

TERMS
- ☐ vulva
- ☐ mons pubis
- ☐ symphisus pubis
- ☐ labia majora
- ☐ labia minora
- ☐ clitoris
- ☐ urethral meatus
- ☐ paraurethral glands
- ☐ vulvovaginal glands
- ☐ perineum
- ☐ episiotomy

- ☐ vagina
- ☐ rugae
- ☐ uterus
- ☐ perimetrium
- ☐ myometrium
- ☐ endometrium
- ☐ fundus
- ☐ corpus
- ☐ isthmus
- ☐ lower uterine segment
- ☐ cervix
- ☐ internal os

- ☐ external os
- ☐ cervical canal
- ☐ fallopian tubes
- ☐ peristalsis
- ☐ ovaries
- ☐ bony pelvis
- ☐ false pelvis
- ☐ true pelvis
- ☐ diagonal conjungate
- ☐ cephalopelvic disproportion

EXTERNAL REPRODUCTIVE ANATOMY

The female external reproductive organs are collectively called the **vulva**. They are the mons pubis, labia majora, labia minora, clitoris, urethral meatus, paraurethral and vulvovaginal glands, and the perineal body. (See Figure 1-1.)

The **mons pubis** is the fatty tissue over the **symphysis pubis** and is usually covered with hair. It cushions the symphysis pubis during conventionally positioned intercourse.

The **labia majora** are two rounded folds of fatty, connective tissue, covered with pubic hair, that extend from the mons pubis to the perineum. They protect the vaginal opening.

The **labia minora** are narrow folds of hairless skin located within the labia majora, highly vascular and rich in nerve supply. They are highly sensitive and swell in response to erotic stimulation.

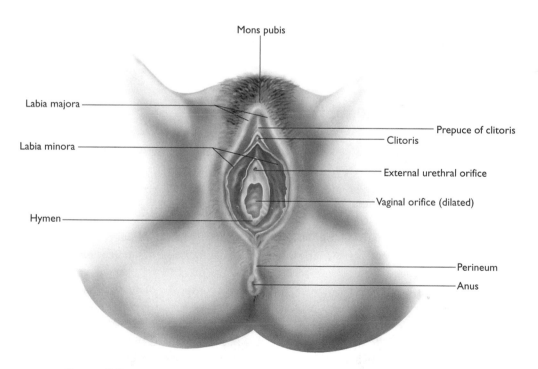

Figure 1-1 External female reproductive anatomy.

The **clitoris** is an erectile organ located beneath the arch of the pubic bone within the folds of the labia. It is extremely sensitive to touch, pressure, and temperature. Its function is sexual stimulation.

The **urethral meatus** is the urinary opening of the urethra. It has a puckered or slit-like appearance, and is located about 1 in. (2.5 cm) below the clitoris.

The **paraurethral glands** (also called Skene's glands) are located inside the urethral meatus and produce mucus for lubrication. These secretions lubricate the vaginal vestibule and make sexual intercourse easier.

The **vulvovaginal glands** (also called Bartholin's glands) are located at the base of each of the labia minora, near the vaginal opening. These glands secrete clear, thick mucus that enhances sperm viability and motility.

The **perineum** is the area between the vagina and the anus. This muscular tissue stretches during childbirth and may be the site of an **episiotomy** or a laceration.

An **episiotomy** is an incision made in the perineum to enlarge the vaginal opening during delivery. It is done to prevent tearing of the perineum.

An episiotomy is an incision made in the perineum to enlarge the vaginal opening during delivery. It is done to prevent tearing of the perineum.

INTERNAL REPRODUCTIVE ANATOMY

The female internal reproductive organs are the fallopian tubes, ovaries, vagina, and uterus. (See Figure 1-2.)

The **vagina** or birth canal is a thin-walled, tubular structure that extends from the vulva to the uterus. It is made of smooth muscle capable of stretching during childbirth and is lined with a glandular mucus membrane arranged in folds called **rugae**. The vagina is a passageway for blood flow during menstruation, sperm during intercourse, and the fetus during delivery.

The **uterus** is a hollow, thick-walled organ composed of an outer layer called the **perimetrium**, a muscle layer called the **myometrium**, and an inner layer called the **endometrium**. The uterus has four parts: the fundus, corpus or body, isthmus, and cervix. It lies behind the symphysis pubis between the bladder and the rectum and above the vagina.

When a woman is not pregnant, her uterus is the shape and size of an

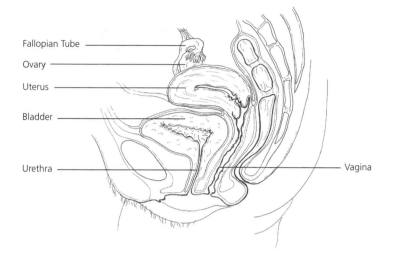

Fallopian Tube

Ovary

Uterus

Bladder

Urethra

Vagina

Figure 1-2 Internal female reproductive anatomy.

upside-down pear. During pregnancy, the uterus stretches to contain the fetus, placenta, membranes, and amniotic fluid.

The **fundus** is the upper rounded portion above the insertion point of the fallopian tubes.

The **corpus** is the main portion of the uterus, located between the fundus and the cervix.

The **isthmus** joins the corpus to the cervix. It is called the **lower uterine segment** during pregnancy.

The **cervix** is divided into the **internal os**, the **canal**, and the **external os**.

The **cervical canal** is a passageway for menstrual flow and sperm. It connects the vagina to the uterine cavity. It is able to dilate to a diameter large enough to allow the fetus to move into the vagina.

During a vaginal exam, the amount of cervical dilation is determined by palpation.

The **fallopian tubes**

 Peristalsis is the coordinated contractions of smooth muscle that occurs like a wave through hollow tubes in the body.

* are a passageway for the sperm to meet the egg.
* move the egg toward the uterus by **peristalsis** and the wavelike movement of a hairlike fringe called cilia.
* secrete nutrients to support the egg during transport.

Peristalsis is the coordinated contractions of smooth muscle that occurs like a wave through hollow tubes in the body.

The fallopian tubes extend from the upper portion of each side of the uterus to the ovaries. Each tube is divided into three parts—the isthmus, ampulla, and infundibulum or fimbria.

The ampulla is the usual site of fertilization.

The **ovaries** are two almond-shaped glandular organs on each side of the pelvic cavity. Their functions are ovulation and the production of estrogen and progesterone. Chapter 2 describes ovarian functions in detail.

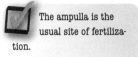
The ampulla is the usual site of fertilization.

BONY PELVIS

The female **bony pelvis** supports and protects the pelvic contents and forms a relatively fixed structure for the birth passage. The components are the iliac crest, the anterior superior iliac spines, the ischial spines, the ischial tuberosities, the symphysis pubis joint, the subpubic arch, the sacrum, and the coccyx. (See Figure 1-3.)

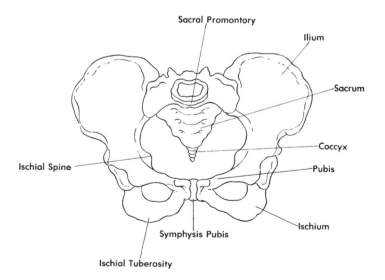

Figure 1-3 Structure of the female bony pelvis.

The **false pelvis** is the shallow cavity above the inlet and is bounded by the iliac crests, the lumbar vertebrae, and the lower abdominal wall above the symphysis pubis.

The **true pelvis** is made up of the inlet, the midpelvis, and the outlet.

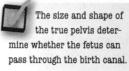 The size and shape of the true pelvis determine whether the fetus can pass through the birth canal.

The size and shape of the true pelvis determine whether the fetus can pass through the birth canal.

The **diagonal conjungate** is the measurement of the inlet from the bottom of the symphysis pubis to the tip of the sacral promontory. The midpelvis measure is the distance (bispinous diameter) between the right and left ischial spines. This is the smallest diameter of the pelvis. The clinical indication that the inlet is large enough for the fetus to enter the true pelvis is the mechanism of labor called engagement. See Chapter 18 for a discussion of the mechanisms of labor.

The outlet is bordered anteriorly (above in front) by the pubic arch and posteriorly (behind) by the distance between the right and left ischial tuberosities.

Pelvic dimensions too small for vaginal birth are called **cephalopelvic disproportion (CPD)**, and require delivery by cesarean section.

What is a cesarean section? Delivery through an incision into the uterus. **See Chapter 52.**

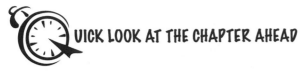 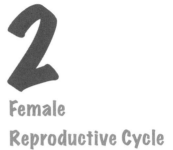

QUICK LOOK AT THE CHAPTER AHEAD

The female reproductive cycle (Figure 2-1) has two components that occur simultaneously:

- The **ovarian cycle** involves the maturation of an egg for ovulation.

- The **menstrual cycle** involves changes in the endometrium of the uterus to prepare for implantation of a fertilized egg.

These cycles are influenced by hormones in the hypothalamic-pituitary-ovarian feedback mechanism.

An understanding of the reproductive cycle is important for the perinatal nurse's role with childbearing families.

Perinatal refers to the time during pregnancy, labor, birth, and one month after birth.

2

Female Reproductive Cycle

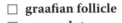

TERMS

- ☐ **graafian follicle**
- ☐ **corpus luteum**
- ☐ **follicular phase**
- ☐ **luteal phase**
- ☐ **menstrual phase**
- ☐ **proliferative phase**
- ☐ **mittelschmerz**
- ☐ **spinbarkeit**
- ☐ **secretory phase**
- ☐ **ischemic phase**
- ☐ **human chorionic gonadotropin (hCG)**
- ☐ **human placental lactogen (hPL)**
- ☐ **human chorionic somatomammotropin (hCS)**
- ☐ **relaxin**

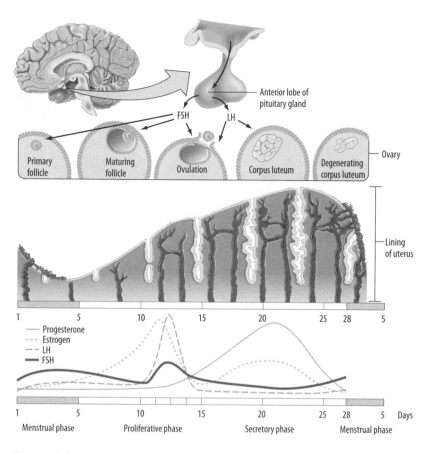

Figure 2-1 The female reproductive cycle.

HYPOTHALAMIC-PITUITARY-OVARIAN MECHANISM

A feedback loop controls ovarian function. During menstruation, estrogen levels are low. These low levels trigger the hypothalamus to send gonadotropin-releasing hormone to the anterior pituitary. The anterior pituitary responds by secreting follicle-stimulating hormone (FSH) and luteinizing hormone (LH). FSH stimulates the ovary to mature one follicle, called the **graafian follicle**. LH stimulates ovulation—the release of the mature egg from the graafian follicle. The ruptured follicle (the **corpus luteum**) secretes both estrogen and progesterone. If the egg is not fertilized, the corpus luteum disintegrates, lowering circulating levels of estrogen and progesterone. Low levels of estrogen initiate menstruation, and another cycle begins.

During each menstrual cycle, usually only one follicle ripens and it is called the graafian follicle after the Dutch physician, Regnier de Graaf, who first described it.

 During each menstrual cycle, usually only one follicle ripens, and it is called the graafian follicle after the Dutch physician, Regnier de Graaf, who first described it.

 ## OVARIAN CYCLE

On day 1 of the menstrual cycle, several follicles in the ovary are maturing. Usually one primary follicle (the graafian follicle) completes maturation during a cycle. This **follicular phase** ends with ovulation, the release of the egg from the graafian follicle. The phase may last 7 to 22 days.

The **luteal phase** begins with ovulation. The ruptured graafian follicle develops into the corpus luteum and secretes estrogen and progesterone. These hormones prepare the lining of the uterus to receive the egg if it is fertilized. The length of this phase is less variable and usually lasts 14 days. If conception does not occur, this phase ends when menstruation begins.

MENSTRUAL CYCLE

There are four phases of the menstrual cycle: menstrual, proliferative, secretory, and ischemic. The **menstrual phase** lasts usually 2 to 8 days, with a total blood loss averaging 30 ml. During this phase the endometrial lining is shed, estrogen levels are low, and cervical mucus is scanty, thick, and opaque.

The **proliferative phase** begins when the lining of the uterus thickens, and continues until ovulation occurs. Estrogen levels peak just before ovulation.

Occasionally ovulation is accompanied by midcycle pain called **mittelschmerz.**

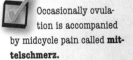 Occasionally ovulation is accompanied by midcycle pain called **mittelschmerz.**

At the end of this phase, the cervix softens and relaxes to admit sperm. During ovulation, cervical mucus becomes more plentiful, has a thinner and more stretchy consistency, and forms columns to facilitate the transport of sperm into the uterus.

The stretchy property of cervical mucus is called **spinbarkeit.**

The **secretory phase** follows ovulation. Estrogen drops sharply and progesterone increases significantly. The blood supply of the entire uterus increases. The uterus is prepared for implantation.

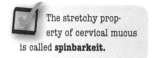

The stretchy property of cervical mucus is called **spinbarkeit.**

The **ischemic phase** begins if fertilization and implantation do not occur. Because the corpus luteum is disintegrating, estrogen and progesterone fall. Small blood vessels constrict and rupture, with blood escaping into the uterus. Menstruation begins.

HORMONAL CHANGES WITH PREGNANCY

When fertilization takes place and pregnancy begins, other hormonal changes occur. Several hormones are necessary to maintain pregnancy: progesterone, estrogen, human chorionic gonadatropin, human placental lactogen, and relaxin. Most of them are secreted initially by the corpus luteum, but as the placenta develops, it gradually increases production of these hormones. If the corpus luteum stops functioning before then, spontaneous abortion will occur.

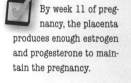

By week 11 of pregnancy, the placenta produces enough estrogen and progesterone to maintain the pregnancy.

By the week 11 of pregnancy, the placenta produces enough estrogen and progesterone to maintain the pregnancy.

Progesterone is essential to maintaining pregnancy. It causes the lining of the uterus to become thicker, inhibits premature contraction of the uterus, and initiates development of the breast for lactation. Estrogen is responsible for enlarging the uterus and breasts and increasing vascularity, especially in the capillaries of the placenta at the end of pregnancy.

Human chorionic gonadotropin (**hCG**) is produced by cells in the fertilized ovum that will become the placenta, and prevents disintegration of the corpus luteum at the end of the menstrual cycle. It also causes the corpus luteum to continue to secrete progesterone and estrogen until the placenta is developed enough to take over this function. It can be detected in maternal blood when implantation occurs, usually 8 to 10 days after fertilization, and in maternal urine at the time of the first missed menstruation. The presence of hCG is the basis for pregnancy testing of urine and blood.

Human placental lactogen (hPL), also called human chorionic somatomammotropin (hCS), is produced by the placenta. This hormone is an antagonist to insulin, increases the amount of free fatty acids avail-

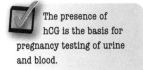

The presence of hCG is the basis for pregnancy testing of urine and blood.

able for metabolic needs, and decreases maternal metabolism of glucose. These changes ensure that nutrients are available for the fetus. Levels of hPL rise with placental growth.

Relaxin is produced primarily by the corpus luteum early in pregnancy, but small amounts are secreted by the placenta and uterus during pregnancy. It is detectable in maternal blood serum at the time of the first missed menstrual period. Like progesterone, relaxin also decreases uterine contractility, thus helping maintain the pregnancy.

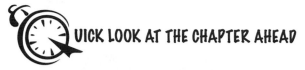

The primary function of the male reproductive system (Figure 3-1) is to create and deposit sperm in the female vagina during sexual intercourse so that fertilization can occur.

The external male reproductive organs are the penis, the glans, and the scrotum. The scrotum protects the testes and the sperm by regulating their temperature.

Sexual stimulation causes the penis to become erect. At sexual climax, rhythmic contractions of the penile muscles expel (ejaculate) semen containing sperm.

The internal male reproductive organs (gonads) are the testicles (testes), the epididymis, vas deferens, ejaculatory ducts, urethra, seminal vesicles, prostate, bulbourethral glands, and urethral glands.

Semen or seminal fluid from the testes is composed of sperm and the secretions from the accessory glands.

The head of a sperm contains the genetic material. The tail is essential for motility.

In the average ejaculate there are about 100 million sperm per milliliter. Once ejaculated, sperm can live only 2 to 3 days in the female genital tract.

The nurse needs to know male anatomy and physiology to understand human reproduction.

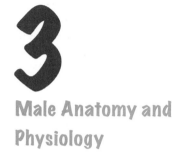

3

Male Anatomy and Physiology

TERMS
- [ ] penis
- [ ] glans
- [ ] foreskin
- [ ] erection
- [ ] ejaculate
- [ ] scrotum
- [ ] gonads
- [ ] testes
- [ ] epididymis
- [ ] vas deferens
- [ ] male accessory glands
- [ ] seminal vesicles
- [ ] prostate
- [ ] bulbourethral glands
- [ ] urethral glands
- [ ] semen

EXTERNAL STRUCTURES

The penis is part of both the urinary and the reproductive systems. Urine is expelled through the urethra.

The **penis** is a cylindrical, pendulous organ suspended from the front and side of the pubic arch. It consists of a body called the shaft and a cone-shaped end called the **glans**. The penis is composed mainly of erectile tissue covered with skin.

The glans is covered with a movable hood called the **foreskin** or prepuce, which may be surgically removed or circumcised.

Sexual stimulation of the parasympathetic nerves causes the blood vessels of the penis to become engorged. This causes the penis to elongate, thicken, and stiffen, and normally point upward, a process called **erection**. At sexual climax, forceful rhythmic contractions of the penile muscles expel or **ejaculate** semen containing sperm.

The **scrotum** is a pouch that hangs in front of the anus and behind the penis. It contains two testes and the epididymis. The function of the scrotum is to protect the testes and the sperm by maintaining a fairly constant temperature, lower than the rest of the body.

The scrotum is sensitive to touch, pressure, temperature, and pain.

The penis is part of both the urinary and the reproductive systems. Urine is expelled through the urethra.

The glans is covered with a movable hood called the **foreskin** or prepuce, which may be surgically removed or circumcised.

Sexual stimulation of the parasympathetic nerves causes the blood vessels of the penis to become engorged. This causes the penis to elongate, thicken, and stiffen, and normally point upward, a process called **erection**. At sexual climax, forceful rhythmic contractions of the penile muscles expel or **ejaculate** semen containing sperm.

The function of the scrotum is to protect the testes and the sperm by maintaining a fairly constant temperature, lower than the rest of the body.

INTERNAL STRUCTURES

The male internal reproductive organs are called **gonads** and include

- the testes or testicles
- a system of ducts including the epididymis, vas deferens, ejaculatory duct, and the urethra
- accessory glands including the seminal vesicles, prostate gland, bulbourethral glands, and urethral glands.

The **testes** are two oval-shaped glandular organs that produce sperm and testosterone. Sperm production is the result of complex neural and hormonal control. As in the female reproductive system, the hypothalamus secretes factors that stimulate the anterior pituitary to release FSH and LH. These hormones cause the testes to secrete testosterone, which maintains the production of sperm and seminal fluid. Testosterone is also responsible for the development of secondary male characteristics and is thought to stimulate aggressiveness and sexual drive.

> Testosterone is also responsible for the development of secondary male characteristics and is thought to stimulate aggressiveness and sexual drive.

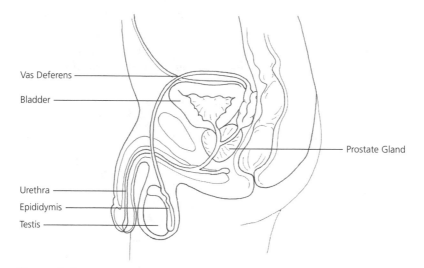

Figure 3-1 The male reproductive anatomy.

The male system of ducts begins with the **epididymis**, a convoluted tube about 13 to 20 feet long that lies behind each testis. It serves as a reservoir for sperm for 2 to 10 days. As the sperm are transported through the epididymis, they become mobile and capable of fertilizing an ovum.

The **vas deferens** is about 18 inches long and connects the epididymis to the prostate gland. The end of each vas deferens expands to form a terminal ampulla, which unites with the seminal vesicle duct to form the ejaculatory duct that enters the prostate gland. The main function of the vas deferens is to transport sperm from the epididymis into the urethra. The male urethra is a duct for passage of both semen and urine.

The **male accessory glands** are structures that secrete components of the seminal fluid in an ordered sequence.

The **seminal vesicles** are glands situated above the prostate gland that secrete clear, thick, alkaline fluid. During ejaculation this fluid combines with sperm in the ejaculatory ducts and provides an environment suitable for sperm motility and metabolism.

The **prostate** gland surrounds the neck of the bladder and the urethra. It secretes a thin, milky, alkaline fluid. This fluid protects the sperm from the acidity of the vagina and the male urethra. An acidic environment destroys sperm.

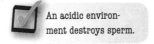 An acidic environment destroys sperm.

The **bulbourethral glands** are on either side of the urethra. They secrete a clear, thick, alkaline fluid. This fluid enhances sperm motility by lubricating the penile urethra during sexual excitement, and neutralizes the acid in the male urethra and the vagina.

The **urethral glands** are small mucus-secreting glands throughout the lining of the penile urethra that contribute to the volume of the seminal fluid.

Semen or seminal fluid is ejaculate, composed of sperm and the secretions from all of the accessory glands. Sperm have two parts: the head and the tail. The head contains the genetic material; the tail is essential for motility.

Sperm have two parts: the head and the tail. The head contains the genetic material; the tail is essential for motility.

Sperm may be stored in the male genital tract for up to 42 days, depending primarily on the frequency of ejaculation. Once ejaculated, sperm can live only 2 to 3 days in the female genital tract. In the average ejaculate there are about 100 million sperm per milliliter.

In the average ejaculate there are about 100 million sperm per milliliter.

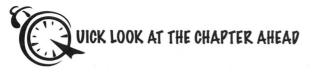

Non-pharmacological methods of contraception are abstinence, fertility awareness (the rhythm method), condoms, diaphragm, and female and male sterilization by tubal ligation or vasectomy.

Couples may choose these methods to avoid the side effects of hormones, contained in the pharmacological methods.

It is important for perinatal and women's health nurses to assist couples in making decisions about methods of contraception. They can discuss the contraceptive method, advantages, disadvantages, risk factors, and contraindications with clients and their partners.

Information to assist with decision making includes medical and obstetrical history, age parity, religion, educational level, socioeconomic level, smoking habits, comfort with touching one's body, frequency of sexual activity, and number of partners.

Other factors to consider are effectiveness and safety of the method, side effects, convenience of use, cost, and preferences of the couple.

4

Contraception: Non-Pharmacological Methods

TERMS
- [ ] abstinence
- [ ] fertility awareness methods
- [ ] condoms
- [ ] diaphragm
- [ ] tubal ligation
- [ ] vasectomy

Abstinence from sexual intercourse is the only method that is 100% effective against pregnancy. It requires commitment, self-control, and agreement by both partners. Counseling should include discussion of alternative ways of expressing intimacy with a partner.

 Abstinence may be unacceptable to the couple and cause relationship problems.

Fertility awareness methods, also called natural family planning, are based upon an understanding of the menstrual cycle and ovulation. (See Table 4-1.) These methods rely upon the understanding that ovulation occurs approximately 14 days before the onset of menses, egg life is approximately 24 hours, and sperm life is about 48 to 72 hours. Fertility awareness methods require careful record keeping for at least 6

Table 4-1 Fertility Awareness Methods

Method	Description	Period of Abstinence
Calendar or rhythm method	The woman needs to collect data about the length of her menstrual cycles for at least 6 months. On a calendar, she would record the first day of her menses and determine the length of each cycle. By subtracting 18 days from the shortest cycle and 11 days from the longest cycle, a woman can estimate her fertile period.	Abstain from intercourse during the estimated fertile period.
Cervical mucus method	The woman evaluates her cervical mucus for changes in stretchiness, wetness, color, and clearness. Ovulation is predicted on the condition of the mucus.	Abstinence during the fertile period when cervical mucus is wet, clear, and stretchable.
Basal Body Temperature (BBT)	The woman measures her basal body temperature every morning before any activity and records it on a graph. There is a drop prior to ovulation and a rise in temperature after ovulation occurs.	Abstain from intercourse for several days before the expected time of ovulation and for 3 days after ovulation.
Symptothermal method or Combination method	The woman evaluates and records cycle days, cervical mucus changes, increased libido, abdominal bloating, mittelschmerz (midcycle abdominal pain), and basal body temperature to determine ovulation time.	Abstinence for several days before and 3 days after ovulation.

months on length of menstrual cycle, basal body temperature, and consistency of vaginal mucus. Some period of abstinence each month is required to avoid fertile periods of the cycle. Partners need to be cooperative and supportive.

Advantages of fertility awareness methods are that they are free, have no side effects, are preferred by couples whose religious beliefs prohibit them from using other methods, and are also useful for planning a pregnancy.

Male and female **condoms** are barrier methods of preventing pregnancy and sexually transmitted diseases. They should be used in combination with spermicidal foam to increase effectiveness.

Fertility aware-ness methods require careful record keeping for at least 6 months on length of menstrual cycle, basal body temperature, and consistency of vaginal mucus.

Some period of absti-nence each month is required to avoid fertile periods of the cycle. Partners need to be cooperative and supportive.

Male and female condoms should not be used together.

Male condoms are small, lightweight, disposable, and inexpensive. Female condoms are much larger in size and more expensive than male condoms.

Male condoms are placed over an erect penis with room at the tip for the deposit of semen. Immediately after ejaculation, the penis should be withdrawn while holding the condom in place.

Condoms decrease sensation, can be messy, and can break or slip.

The female condom can be inserted into the vagina up to 8 hours before intercourse and is held in place by inner and outer rings. Condoms decrease sensation, can be messy, and can break or slip.

 Sensitivity to latex can cause severe allergic reactions.

Condoms are recommended to prevent sexually transmitted diseases for couples who are not in long-standing, mutually monogamous relationships.

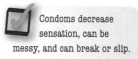 Condoms are recom-mended to prevent sexually transmitted diseases for couples who are not in long-standing, mutually monogamous relationships.

The **diaphragm** is another barrier method. It is a round flexible device that covers the cervix. It must be fitted for size by a health care provider. A diaphragm is inserted into the vagina up to 6 hours before intercourse. It is used with spermicidal jelly or cream and must remain in place for at least 8, but no more than 24 hours after intercourse.

Use of the diaphragm may increase the risk of urinary tract infections from pressure on the urethra and the risk of toxic shock syndrome if used for a prolonged period during menses.

Tubal ligation or female sterilization is a surgical procedure in which both fallopian tubes are tied, cut, or blocked in order to prevent conception. About half of the procedures are done in the immediate postpartum period because access to the fallopian tubes is much easier at this time. The procedure does not affect hormonal levels or sexuality.

Women should be informed that tubal ligation is considered a permanent procedure; attempts to reverse it surgically are often unsuccessful. Only women who are certain that they do not want more children should undergo the procedure.

Vasectomy or male sterilization is a surgical procedure in which the vas deferens is cut and tied or cauterized. Sterility is achieved after sperm has cleared the ducts through numerous ejaculations. A sperm count is then done to determine effectiveness.

Some men may have psychological reservations about having this procedure performed. It may interfere with their feelings of manhood.

Vasectomy should be considered permanent, although it is sometimes successfully reversed.

 Vasectomy should be considered permanent, although it is sometimes successfully reversed.

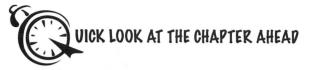
Most pharmacological methods prevent ovulation through hormonal influence, and the copper IUD interferes with sperm motility.

The contraceptive skin patch contains a combination of estrogen and progestin. Oral contraceptive pills contain a combination of estrogen and progestin or progestin only. A vaginal ring, a small, flexible ring inserted into the vagina, contains estrogen and progestin. They all inhibit the release of an egg and change cervical mucus.

A single rod implant inserted under the skin of the upper inner arm releases synthetic progesterone to prevent ovulation for about three years.

Depo-Provera, an intramuscular injection containing synthetic progesterone, suppresses ovulation and produces cervical mucus that decreases sperm motility.

An intrauterine device (IUD) decreases sperm motility and initiates an inflammatory response in the endometrium. IUDs are recommended only for women with children.

Emergency contraception (EC) is used to prevent pregnancy after unprotected intercourse.

Research and development on other methods of contraception include new spermicidal products, hormonal methods to decrease sperm production in males, and female sterilization through the use of quinacrine.

5

Contraception: Pharmacological Methods

TERMS
- [ ] side effects
- [ ] contraindications
- [ ] oral contraceptive pills
- [ ] contraceptive skin patch
- [ ] vaginal ring
- [ ] single rod implant
- [ ] Depo-Provera
- [ ] intrauterine device (IUD)
- [ ] emergency contraception

21

Couples may choose pharmacological methods because they are very effective, separate from the act of intercourse, convenient, and private.

Couples may choose pharmacological methods because they are very effective, separate from the act of intercourse, convenient, and private.

Side effects of oral contraceptive and other hormonal contraceptives range from breakthrough bleeding, headache, nausea, breast tenderness, acne, depression, fatigue, and weight gain, to thrombophlebitis, pulmonary embolism, and cerebrovascular accident.

Contraindications (reasons not to use) include pregnancy, breast or other estrogen-dependent cancer, recurrent chronic cystic mastitis, a history or presence of thrombophlebitis or thromboembolic disorders, cerebral vascular or coronary artery disease, myocardial infarction, serious liver disease, gall bladder disease, hypertension, diabetes, hyperlipidemia, heavy smoking, undiagnosed abnormal vaginal bleeding, and women over age 40.

 More than half of the women who use hormonal methods discontinue their use in the first year because of side effects such as bleeding, nausea, weight gain, breast tenderness, or headache.

Newer methods of contraception such as the transdermal patch, vaginal ring, single rod implant, and the intrauterine device have fewer side effects and require less supervision by a health care provider.

The use of hormonal contraceptives is associated with an increased risk of cardiovascular side effects, especially in women over 35 years of age and women who smoke.

It is strongly advised that women not smoke while using hormonal contraceptive therapies.

Oral contraceptive pills contain a combination of estrogen and progestin or progestin only. These hormonal medications inhibit the release of an egg and change cervical mucus. Although there are several brands and varieties of oral contraceptives, all must be prescribed by a health care provider.

Although there are several brands and varieties of oral contraceptives, all must be prescribed by a health care provider.

Some packets contain 28 pills, of which 21 have hormones and 7 are placebos. Other packets contain 21 pills. A woman is instructed to take one pill daily.

If one pill is missed, it is taken as soon as remembered. The next pill is taken as usual.

If two pills are missed, the woman takes a pill every 12 hours until she is caught up, then she continues through the cycle. Backup contraception is recommended for the next week.

If more than two pills are missed, emergency contraception, discussed later, should be considered.

Women on oral contraceptives should contact their health care provider if they experience severe side effects. (See Table 5-1.)

A woman is instructed to take one pill daily.
• If one pill is missed, it is taken as soon as remembered. The next pill is taken as usual.
• If two pills are missed, the woman takes a pill every 12 hours until she is caught up, then she continues through the cycle. Backup contraception is recommended for the next week.
• If more than two pills are missed, emergency contraception should be considered.

The **contraceptive skin patch** contains a combination of estrogen and progestin. One patch is placed on the abdomen, buttocks, upper outer arm, or upper torso, but not the breast. It is replaced each week for 3 weeks, rotating sites; then it is not used for 1 week to allow for menstruation. The 28-day cycle is then repeated.

A **vaginal ring** is a small, flexible ring containing estrogen and progestin inserted deep into the vagina for 3 out of every 4 weeks. A new ring is used for each 4-week cycle. A vaginal ring does not need to be removed for intercourse, but may be taken out for up to 3 hours if it interferes with sexual sensation.

A vaginal ring does not need to be removed for intercourse, but may be taken out for up to 3 hours if it interferes with sexual sensation.

Table 5-1 ACHES: Serious Side Effects of Oral Contraceptives

A	Abdominal pain
C	Chest pain or shortness of breath
H	Severe headaches
E	Eye problems such as dizziness, vision loss, or blurring of vision
S	Severe leg pain or swelling

Hatcher, R.A., Zieman, M., Cwiak,C., Darney, P.D., Creinin, M.D., & Stosur, H.R. (2004). *A pocket guide to managing contraception.* Tiger, GA: Bridging the Gap Foundation.

A **single rod implant** can be inserted under the skin of the upper inner arm. Synthetic progesterone is released to prevent ovulation for about 3 years.

Depo-Provera is an intramuscular injection containing synthetic progesterone, given every 3 months. It suppresses ovulation and produces thick cervical mucus that decreases sperm motility. It is very effective, convenient, private, and inexpensive compared to other methods.

> With the use of Depo-Provera, menstrual bleeding is usually diminished or may be absent; clear explanations of this side effect are important.

> When Depo-Provera is discontinued, there may be a delay in fertility for 9 to 10 months.

An **intrauterine device (IUD)** provides contraception by decreasing sperm motility and initiating an inflammatory response in the endometrium. It contains copper or progesterone, and is inserted into the uterus by a health care provider. It is highly effective, provides continuous contraceptive protection, and is relatively inexpensive over time.

Side effects include increased bleeding and cramping during menstruation and irregular menstrual cycles. Complications are uterine perforation, pelvic inflammatory disease, and expulsion of the IUD. Newer IUDs reduce these side effects and complications. Nurses should teach the woman to look for and report any early warning signs of complications. (See Table 5-2.)

> Nurses should teach the woman to look for and report any early warning signs of complications.

Table 5-2 PAINS: Serious Side Effects of Intrauterine Devices

P	Period late; abnormal spotting or bleeding
A	Abdominal pain; pain during sexual intercourse
I	Infection exposure; STIs
N	Not feeling well; fever and chills
S	String missing, shorter, or longer

Hatcher, R.A., Zieman, M., Cwiak, C., Darney, P.D., Creinin, M.D., & Stosur, H.R. (2004). *A pocket guide to managing contraception.* Tiger, GA: Bridging the Gap Foundation.

IUDs are not recommended for women who have not had children, or with a history of pelvic inflammatory disease, or who have multiple sexual partners.

If pregnancy occurs with an IUD in place, there is an increased risk for miscarriage and premature labor.

Emergency Contraception (EC)

Emergency contraception is used to prevent pregnancy after unprotected intercourse. There are three options:

- insertion of a copper IUD
- ingestion of high-dose progesterone-only pills (POP), also known as Plan B
- ingestion of a high-dose combination of oral contraceptive pills (COC).

The IUD is used if a woman intends to continue this contraceptive method. The oral medications are available by prescription only, but several medical, nursing, and public health organizations have recommended that Plan B be approved by the FDA for over-the-counter use.

The oral medications are taken as two doses. The first dose is taken as soon as possible within 72 hours of unprotected intercourse; the second dose is taken 12 hours later.

Emergency contraceptive pills inhibit ovulation if taken before it occurs, and decrease the tubal transport of sperm. The main side effects of the pills are nausea and vomiting.

> The IUD is used if a woman intends to continue this contraceptive method.

> The oral medications are available by prescription only, but several medical, nursing, and public health organizations have recommended that Plan B be approved by the FDA for over-the-counter use.

Deep vein thrombosis has occurred in women using COCs as emergency contraceptives.

Since oral emergency contraceptive pills have become available in the United States, the rate of abortion has decreased.

Since oral emergency contraceptive pills have become available in the United States, the rate of abortion has decreased.

Research and Development

Research and development on other methods of contraception include new spermicidal products, hormonal methods to decrease sperm production in males, and female sterilization through the use of quinacrine.

Hormonal methods for males include administration of testosterone alone or combined with progestin, using injections, transdermal patches, and pellet implants. Side effects are oily skin, acne, mild gynecomastia, and increased fat mass.

Quinacrine sterilization is a nonsurgical technique. Quinacrine pellets are inserted into the uterine cavity, similarly to IUD insertion. Insertion must be done on day 6 to day 12 of the menstrual cycle to minimize the risk of doing it during a pregnancy. Some quinacrine migrates to the fallopian tubes, causing inflammation and scarring that blocks the tubes. Two insertions are done a month apart to ensure complete blockage of the tubes.

PART I · QUESTIONS

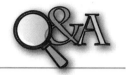

1. What part of the uterus will a nurse directly assess for dilation in a laboring client?
    a. Cervix
    b. Isthmus
    c. Corpus
    d. Fundus

2. What term identifies a measurement of the midpelvis?
    a. Pubic arch
    b. Diagonal conjugate
    c. Bispinous diameter
    d. Ischial tuberosities

3. What happens under the influence of follicle-stimulating hormone (FSH) and luteinizing hormone (LH)?
    a. Menstrual cycle begins.
    b. Ovulation occurs.
    c. Graafian follicle degenerates.
    d. Secretory phase ends.

4. What hormone indicates that a woman is pregnant?
    a. Estrogen
    b. Progesterone
    c. Luteinizing hormone
    d. Human chorionic gonadotropin

5. What statement by a client would indicate that a diaphragm is not the best contraceptive choice for her?
    a. "My boyfriend says that it is a woman's job to keep herself from getting pregnant."
    b. "I am not sure that I want to mess up my body taking those hormones."
    c. "My mother always taught me not to touch myself down there."
    d. "I have a hard time remembering to take my vitamins every day."

6. What structure is interrupted in the male sterilization procedure?
   a. Epididymis
   b. Vas deferens
   c. Seminal vesicle
   d. Bulbourethral gland

7. Which statement by a woman would indicate to the nurse that further teaching about fertility awareness is needed?
   a. "Eggs live a lot longer that sperm. Sperm live about 2 to 3 hours."
   b. "There will be a drop in my temperature before ovulation."
   c. "Ovulation usually happens 14 days before my next period begins."
   d. " I am fertile when the cervical mucus is wet, clear, and stretchable."

8. A woman who is receiving Depo-Provera reports breast tenderness, weight gain, and leg pain. What would be the most appropriate response for the nurse to give this client?
   a. "Many women have these side effects with this medication."
   b. "Report the symptoms to your health care provider."
   c. "That is normal. Don't worry about it."
   d. "These symptoms should go away after a few months."

9. What advice should the nurse give a woman who reports missing one oral contraceptive pill?
   a. "You should use backup contraception for the next week."
   b. "That is OK, just take the next one at the usual time."
   c. "You might need to get a prescription for emergency contraception."
   d. "Take the pill now and take the next one at the usual time."

10. Which contraceptive method would be recommended only for women who have had children?
    a. Vaginal ring
    b. Diaphragm
    c. Intrauterine device
    d. Symptothermal method

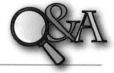

PART I · ANSWERS AND RATIONALES

1. **The answer is a.** The cervix is the part of the uterus that dilates in labor. It can be felt during a vaginal exam. The other answers list the portions of the uterus that are not directly accessible.

2. **The answer is c.** The bispinous diameter is the distance between the ischial spines. The plane of the midpelvis is at the level of the ischial spines. The diagonal conjugate is the measurement of the inlet of the pelvis. The pubic arch and the ischial tuberosities are the borders of the pelvic outlet.

3. **The answer is b.** Both follicle-stimulating hormone (FSH) and lutenizing hormone (LH) must be present for ovulation to occur. FSH and LH are not being secreted when the menstrual cycle begins. The graafian follicle changes into the corpus luteum after ovulation; the corpus luteum will degenerate if pregnancy does not occur. When estrogen and progesterone decrease, the secretory phase ends.

4. **The answer is d.** Human chorionic gonadotropin (hCG) is the hormone needed to maintain the corpus luteum during pregnancy. The fertilized ovum produces hCG. The other hormones listed do not indicate pregnancy.

5. **The answer is c.** Using a diaphragm requires a woman to be comfortable with touching her genitals and inserting a finger into her vagina to check for proper placement. The other answers indicate factors that would make the diaphragm a good choice for this client.

6. **The answer is b.** The vas deferens in the structure that is cut and tied or cauterized during a vasectomy. The other structures are not affected by a vasectomy.

7. **The answer is a.** Fertility awareness relies on a woman's understanding the menstrual cycle and ovulation, as well as knowledge about the life span of the egg and sperm. Sperm life is longer than egg life—between 48 and 72 hours. The other answers indicate an accurate understanding of fertility awareness methods.

8. **The answer is b.** Side effects that should be reported to a health care provider are those covered by the acronym ACHES. Leg pain is one such symptom. The other answers do not acknowledge the seriousness of the symptoms being reported.

9. **The answer is d.** When one oral contraceptive pill is not taken, the woman should take the pill as soon as she remembers and then continue with the usual routine. Backup contraception is suggested if two pills are missed; emergency contraception should be considered if more than two pills are missed.

10. **The answer is c.** Because the intrauterine device increases the risk of pelvic inflammatory disease, which may lead to infertility, it is not recommended for women who have not had children. The other methods given as options do not influence fertility after discontinuance and may be used by any woman.

II

Psychosocial Aspects of Childbearing

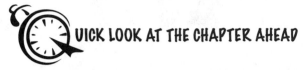

The time of pregnancy, birth, and return to a non-pregnant state is called the "childbearing year." The transition to parenthood begins during pregnancy and takes place over time after the birth.

Family is defined as "a group of people related by blood, marriage, or adoption living together." Two structures are family of origin and family of procreation. Family members perform a variety of roles. The family responds to the pregnancy according to their families of origin, cultural beliefs and practices, and societal expectations.

The modern U.S. family is smaller, giving new parents less experience with childrearing practices. More families have both parents working; experience increased mobility; fall below the poverty level; are homeless; have one parent; experience more violence; and need educational and support services.

The nurse needs to understand concepts related to the family and the interactions of its members in order to provide appropriate care.

6

The Family During the Childbearing Year

TERMS

- ☐ family of origin
- ☐ family of procreation
- ☐ stages of development
- ☐ transition to parenthood
- ☐ societal factors

DEFINITIONS OF FAMILY

According to the U.S. Census Bureau (2000), family is defined as "a group of people related by blood, marriage, or adoption, living together." Current definitions of family recognize that family members are not always legally related and may not always live in the same household. Instead, family is perceived as people who give support and share common goals concerning the family's well-being. The people who will be supportive of a woman throughout the childbearing year are her family.

The people who will be supportive of a woman throughout the childbearing year are her family.

TYPES OF FAMILIES

Families come in many types, and members of the family may change over time. There are two basic family structures: family of origin and family of procreation. **Family of origin** refers to the family into which a person is born, and **family of procreation** is the family a person chooses to establish. (See Table 6-1.)

FAMILY FUNCTIONS

The family performs certain tasks to meet the needs of individual family members.

- Food, clothing, shelter, safety, and health care are the physical needs of the family.
- Families are the first teachers; children learn many things before they enter school.
- Socialization of children and other family members to the expectations of the family and community occurs within the family.
- Decisions about use of time, financial resources, material goods, and space are made within the family, and priorities are usually set based upon fairness to all members.
- Work is divided and roles are defined within the family unit.
- Most family members support each other in times of crisis.

Family members function in a variety of roles. Some task-oriented roles are financial manager, wage earner, problem solver, decision maker, nurturer, health manager, and homemaker. Some roles are defined by relationship, such as spouse, mother, father, daughter, son, sister, and brother.

FAMILY DEVELOPMENTAL STAGES

The family passes through predictable **stages of development** based on the age of the oldest child. Family stages begin with a couple forming a relationship and end with the death of both members of the couple.

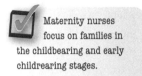

Maternity nurses focus on families in the childbearing and early childrearing stages.

Maternity nurses focus on families in the childbearing and early childrearing stages. (See Table 6-2.)

FAMILY RESPONSES TO CHILDBEARING

Having a child is a turning point in the life of a family. The way that the family responds to the reality of the pregnancy is influenced by experiences in their families of origin, cultural beliefs and practices, and societal expectations. Some of the areas in which members of the family might view pregnancy as a challenge are

- accepting the role of mother or father
- incorporating the baby as a new family member
- changing financial needs
- altering family dynamics.

The commitment to parent a child is a developmental milestone for an adult and can be a time of growth or difficulty. Toward the end of the pregnancy, the mother and father prepare for parenthood by taking classes, buying the layette, and getting an infant care area ready.

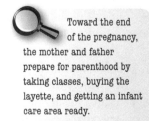

Toward the end of the pregnancy, the mother and father prepare for parenthood by taking classes, buying the layette, and getting an infant care area ready.

The **transition to parenthood** begins during pregnancy and takes place over time after the birth.

Table 6-1 Types of Families

Type	Description
Nuclear	Married mother, father, and their biological children. Most classic family theories are based on this family structure.
Cohabitation	An unmarried man and woman who live together. There may be children from this relationship.
Extended	Multiple generations of a family living together. May include grandparents, aunts, uncles, and cousins.
Single parent	One parent living with children. In most situations, the single parent is the mother.
Blended/Stepfamily	A parent with children marries another person with or without children.
Communal	Groups of people who have chosen to live together as an extended family.
Gay or Lesbian	Individuals of the same sex living together as partners. There may or may not be children.
Foster	A legal arrangement is made for children to be cared for by someone outside their family.
Informal fostering	Grandparents, aunts, or uncles assume responsibility for child-rearing.
Adoptive	A legal arrangement in which adults unrelated to the child become the parents of that child.

Table 6-2 Duvall's Family Developmental Stages

Stage	Description
1 - Marriage	A couple forms a commitment to each other
2 - Early Childbearing Family	Begins with the birth or the adoption of the first baby and ends when the first child becomes 2 years of age
3 - Family with Preschool Children	When the first child is between the ages of 2 and 5 years
4 - Family with School-Age Children	When the first child is between the ages of 6 and 12 years
5 - Family with Adolescent Children	When the first child is 13 years old to when the child leaves home
6 - Launching Family	Begins when the oldest child leaves home and ends when the youngest child leaves home
7 - Family of Middle Years	The family returns to a two-partner relationship
8 - Family of Older Age	Begins with the retirement of the first member of the couple and ends with the death of both members of the couple

Adapted from Hockenberry, M., Wilson, D., Winkelstein, M.L., & Kline, N.E. (2003). *Wong's nursing care of infants and children* (7th ed.). St Louis, MO: Mosby.

THE MODERN FAMILY

Some **societal factors** in current family life in the United States influence the childbearing experiences of families.

- The modern family is smaller, giving new parents less experience with childrearing practices.
- More families have both parents working.
- Quality child care may be difficult to obtain.
- The number of roles required of women is greater.
- Families experience increased mobility as members move from place to place, providing less family support.
- More families fall below the poverty level, resulting in less prenatal care and inadequate nutrition.
- There is more homelessness, particularly in families headed by women.
- There are more one-parent families as a result of an increased divorce rate and societal acceptance of single parenthood.
- A pregnancy may precipitate or increase violence within a family.
- Some families are taking more responsibility for their health, prompting a need for more educational and support services.

ASSESSMENT OF THE FAMILY

Assessment of the family by the nurse is necessary in order to understand how the family interacts with each other and with their community. Tools have been developed to assess family structure, family health history, and interactions within the family.

Assessment of the family by the nurse is necessary in order to understand how the family interacts with each other and with their community. Tools have been developed to assess family structure, family health history, and interactions within the family.

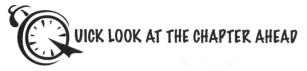

QUICK LOOK AT THE CHAPTER AHEAD

The family is part of a larger group—the community.

The community assists the modern childbearing family to meet its needs, providing support usually given by the extended family.

The community helps the family purchase food, clothing, and household goods, and provides housing, safety, health care needs, and opportunities for education, socialization, and leisure.

During the childbearing year, the woman receives care from the community: prenatal care, home visits, time off from work for health care visits, and child-care resources.

The nurse assesses community resources and evaluates the family's ability to access them.

The nurse needs to understand the relationship between a family and its community in order to provide appropriate care to individuals within a family.

1

The Childbearing Family Within the Community

TERMS
- [ ] **community**
- [ ] **support network**
- [ ] **windshield survey**

MODEL FOR COMMUNITY AS A PLACE OF SUPPORT

A model for the community as a place of support depicts the community helping the family meet its needs. (See Figure 7-1.) At the center of the circle is the family. Six categories of family needs are the wedges in the larger circle surrounding the family. Selected community services that will help the family meet its needs are listed in each category. The line between the family and the needs is open to indicate that the family must be able to access community services to meet their needs.

Community is usually referred to as a limited geographic area in which residents interact as they perform their daily activities.

> **Community** is usually referred to as a limited geographic area in which residents interact as they perform their daily activities.

The health of the individuals within the community is related to the presence of certain factors. For example, air and water quality, protection by police and fire departments, and rate of unemployment are areas in which the community influences the health of the individual.

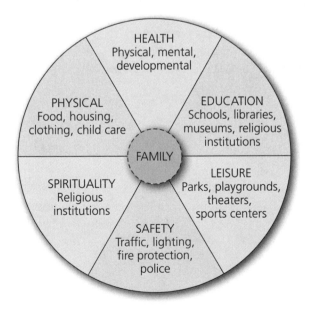

Figure 7-1   Model of community support.

COMMUNITY AS A PLACE OF GENERAL SUPPORT FOR FAMILIES

The childbearing family members may be away from their extended family and have little experience in childrearing practices. The community can provide some of the support usually given by the extended family.

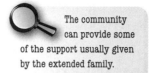
The community can provide some of the support usually given by the extended family.

The community is more than official agencies; it is also the **support network** of friends, neighbors, co-workers, and religious institutions.

The community helps the family perform its tasks in several ways:

- Places for the family to purchase food, clothing, and household goods
- A variety of housing options
- Safety features, such as police and fire departments, traffic regulations, sidewalks, adequate lighting of public spaces (streets and shopping centers), and appropriate places for recreation
- Health care needs in office, clinic, school, workplace, and hospital settings
- Education, socialization, and leisure at schools, libraries, religious institutions, and cultural or recreational facilities

COMMUNITY SUPPORT FOR THE CHILDBEARING FAMILY

The childbearing year lasts 10.5 months; unless there are complications, the woman is only in the hospital for 3 to 4 days. The rest of the time she is receiving care in the community.

The pregnant woman receives prenatal care from health care providers such as physicians, nurse practitioners, or nurse midwives in office or clinic settings. Many women receive home visits by nurses to assess mother and baby as part of their routine postpartum health care.

Before and after the baby's birth, the work setting may provide time off for health care visits, health education classes, maternity and family leave, facilities for the breastfeeding mother to pump and store her breastmilk, and child-care resources. One of the most

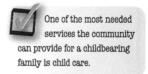
One of the most needed services the community can provide for a childbearing family is child care.

needed services the community can provide for a childbearing family is child care.

When a childbearing woman has problems during pregnancy or postpartum, she needs special services from the community. If there is a complication, many women remain at home rather than being hospitalized. The at-home services the family might need from the community include cooking, cleaning, financial assistance, equipment, and counseling, as well as health care.

COMMUNITY ASSESSMENT

In order to know if the community is going to be able to help a particular family, the nurse needs to make some assessment of the community. The ideal would be to visit the community and conduct a direct **windshield survey** of housing, open spaces, transportation, shopping areas, signs of decay, and characteristics of the residents.

The most practical approach to assessing a community is by asking the family questions about their neighborhood, what resources are available to them, and how they might access those services within their community. (See Table 7-1.)

By asking questions of the family, the nurse can raise their awareness of what is available and how they might use it, and can evaluate the family's ability to access community services. Factors to consider are transportation, cost, and convenience.

A windshield survey is when one drives around and looks at the community.

The most practical approach to assessing a community is by asking the family questions about their neighborhood, what resources are available to them, and how they might access those services within their community.

By asking questions of the family, the nurse can raise their awareness of what is available and how they might use it, and can evaluate the family's ability to access community services. Factors to consider are transportation, cost, and convenience.

Table 7-1 Community Assessment Questions

Topic	Suggested Questions
Home	Describe your house or apartment. Is there anything about your living arrangements that will make it difficult for you to take care of the baby?
Neighborhood	Do you live in a city, suburb, or the country? Describe your neighborhood.
Safety	How safe do you feel in your home and neighborhood? Are there sidewalks? How busy are the streets? What kind of lighting is there? How far away are the police and fire departments?
Transportation	What means of transportation are available in the community? What do you use for transportation?
Health	Where does your family go for health care? Where is the closest place to go for emergencies? Where do you get your medications?
Shopping	Where is the closest place to buy food, clothing, and household items? Where do you do most of your shopping?
Child care	Are there child-care resources in your community? Do you plan to use them?
Education	Where are the closest schools and libraries? What experiences have you had using them?
Leisure	Where are the closest recreational facilities: parks, playgrounds, gyms, museums, theaters, and sports centers? What experiences have you had using them?
Spirituality	Where do you and your family go for experiences that bring inner peace?

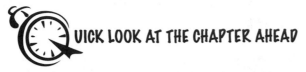

Cultural beliefs and practices determine how the woman will respond to her care during the child-bearing year. The nurse needs to be open to the cultural beliefs and practices of each family.

When client and nurse do not speak the same language, interpreters are preferred.

In providing perinatal care, it is impossible to avoid invading intimate space for physical examinations, urinary catheterizations, breastfeeding assistance, and comforting. Explanations to client and family and respect for modesty are ways to reduce anxiety about intrusion into intimate space. Asking permission prior to touching a client is culturally competent nursing care.

Some cultures may not accept modern technological advances, practice long-term planning, or follow schedules. The nurse needs to appreciate differences in time orientation.

In traditional families, male and female activities are defined by gender. In modern families, they tend to be shared.

Cultural restrictions on women and children may limit their activities with people outside the family.

The acceptance of health care recommendations may be influenced by the client's sense of control over the situation.

The meaning of food varies among cultures and eating has strong social significance. To insure adequate nutrition, exploring dietary preferences during the perinatal period is vital.

8

Culturally Competent Perinatal Care

TERMS
- [ ] communication
- [ ] translators
- [ ] interpreters
- [ ] space and touch
- [ ] time orientation
- [ ] social organization
- [ ] environmental control
- [ ] nutrition
- [ ] spiritual beliefs and practices

Spiritual beliefs and practices that do not increase risk to the mother or baby should be respected. If there is any health risk, explanations should be given and compromises explored.

The nurse needs to understand how cultural beliefs and practices may affect the family's acceptance of health care recommendations. Respect for the client's culture is essential for providing culturally competent perinatal care. (See Table 8-1.)

In the United States, the current dominant ethnic group of western European descent will be less than 50% of the total population by 2050. Although patients are ethnically and culturally diverse, the nursing profession is less so. Consequently, the nurse is more likely to be of a culture different from the family for whom care is being provided.

Table 8-1 Definitions Pertinent to Cultural Competence

Term	Definition
Cultural competence	Understanding and appreciation of cultural differences and ability to adapt clinical skills and practices to meet the needs of the individual client
Enthnocentrism	Belief that one's own beliefs and practices are the only correct way of doing things; therefore, different beliefs and practices are incorrect
Stereotyping	Oversimplified assumption that all members of a particular group share the same values, beliefs, and practices
Generalizing	Using knowledge about a specific cultural group as a basis for assessing an individual within the culture
Acculturation	Process of modifying one's own culture in response to contact with another culture
Assimilation	Incorporation of the characteristics of the dominant culture into one's own values, beliefs, and practices
Spirituality	Beliefs and practices giving meaning to life and providing strength to the individual

CULTURAL CONSIDERATIONS

Some areas in which beliefs and practices may vary among cultural groups include communication, space and touch, time orientation, social organization, environmental control, nutrition, and spirituality.

Communication

Communication includes primary language spoken, voice volume and tone, eye contact, facial expressions, and hand gestures. In some cultures, loud voice volume and tone, as well as hand gestures, may indicate anger or hostility. Sometimes facial expressions showing teeth may be considered as aggression. Not making eye contact with a person of authority is considered a sign of respect in some cultures: direct eye contact may be viewed as confrontational.

When client and nurse do not speak the same language, translators or interpreters may be used. **Translators** restate the exact words with no interpretation of their meaning; **interpreters** provide the meaning of the information without direct translation of all the words.

In order to be sure that the patient understands the information, interpreters in the health care field are preferred.

> When client and nurse do not speak the same language, translators or interpreters may be used. **Translators** restate the exact words with no interpretation of their meaning; **interpreters** provide the meaning of the information without direct translation of all the words.

Clients who have limited proficiency in the dominant language may nod or say "yes" during explanations; however, such affirmation should not be perceived by the nurse as the client's fully understanding the information being given.

Space and Touch

Clients of differing cultures may regard **space and touch** in a variety of ways. Space refers to the distance with which a person is comfortable for certain interactions. Intimate space is up to 18 in. around the body; personal space is from 18 in. to 4 ft, and social space is more than 4 ft.

In providing perinatal care, it is impossible for the nurse to avoid invading intimate space for physical examinations, urinary catheterizations, breastfeeding assistance, and comfort. Explanations to the client and family and respect for modesty are ways the nurse can reduce anxiety about intrusion into intimate space.

Touch is a form of nonverbal communication and is used in caregiving activities such as assessments, procedures, and comfort. Touch may have different significance among families of diverse cultures.

Asking permission prior to touching a client is one way for the nurse to practice culturally competent nursing care.

> In providing perinatal care, it is impossible for the nurse to avoid invading intimate space for physical examinations, urinary catheterizations, breastfeeding assistance, and comfort. Explanations to the client and family and respect for modesty are ways the nurse can reduce anxiety about intrusion into intimate space.

> Asking permission prior to touching a client is one way for the nurse to practice culturally competent nursing care.

Time Orientation

Time orientation is having a focus on the past, present, or the future. Cultures that focus on the past are more likely to adhere to tradition and may not accept modern technological advances.

In a present-oriented culture, the focus is on the current situation. Acceptance of long-term health care recommendations or planning may be difficult.

> Cultures that focus on the past are more likely to adhere to tradition and may not accept modern technological advances.

In future-oriented cultures, the focus is on planning for the future, and health promotion activities are more readily accepted. Although individual cultural groups may have a predominate time orientation, elements of all orientations usually exist in families living in the United States because of acculturation.

Another aspect of time is adherence to a set schedule. This may affect health care behaviors such as being on time for appointments, taking medications at specified times, or following an immunization schedule.

The nurse needs to appreciate differences in time orientation in order to be nonjudgmental about a family's concern for the well-being of its members.

>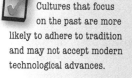
> The nurse needs to appreciate differences in time orientation in order to be nonjudgmental about a family's concern for the well-being of its members.

Social Organization

Social organization refers to roles within the family and relationships of the family with the outside world. Some cultures are patriarchal, with a male as the chief decision-maker. Other cultures are matriarchal with a female as the chief decision-maker. In more traditional families, child care and household chores are defined by gender. In modern childbearing families, decision making and household chores tend to be shared between male and female partners.

Interaction of family members with the outside community is affected by cultural beliefs about gender roles and behaviors. Restrictions on women and children may limit their activities with people outside the family. The type of community associations and clubs to which the family may belong are influenced by culture and socioeconomic status.

There may be behaviors that are required or prohibited associated with the perinatal period. For example, in some cultures, it is believed that the fetus may strangle in the umbilical cord if the pregnant woman reaches over her head. In the Mexican culture, wearing a metal object on the abdomen during pregnancy is believed to prevent birth defects. In Vietnamese culture, washing the infant's head during the bath may be upsetting to the family because of taboos against touching the head.

> There may be behaviors that are required or prohibited associated with the perinatal period. For example, in some cultures, it is believed that the fetus may strangle in the umbilical cord if the pregnant woman reaches over her head. In the Mexican culture, wearing a metal object on the abdomen during pregnancy is believed to prevent birth defects. In Vietnamese culture, washing the infant's head during the bath may be upsetting to the family because of taboos against touching the head.

Environmental Control

Environmental control is the perception of one's ability to control destiny. This includes a definition of health, causative factors for illness, and practices to promote health and treat illness. The acceptance of health care recommendations may be influenced by the client's sense of control over the situation. If a family believes that they have control over the future of their health, they are more likely to seek health care and engage in health promotion behaviors.

Nutrition

Nutrition has broader implications than meeting the body's dietary needs. The meaning of food varies among cultures and eating has strong social significance.

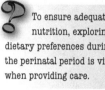 The meaning of food varies among cultures and eating has strong social significance.

Foods may be used to convey love and acceptance, to promote health, and to treat disease. Withholding certain types of food may be culturally prescribed in certain health or illness conditions. In several cultures, there is meaning to hot and cold foods and beverages as a way to restore balance to the body. Celebrations and rituals in which food is a component are in every culture.

To ensure adequate nutrition, exploring dietary preferences during the perinatal period is vital when providing care.

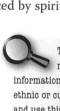 To ensure adequate nutrition, exploring dietary preferences during the perinatal period is vital when providing care.

Spiritual Beliefs and Practices

Most members within a particular ethnic group share common **spiritual beliefs and practices**. Religious or spiritual meaning might be associated with prayer or meditation, holy writings, and religious objects such as pictures, prayer beads, altars, and amulets. Specific rituals surrounding significant life events such as birth, illness, and death may provide comfort. Other aspects of culture such as nutrition, social organization, and environmental control are influenced by spiritual beliefs and practices.

Health care providers need to explore with the family how their spiritual beliefs are related to health care practices before making health promotion recommendations.

The nurse needs to seek out information about individual ethnic or cultural groups and use this as the basis for collecting data about a particular family. (See Table 8-2.)

Health care providers need to explore with the family how their spiritual beliefs are related to health care practices before making health promotion recommendations.

The nurse needs to seek out information about individual ethnic or cultural groups and use this as the basis for collecting data about a particular family.

Every member of an ethnic group does not necessarily adhere to the same beliefs and practices. However, information about the culture is a basis for discussion and asking pertinent questions. It is important to avoid stereotypic thinking. Practices that do not increase risk to the mother or baby should be respected. If there is any health risk, explanations should be given and compromises explored.

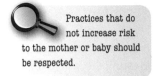

Practices that do not increase risk to the mother or baby should be respected.

Table 8-2 Questions for Assessing Cultural Variations in Perinatal Care

Perinatal Period	Questions
Antepartum	What is the significance of this pregnancy and child to the family? Is this pregnancy planned and desired? What significance is placed on the gender of the child? Is this a first child or first grandchild? What changes in the status of the woman will occur because of this pregnancy? Is pregnancy viewed as something that requires medical intervention? What are pregnant women supposed to eat or drink? What are pregnant women supposed to do or avoid?
Intrapartum	Who is supposed to be present during birth? Who will deliver the baby? How is the woman allowed to express her pain in labor? What position is best for labor and birth? What comfort measures are desired? Is there a special way to dispose of the placenta and umbilical cord?
Postpartum	What food is the woman supposed to eat or drink? What kind of activities is the woman allowed to do? How active is the mother in the newborn's care? When does the woman start breastfeeding? How are heat and cold used to promote comfort? How long does the recovery from the birth last?
Newborn	What is the significance of naming the baby? When is the baby named? How might bonding behaviors be different? How are infant care procedures different: feeding, bathing, dressing, or umbilical cord care? What spiritual practices are important: circumcision, baptism, blessings, or last rites?

PART II • QUESTIONS

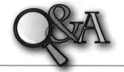

1. A family consists of a 32-year-old woman married to a 35-year-old man, the woman's 6-year-old daughter from a previous relationship, the couple's 3-year-old son, and a newborn daughter. What type of family is this?
    a. Adoptive
    b. Blended
    c. Extended
    d. Nuclear

2. The members of a family include a 3-year-old son, 7-year-old twin daughters, and a 28-year-old single mother. In what developmental stage is this family?
    a. Early childbearing family
    b. Family with preschool children
    c. Family with school-age children
    d. Launching family

3. The children in a family attend a local public school. With what family function is the community assisting?
    a. Distribution of resources
    b. Division of labor
    c. Meeting physical needs
    d. Socialization of the children

4. In the hospital, a nurse is discussing child care with a postpartum woman. What would be the most appropriate way to collect information about community services available to the woman?
    a. Ask the woman questions
    b. Look in the telephone book
    c. Review the community's website
    d. Visit the community

5. The nurse is helping a postpartum woman to breastfeed. What nursing action would be most appropriate with regard to invasion of intimate space?
    a. Ask to loosen her clothing
    b. Explain actions before touching her
    c. Pull the curtain around the bed
    d. Shut the door to the room

6. A newly delivered woman is transferred to the postpartum unit. Which of the following remarks by the nurse would reflect the most awareness of the client's culture?
   a. "Do you need help to go to the bathroom?"
   b. "I will help you into the nursery to see the baby's bath."
   c. "Taking a shower would make you feel better."
   d. "Would you prefer your water iced or room temperature?"

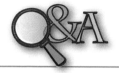

PART II · ANSWERS AND RATIONALES

1. **The answer is b.** The family in the question fits the description of a blended/stepfamily. The other options are not accurate.

2. **The answer is c.** The developmental stage of a family depends on the age of the oldest child. The 7-year-old twin daughters are school age.

3. **The answer is d.** The community helps the family to meet its needs. Much of the socialization and education of children takes place in schools. Although schools play a part in meeting the physical needs of children, it is not their primary function. The other options are not appropriate.

4. **The answer is a.** Although the nurse may do any of these activities, the one that is most readily available and would reveal what the client knows about her community already would be option a. Options b and c might be done after determining the woman's knowledge about her community. Option d is not realistic for a hospital-based nurse.

5. **The answer is b.** Breastfeeding assistance is an activity that puts the nurse in the intimate space of the woman. Explanations and respect for modesty reduce anxiety associated with intrusion into intimate space. In option a the nurse is not invading intimate space. Options c and d are actions to respect privacy, but do not specifically address intimate space.

6. **The answer is d.** Allowing the patient to make a choice and being aware of cultural differences with respect to hot and cold beverages are reflected in option d. Options a, b, and c reflect assumptions by the nurse about postpartum behaviors and do not take possible cultural differences into consideration.

III

Antepartum Period: The Pregnant Client

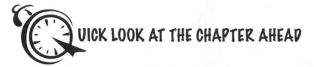

The pre-embryonic stage is the first 14 days of a pregnancy. The embryonic stage occurs between the third and the eighth week of gestation. The fetal stage is the period between week 9 of gestation and birth. About week 24, when the fetus weighs about 500 g, it is considered to be viable, capable of survival outside the uterus.

The placenta is the organ where metabolic and nutrient exchange between the maternal and fetal circulations takes place. The umbilical cord connects the fetal circulatory system to the placenta through two arteries and one vein. The two fetal membranes are the outer chorion and the inner amnion. Amniotic fluid protects the fetus from injury, helps maintain fetal temperature, and provides a medium for fetal movement.

During the embryonic and fetal stages, organ formation occurs.

- Brain and central nervous system: week 4 to week 28

- Heart and cardiovascular system: week 4 to week 28

- Lungs and respiratory system: week 6 to week 37

- Musculoskeletal system: week 4 to week 30

- Gastrointestinal system: week 4 to week 16

- Genitourinary system: week 7 to week 12

9

Embryonic and Fetal Development

Development of fetal weight and length:

- At 12 weeks, 45 g and 8 cm

- At 20 weeks, 435 g and 20 cm

- At 24 weeks, 680 g and 28 cm

- At 28 weeks, 1200 g and 35 cm

- At 36 weeks, 1800–2800 g and 45 cm

- At 40 weeks, 3000–3600 g and 50 cm

 Because health practices during pregnancy have a major impact on fetal well-being, knowledge of fetal development can be used by nurses in patient teaching to promote healthy behaviors and avoid possible teratogenic effects on the fetus. Explaining fetal development to prospective parents can promote parental bonding and the perception of the fetus as a developing person.

Teratogenic: causing abnormal development and birth defects.

TERMS
- ☐ **pre-embryonic stage**
- ☐ **blastocyst**
- ☐ **embryonic stage**
- ☐ **fetal stage**
- ☐ **placenta**
- ☐ **diffusion**
- ☐ **chorion**
- ☐ **amnion**

STAGES OF DEVELOPMENT

The **pre-embryonic stage** is the first 14 days of a pregnancy. It begins with conception (fertilization of a mature ovum by a sperm). This takes place in the ampulla of the fallopian tube.

Cell division starts immediately after conception. Over the next week, the fertilized ovum travels through the fallopian tube to the uterus.

Between 7 and 10 days after conception, implantation occurs when the fertilized ovum, now called a **blastocyst**, becomes attached to the wall of the uterus.

Cells now have differentiated into three layers from which all tissues, organs, and organ systems will develop: the ectoderm, mesoderm, and endoderm.

The **embryonic stage** occurs between weeks 3 and 8 of gestation. During this stage, the placenta, membranes, and umbilical cord form. By week 8 of pregnancy, every major organ system and external structure are present.

The embryonic stage is the period of most vulnerability to teratogens.

The **fetal stage** is the period between week 9 of gestation and birth. During this stage, refinement of the systems and development of organ function occur.

When the fetus weighs about 500 g, it is considered to be viable or capable of survival outside the uterus. Viability usually begins at about week 24 of pregnancy.

EMBRYONIC AND FETAL STRUCTURES

The **placenta** is the organ where metabolic and nutrient exchange between the maternal and fetal circulations takes place. It develops at the site of implantation, covers about half of the inside of the uterus at term, and weights approximately 1 lb at term. By week 13 of pregnancy, the placenta is fully formed and functioning.

The placenta produces hormones that are integral to the maintenance of the pregnancy: human chorionic gonadotropin (hCG), human placental lactogen (hPL), estrogen, and progesterone.

In the placenta, the fetal and maternal circulations do not connect directly. Nutrients and gases cross placental membranes through **diffusion**. The umbilical cord connects the fetal circulatory system to the placenta through two arteries and one vein.

Diffusion is the process in which a substance moves from an area of higher concentration to an area of lower concentration.

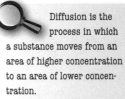

Diffusion is the process in which a substance moves from an area of higher concentration to an area of lower concentration.

There are two fetal membranes: the outer **chorion** and the inner **amnion**. These membranes line the uterus and contain the fetus, the umbilical cord, and the amniotic fluid. The cells of the amnion produce amniotic fluid; however, in the second half of the pregnancy, excretion of fetal urine also contributes to amniotic fluid volume. At term, the amount of amniotic fluid is about 1 liter.

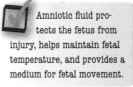

Amniotic fluid protects the fetus from injury, helps maintain fetal temperature, and provides a medium for fetal movement.

Amniotic fluid protects the fetus from injury, helps maintain fetal temperature, and provides a medium for fetal movement.

MAJOR MILESTONES IN FETAL DEVELOPMENT

During the embryonic and fetal stages, organ formation occurs. (See Figure 9-1.)

Brain and Central Nervous System

By week 4, the neural tube closes. By week 5, the brain differentiates. By week 12, one half of the size of the fetus is the head, and spontaneous movement of the fetus occurs. By week 20, the fetus is active, with sucking reflex and periods of wake and sleep. By week 28, the nervous system begins to regulate some body functions and body temperature.

Heart and Cardiovascular System

By week 4, a tubular heart beats, major veins are completed, and primitive red blood cells circulate. By week 6, chambers of the heart are present. By week 8, development of the heart is essentially complete and a heart beat is audible by Doppler technology. Between weeks 16 and 20, the fetal heart beat is audible by a specialized stethoscope called a fetoscope. By week 28, the fetal heart rate accelerates in response to fetal movement.

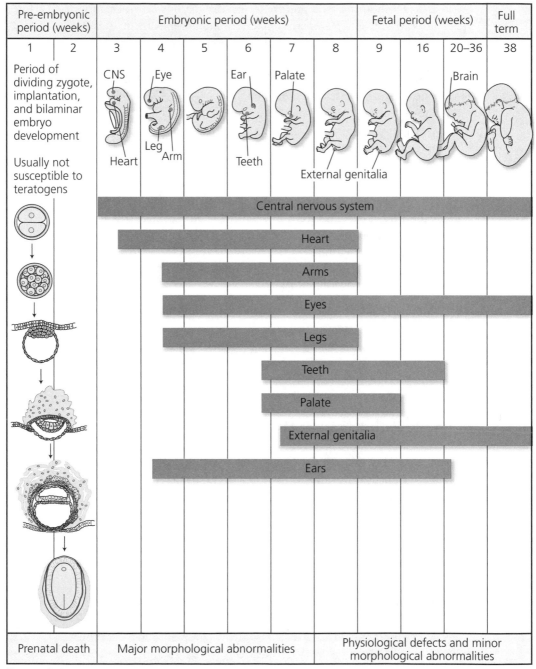

Figure 9-1 Critical periods of organogenesis.

Lungs and Respiratory System

By week 6, the trachea, bronchi, and lung buds are present. By week 7, the diaphragm has formed. Between weeks 13 and 16, the lungs are fully shaped. By week 24, alveoli are developing, primitive respiratory movements begin, surfactant production begins, and gas exchange is possible. By week 37, the lecithin/sphingomyelin (L/S) ratio is greater then 2:1, indicating lung maturity.

Musculoskeletal System

By week 4, there are noticeable limb buds. By week 6, there is a primitive skeletal shape forming. By week 12, the limbs are long and slender with all the fingers and toes. Spontaneous movements are present by week 13, but may not be detected by the mother until weeks 16 to 18. By week 30, bones are fully developed, but soft and flexible.

Gastrointestinal System

By week 4, the respiratory and upper digestive tracts have separated to form the esophagus and trachea. By week 16, the mouth and palate are completely formed. By week 20, the fetus begins to suck and swallow amniotic fluid; however, these reflexes are not mature until about week 32. Meconium, consisting of cellular wastes, bile, and fats, forms in the intestine starting at week 16.

Genitourinary System

By week 7, the lower gastrointestinal and the genitourinary tracts separate. By week 8, external genitalia are present. Sex is distinguishable by observation at week 12. Rudimentary kidneys are present by week 4. Urine production begins by week 12.

Weight and Length

- At 12 weeks, the fetus weighs about 1.5 ounce (45 g) and is about 3 in. (8 cm) in length.
- At 20 weeks, fetal weight is about 1 lb (435 g) and length is about 8 in. (20 cm).

- At 24 weeks, fetal weight is about 1.5 lb (680 g) and length is 11 in. (28 cm).
- By 28 weeks, the fetus weighs about 2.5 lb (1200 g) and is about 14 in. (35 cm).
- At 36 weeks, average fetal weight is 5 to 6 lb (1800–2800 g) and length is 18 in. (45 cm).
- At 40 weeks, average fetal weight is 6.5 to 8 lb (3000–3600 g) and length is 20 in. (50 cm).

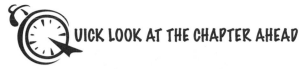

Pregnancy is a time of numerous maternal physical changes that occur to meet the demands of the growing fetus and to prepare for birth and lactation.

The uterus increases 20 times. The cervix softens, becomes more vascular, and produces increased mucus. A mucus plug seals the cervix. Egg production stops in the ovaries. The vagina increases in vascularity, the mucosa thickens, and connective tissue loosens. Vaginal secretions become more acidic.

Glandular tissue and fat deposits increase in the breasts. Colostrum, a precursor to breastmilk, is produced.

Blood volume and cardiac output increase 30 to 50%; stroke volume increases 50%. Blood pressure usually lowers, then rises to baseline in the third trimester. Hemodilution can lead to physiologic anemia of pregnancy. Clotting factors increase.

The lungs adjust to provide increased amounts of oxygen. The diaphragm is displaced upward. The ribs flare out slightly and lungs expand laterally. Tidal volume increases 30 to 40%, total oxygen consumption increases 20%, and the respiratory rate increases.

The kidneys increase renal plasma flow 30 to 50%, glomerular filtration rate 50%, and urine output 25%. Within the kidney the renal pelvis dilates and the ureters elongate and twist. Urinary stasis occurs.

10

Maternal Physical Adaptations to Pregnancy

TERMS
- [ ] **mucus plug**
- [ ] **colostrum**
- [ ] **physiologic anemia of pregnancy**
- [ ] **linea nigra**
- [ ] **melasma**
- [ ] **striae gravidarum**

The bladder increases in capacity and decreases in tone. The smooth muscle of the stomach and intestines relax. The ligaments and joints of the pelvis soften and relax.

The woman's center of gravity changes. The enlarging uterus may cause diastasis recti, the separation of the rectus muscles of the abdominal wall.

Skin pigmentation changes. Stretch marks may appear on the abdomen, breasts, thighs, and hips. Almost all aspects of the endocrine system increase. Resistance to infection decreases.

 Understanding normal physiologic changes of pregnancy will assist the nurse to differentiate between normal and abnormal findings.

 Pregnant women require explanations about physical adaptations to pregnancy in order to incorporate these changes into their body image. (See Figure 10-1.)

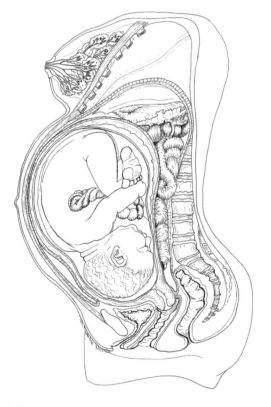

Figure 10-1 Anatomical changes in the third trimester of pregnancy.

REPRODUCTIVE SYSTEM

The uterus will increase 20 times in size as it stretches to accommodate the growing fetus. In response to increasing estrogen levels, the cervix softens, becomes more vascular, and produces increased mucus. A **mucus plug** seals the cervix, preventing infection from entering the uterus.

The elevated estrogen and progresterone levels during pregnancy prevent egg production in the ovaries. Increased estrogen levels prepare the vagina for birth by increasing vascularity, thickening the mucosa, and loosening connective tissue. Vaginal secretions become more acidic, decreasing the risk of bacterial infection, but increasing the risk of yeast infection.

High estrogen levels prepare the breasts for lactation by increasing the amount and size of glandular tissue and fat deposits. **Colostrum**, a precursor to breastmilk, is produced by week 16 of pregnancy.

CARDIOVASCULAR SYSTEM

By week 28 of pregnancy, the heart and blood vessels have adapted to accommodate additional maternal and fetal circulations. Blood volume and cardiac output have increased by 30 to 50%, while stroke volume has increased by 50%. Blood pressure usually drops during

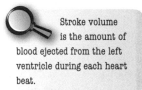
Stroke volume is the amount of blood ejected from the left ventricle during each heart beat.

pregnancy because of vasodilation of the blood vessels from progesterone. The lowest blood pressure level occurs during the second trimester, and gradually returns to baseline during the third trimester.

Hemoglobin and hematocrit decrease in relation to plasma volume because red blood cell (RBC) production increases less rapidly than plasma volume.

This hemodilution can lead to **physiologic anemia of pregnancy**. Hemoglobin less than 11 g/dL or hematocrit less than 35% is considered indicative of anemia. Clotting factors increase, placing the woman at risk for the development of thromboses and alterations in coagulation.

The white blood cell (WBC) count at the end of pregnancy may range from 6000 to 16,000 in labor, and early postpartum WBC count may reach 30,000 without being indicative of infection.

RESPIRATORY SYSTEM

To meet the increased metabolic needs of the mother and fetus, the lungs must adjust to provide increased amounts of oxygen. As the uterus enlarges, the diaphragm is pushed upward, decreasing the length of the lungs. To

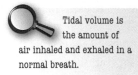
Tidal volume is the amount of air inhaled and exhaled in a normal breath.

compensate for this, the ribs flare out slightly and lungs expand laterally. Tidal volume increases by 30 to 40%, total oxygen consumption increases 20%, and respiratory rate increases by 1 to 2 breaths per minute.

Because estrogen increases vascularity, nasal congestion and nasal stuffiness are common. Nosebleeds may occur.

URINARY SYSTEM

The kidneys must excrete waste products for both mother and fetus. Renal plasma flow increases by 30 to 50%, glomerular filtration rate increases by 50%, and urine output increases by 25%. Structural changes within the kidney include dilation of the renal pelvis and elongation and twisting of the ureters.

Glomerular filtration rate is the rate at which the blood is filtered across the capillaries in the part of the kidney called the glomerulus.

Urinary stasis occurs and increases the risk of pyelonephritis. Pyelonephritis is an infection in the kidneys.

The bladder increases in capacity and decreases in tone due to the influence of progesterone. The enlarging uterus puts pressure on the bladder, resulting in more frequent urination.

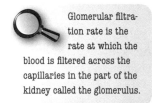
The enlarging uterus puts pressure on the bladder, resulting in more frequent urination.

Urinary stasis in the bladder can lead to bladder infection that may ascend to the kidney.

GASTROINTESTINAL SYSTEM

Changes in the gastrointestinal system contribute to many discomforts of pregnancy. Nausea and vomiting in the first trimester are associated with increased human chorionic gonadotropin (hCG) levels of early pregnancy. The smooth muscle of the stomach and intestines relaxes from elevated progesterone levels, causing delayed gastric emptying, heartburn, and constipation. Displacement of these organs during the second half of pregnancy creates pressure on blood vessels below the uterus, resulting in increased risk for hemorrhoids.

MUSCULOSKELETAL SYSTEM

The hormones relaxin and progesterone soften and relax the ligaments and joints of the pelvis during pregnancy to facilitate birth, but may cause discomfort and a waddling gait. The center of gravity changes with the enlarging uterus, resulting in changes in posture, such as increased lordosis. The enlarging uterus may cause diastasis recti, the separation of the rectus muscles of the abdominal wall. This may persist in the postpartum period until the muscle tone of the abdomen is regained.

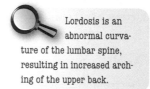

Lordosis is an abnormal curvature of the lumbar spine, resulting in increased arching of the upper back.

INTEGUMENTARY SYSTEM

Changes in skin pigmentation occur, due to the increased amount of hormones during pregnancy:

- **Linea nigra** is a darkening line up the center of the abdomen from the symphysis pubis to above the umbilicus.
- **Melasma**, commonly called "mask of pregnancy," is a darkening of the skin on the cheeks, forehead, and nose.
- Because the skin stretches to accommodate the enlarging uterus, **striae gravidarum,** or stretch marks, may occur on the abdomen, breasts, thighs, and hips.

After birth, when the hormones return to nonpregnant levels, these skin changes regress but may not entirely disappear.

ENDOCRINE SYSTEM

Almost all aspects of the endocrine system increase during pregnancy, including hormone production by the pituitary, thyroid, parathyroid, and adrenal glands. The greatest change in this system is the addition of the placenta as an endocrine organ.

IMMUNOLOGICAL SYSTEM

The immune system changes to prevent rejection of the fetus. There is decreased resistance to infection as a result of a decrease in immunoglobulin G levels and T-cell function. However, the increase in WBC production may counteract these deficiencies.

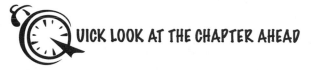
In preparing to become a couple with a child, the expectant family must deal with many changes. Behaviors used to express psychological responses can vary by culture. Childrearing behaviors must be blended from both families.

The woman experiences various emotions and incorporates her role as a mother into her self-concept by her acceptance of pregnancy and anticipation of birth. Her body image dramatically changes with alterations in physical appearance associated with the enlarging uterus.

Expectant fathers often experience ambivalence, acceptance of the fetus as an individual and of his partner's changing body, and anticipation of the birth.

Both expectant mother and father may experience changes in sexual desire.

The birth of a new baby results in changes within family structure and dynamics. It is important to prepare expectant siblings in age-appropriate contexts. Advice from the grandparents may or may not be welcome.

The nurse's role is to assess psychological adaptations and to provide anticipatory guidance and education.

11

Family Psychological Adaptations to Pregnancy

TERMS
- [ ] **ambivalence**
- [ ] **acceptance**
- [ ] **bonding**
- [ ] **anticipation**
- [ ] **psychological tasks of pregnancy**
- [ ] **body image**

THE EXPECTANT FAMILY

The expectant family undergoes a developmental challenge in preparing to become a family with a child. There is a need to reorganize tasks, relationships, and decision-making patterns. Both the mother and the father approach the time of pregnancy influenced by culture, family dynamics, and past experiences with pregnancy and parenting. There are many variations in childbearing and childrearing practices within individual families: the expectant couple must negotiate to incorporate behaviors from both their families.

MATERNAL PSYCHOLOGICAL RESPONSES

Psychological changes commonly occur throughout pregnancy as the woman incorporates her role as a mother into her self-concept. In the beginning of pregnancy, a woman may experience a feeling of **ambivalence**. She questions if this is the right time to have a child and may feel anxious about motherhood. **Acceptance** of the idea of pregnancy must occur. This involves viewing the fetus as part of herself and incorporating it into her body image. This usually happens once the pregnancy has been confirmed by a pregnancy test, by early ultrasound, or physical examination.

Additional acceptance of the reality of the fetus and viewing the fetus as a separate individual occur when the woman feels fetal movement, notices the changes in her body, and others validate the pregnancy. This is the beginning of **bonding,** or emotional attachment to the fetus. **Anticipation** of the birth occurs during the third trimester when the woman is ready for the pregnancy to end. This is the time for childbirth preparation classes, buying infant clothes and supplies, and arranging the home for the baby.

The **psychological tasks of pregnancy** have been studied by several theorists, e.g., Reva Rubin, to describe the maternal-fetal relationship that develops during pregnancy. (See Table 11-1.)

During pregnancy women experience various emotions such as mood swings, increased sensitivity, introspection, fear, and a sense of vulnerability.

> The **psychological tasks of pregnancy** have been studied by several theorists, e.g., Reva Rubin, to describe the maternal-fetal relationship that develops during pregnancy.

Table 11-1 Rubin's Maternal Tasks of Pregnancy

Task	Behaviors
Ensures safe passage through pregnancy, labor, and birth	Seeks prenatal care, seeks knowledge, engages in self-care activities, verbalizes real or perceived threats to herself or fetus
Seeks acceptance of this child by others	Seeks support from partner and family, assists siblings to accept the baby
Seeks commitment and acceptance of self as mother to the infant (binding in)	Acknowledges the child as a separate person, verbalizes beginning attachment to the fetus, seeks information about parenting
Learns to give of oneself on behalf of one's child	Changes lifestyle behaviors for the health of the fetus

Adapted from Rubin, R. (1984). *Maternal identity and the maternal experience.* New York: Springer.

The nurse should assess the woman's emotions during pregnancy, reassure her that they are normal, and encourage her to share her feelings with her family. If the emotions during pregnancy interfere with the woman's daily activities, further assessment needs to be done.

The nurse should assess the woman's emotions during pregnancy, reassure her that they are normal, and encourage her to share her feelings with her family. If the emotions during pregnancy interfere with the woman's daily activities, further assessment needs to be done.

Relationships with her family undergo major changes. The woman may reexamine her relationship with her own mother during pregnancy as part of the psychological process of identifying herself as a mother. The dynamics between the couple are altered and the extent of physical and emotional support a woman receives from her partner contributes to her adjustments to pregnancy.

Both partners may experience changes in sexual desire and activity:

- Intercourse may be avoided out of fear of harming the fetus.
- Discomforts of early pregnancy such as nausea, vomiting, or breast tenderness may require alterations in sexual expression.
- During the third trimester, shortness of breath, leg cramps, enlarged abdomen, and leaking of colostrum from the breasts may interfere with sexual activity.

Body image dramatically changes throughout pregnancy, with the alterations in physical appearance associated with the enlarging uterus. The body image the woman had before she became pregnant, the attitude of others toward her changing body, and her feelings about the pregnancy determine whether she will have a negative or positive body image during pregnancy.

PATERNAL PSYCHOLOGICAL RESPONSES

Expectant fathers often experience the same feelings as expectant mothers. Ambivalence, acceptance of the fetus as an individual, acceptance of his partner's changing body, and anticipation of the birth all occur as the expectant father adjusts to his role.

> Ambivalence, acceptance of the fetus as an individual, acceptance of his partner's changing body, and anticipation of the birth all occur as the expectant father adjusts to his role.

The expectant father may have fears about the well-being of his partner and the fetus and may experience anxiety or stress. Also, men may not receive the support and education they need to fully participate in their role as expectant fathers. (See Table 11-2.)

OTHER FAMILY MEMBERS

The birth of a new baby will result in changes within family structure and dynamics. Other children may view the new baby as a threat to their relationships with their parents. Because sibling reactions to a pregnancy depend on stage of development, it is important to prepare expectant siblings in age-appropriate contexts.

> Because sibling reactions to a pregnancy depend on stage of development, it is important to prepare expectant siblings in age-appropriate contexts.

The relationship with the expectant grandparents changes throughout the pregnancy. Grandparents may be uncertain about how much involvement the couple wishes them to have in the life of the new family. Childbearing and childrearing practices may be different between the two generations;

> Childbearing and childrearing practices may be different between the two generations; therefore, advice from the grandparents may not be welcome. There are classes for both siblings and grandparents to prepare them for their new roles in the family.

Table 11-2 Paternal Tasks of Pregnancy

Time Period	Behaviors
First trimester	Verbalizes ambivalence, announces the pregnancy to family and friends, commits to partner and baby
Second trimester	Attends prenatal visits, accepts changes in the woman's altered appearance, verbalizes feelings of being left out, may fear harm of the fetus during sexual intercourse, seeks clarification of role of father
Third trimester	Concerned about financial responsibilities, attends childbirth education classes, prepares home for baby's arrival, may express fears about health of partner and baby

therefore, advice from the grandparents may not be welcome. There are classes for both siblings and grandparents to prepare them for their new roles in the family.

CULTURAL VARIATIONS

Although there are common psychological responses to pregnancy, the behaviors used to express these responses can vary according to culture. Beliefs about male and female roles, the significance of the pregnancy and the child, and view of pregnancy as a normal event or illness will influence the expectant couple.

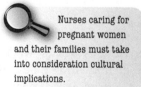

Nurses caring for pregnant women and their families must take into consideration cultural implications.

Nurses caring for pregnant women and their families must take into consideration cultural implications. See Chapter 8 for a discussion of cultural considerations in perinatal care.

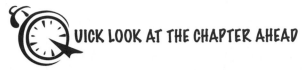

The prenatal visit is an opportunity for education and anticipatory guidance related to pregnancy. The goal of prenatal care is a healthy mother and a healthy baby, through identification of risk factors, assessment for complications, and education of the mother.

Presumptive signs of pregnancy are subjective symptoms reported by a woman. Probable signs of pregnancy are perceived by a health care provider.

Positive signs of pregnancy are fetal heart beat, fetal movement, and visualization of embryo or fetus by ultrasound.

A woman's pregnancy history is described by gravida, the number of times a woman has been pregnant, including the present pregnancy, and para, the number of pregnancies in which she has carried a fetus to viability.

Nagele's Rule is used to calculate the expected date of delivery by taking the first day of the last menstrual period (LMP), subtracting 3 months, and adding 7 days. Fetal measurements taken during ultrasound are also useful in determining gestational age and due date.

At the initial prenatal visit, the pregnant woman is screened for risk factors and given information about behaviors that would contribute to the birth of a healthy baby.

Subsequent visits are monthly until week 28, then biweekly until week 36, then weekly until birth.

12

Assessment for Maternal Well-Being

Changes since last visit are recorded. Physical assessments include blood pressure, weight, fundal height, fetal heart rate, fetal movement, presence of edema, and testing of urine for glucose or protein.

Leopold's maneuvers are performed after week 32 to determine fetal presentation. Additional laboratory tests are completed at different times.

During the prenatal visit at week 36, a vaginal exam is performed to assess for cervical changes in preparation for labor and to collect cultures.

 Nurses need to know normal assessments during pregnancy, signs of complications, and appropriate interventions. Nurses use this information to educate the pregnant woman and her family. **See Part VII for information about risk-factor assessment and complications of pregnancy.**

TERMS
- [ ] presumptive
- [ ] probable
- [ ] positive
- [ ] gravida
- [ ] para
- [ ] viability
- [ ] GTPAL
- [ ] Nagele's rule

SIGNS OF PREGNANCY

Presumptive signs of pregnancy are those subjective symptoms reported by a woman. They include amenorrhea, nausea and vomiting, fatigue, urinary frequency, breast tenderness, and the mother's perception of fetal movement (quickening).

 Presumptive signs of pregnancy may be caused by conditions other than pregnancy.

Probable signs of pregnancy are those perceived by a health care provider and are most likely to be a result of pregnancy:

- Changes in the color and texture of the cervix, lower uterine segment, and vagina
- Braxton-Hicks contractions
- Enlargement of the uterus
- Changes in skin color
- Positive pregnancy tests.

> Braxton-Hicks contractions are uterine contractions that do not cause effacement or dilation.

Positive signs of pregnancy are objective and caused only by pregnancy:

- Fetal heart beat detected by a health care provider
- Fetal movement felt by a health care provider
- Visualization of the embryo or fetus by ultrasound.

NOTATION OF PREGNANCY HISTORY

In her medical records, a woman's pregnancy history is described in terms of gravida and para.

Gravida refers to the number of times a woman has been pregnant, including the present pregnancy.

Para refers to the number of pregnancies during which she carried a fetus to **viability**, usually defined as 24 weeks of pregnancy, regardless of whether or not the fetus was born alive. Determination of para is made on the number of pregnancies, not the number of fetuses.

A more detailed description of pregnancy history uses the **GTPAL** method: **g**ravida, determined as previously stated, and the number of term, preterm, abortions, and living children. The number of abortions includes spontaneous miscarriages as well as termination procedures. Using the GTPAL method of notation, a woman who is 13 weeks pregnant and reports a history of 1 term delivery, 1 preterm delivery of an infant that did not survive, and no abortions or miscarriages, would be identified as gravida 3, term 1, preterm 1, abortions 0, and living 1. This is written as Gravida 3 Para 1-1-0-1.

 ## CALCULATION OF DUE DATE

Nagele's Rule is the common method of determining the expected date of delivery. Nagele's Rule is calculated by taking the first day of the last menstrual period (LMP), subtracting 3 months, and adding 7 days.

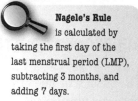
Nagele's Rule is calculated by taking the first day of the last menstrual period (LMP), subtracting 3 months, and adding 7 days.

Fetal measurements taken during an ultrasound are also useful in determining gestation age and due date. Measurement of fundal height, especially between weeks 20 and 31, can be used to estimate the number of weeks of gestation: The height in centimeters from the top of the symphysis pubis to the top of the fundus usually corresponds with weeks of pregnancy.

 ## FIRST PRENATAL VISIT

The initial prenatal visit is the time when pregnant women are screened for risk factors and given information about behaviors that would contribute to the birth of a healthy baby. A detailed history is taken, describing the current pregnancy, past pregnancies, previous medical conditions of the woman and her family, nutrition, and sociocultural factors. Many risk factors can be identified in the history. A good history during the first prenatal visit can direct the caregiver to interventions that are specific to the patient.

A good history during the first prenatal visit can direct the caregiver to interventions that are specific to the patient.

The following assessments are done in the initial physical examination: vital signs, height and weight, and a complete physical assessment with special emphasis on the uterus and pelvis.

Pelvic measurements are estimated to determine if pelvic size is adequate for a vaginal birth.

Initial laboratory studies include

- Urinalysis
- Cervical smears for cancer (PAP test), *chlamydia*, and gonorrhea
- Blood work for a complete blood count (CBC), hemoglobin and hematocrit, blood type and Rh factor, antibody screen, rubella titer, and syphilis.

Additional blood tests may be done, based on the woman's history and the physical examination.

 ## SUBSEQUENT PRENATAL VISITS

The usual schedule of visits is monthly until 28 weeks of gestation, then biweekly until 36 weeks of gestation, then weekly until birth. Visits may be more frequent if needed. A brief interview is conducted about changes that have occurred since the last visit.

The usual physical assessments include blood pressure, weight, fundal height, fetal heart rate, fetal movement, presence of edema, and testing of urine for glucose or protein. Physical assessments during prenatal visits may indicate major complications such as diabetes, hypertensive disorders, inadequate nutrition, or abnormal fetal growth.

> Physical assessments during prenatal visits may indicate major complications such as diabetes, hypertensive disorders, inadequate nutrition, or abnormal fetal growth.

Leopold's maneuvers are performed after 32 weeks gestation to determine fetal presentation.

Laboratory tests are completed at different times in the pregnancy:

- Screening of maternal serum for maternal alpha-fetoprotein (MSAFP), estriol, and hCG is done between weeks 14 and 18 to detect some fetal abnormalities.
- Diabetes screening and a CBC are done between weeks 25 and 28.

Additional laboratory testing may be done if indicated by history or exam.

During the prenatal visit at week 36, in addition to the usual assessments, a vaginal exam is performed to assess cervical changes in preparation for labor and to collect cultures for *chlamydia*, gonorrhea, and group B *streptococcus*. Blood work for syphilis screening is done. HIV or antibody screening is included if indicated.

 ## PRENATAL EDUCATION

The prenatal visit is an opportunity for education and anticipatory guidance related to pregnancy. Topics that need to be addressed include

- health promotion during pregnancy
- dealing with the discomforts of pregnancy
- recognition of possible complications of pregnancy
- preparation for labor and birth
- postpartum decision making.

> The nurse should teach the patient about signs of complications during pregnancy.

Some specific areas include diet and weight gain, exercise, sexual activity, signs and symptoms of complications, types of prenatal classes, anesthesia, contraception, infant feeding type, and choice of infant care provider. (See Table 12-1.)

The nurse should teach the patient about signs of complications during pregnancy.

Table 12-1 Patient Teaching About Complications of Pregnancy

Possible Complication	Danger Signs to Report
Hyperemesis gravidarum	Persistent vomiting
Infection	Fever and chills, burning on urination, diarrhea
Spontaneous abortion or miscarriage	Abdominal cramps, vaginal bleeding
Premature rupture of membranes	Leakage of fluid from the vagina
Premature labor	Menstrual-like cramps, low backache, pelvic pressure, 4 or more contractions in an hour
Hypertensive conditions	Blurred or double vision, spots before the eyes, severe headache, swelling of face or fingers, feeling shaky or jittery, convulsions, upper abdominal pain, decrease in the amount of urine
Placental problems	Vaginal bleeding, sudden or sharp severe abdominal pain
Fetal problems	Diminished or absent fetal movement

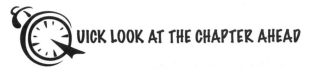
A primary concern during pregnancy is assessing the well-being of the fetus

- indirectly by determining maternal fundal height, weight gain, and serum screenings

- directly by noninvasive measures such as auscultation of fetal heart rate, fetal movement counts, and ultrasound

- or directly by invasive procedures such as chorionic villus sampling and amniocentesis.

Fundal height of the uterus in centimeters is usually equivalent to the number of weeks gestation. Maternal serum screening is done to detect fetal anomalies. Decreased activity in a previously active fetus may indicate that the placenta is not functioning properly.

The fetal heart rate is counted at each prenatal visit. A baseline rate between 120 and 160 beats per minute is considered normal.

Ultrasound uses intermittent high-frequency sound waves to visualize the fetus, placenta, umbilical cord, and amniotic fluid.

A nonstress test measures the response of the fetal heart rate to fetal movement.

A biophysical profile evaluates a fetus at risk for inadequate placental perfusion by measuring fetal heart rate during a non-stress test, body movement, muscle tone, breathing movements, and amniotic fluid volume during an ultrasound examination.

13

Assessment of Fetal Well-Being

In chorionic villus sampling a small amount of chorionic villi is taken by needle from the edge of the developing placenta to test for genetic abnormalities in the fetus.

Amniocentesis is the insertion of an ultrasound-guided needle into the uterine cavity for a sample of amniotic fluid to detect chromosomal abnormalities.

Percutaneous umbilical blood sampling is the collection of fetal blood after 18 weeks of gestation for testing of blood disorders, infection, or genetic disorders.

A contraction stress test evaluates the response of the fetal heart rate to controlled uterine contractions.

 The nurse's role is to gather some of the data, explain medical procedures to the mother and her family, and help them understand the implications of the results of fetal evaluation.

TERMS

- ☐ **fundal height**
- ☐ **quickening**
- ☐ **auscultation**
- ☐ **ultrasound**
- ☐ **nonstress test (NST)**
- ☐ **biophysical profile (BPP)**
- ☐ **chorionic villus sampling (CVS)**
- ☐ **amniocentesis**
- ☐ **percutaneous umbilical blood sampling (PUBS)**
- ☐ **contraction stress test (CST)**

EVALUATION OF FETAL WELL-BEING

Fetal well-being can be assessed indirectly by assessing maternal fundal height, weight gain, and serum; and directly by such noninvasive measures as auscultation of fetal heart rate, fetal movement counts, and ultrasound, or by such invasive procedures as chorionic villus sampling and amniocentesis.

When high-risk situations occur requiring testing beyond routine screenings, the increased anxiety levels of the woman and her family may require additional emotional support and patient education from the nurse or other health care professionals.

Indirect Techniques

Measurement of **fundal height** gives information about the growth of the fetus. From week 20 to week 36 of pregnancy, the height of the uterus in centimeters is usually equivalent to the number of weeks of gestation. (See Figure 13-1.) If growth of the uterus is not consistent with this expectation, further testing is done.

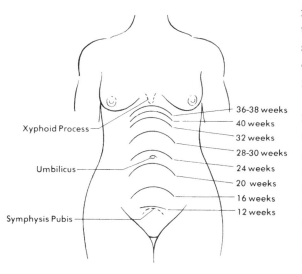

Xyphoid Process

36-38 weeks
40 weeks
32 weeks
28-30 weeks

Umbilicus

24 weeks
20 weeks
16 weeks
12 weeks

Symphysis Pubis

Figure 13-1 Growth of fundus during pregnancy.

Maternal weight gain should follow an expected pattern. Further assessments may be necessary if weight gain is inadequate or excessive. See Chapter 14 on maternal nutrition.

Maternal serum screening for alpha fetoprotein (AFP), estriol, and human chorionic gonadotropin (hCG) is done to detect fetal anomalies such as neural tube defects, Down syndrome or other chromosomal abnormalities, or fetal death.

Fetal movement assessments include **quickening**, when fetal movement is first felt by the pregnant woman, and daily fetal movement counts. Decreased activity in a previously active fetus may indicate that the placenta is not functioning properly and further assessment is needed.

Direct Techniques

The fetal heart rate is checked at each prenatal visit. A baseline rate between 120 and 160 beats per minute is considered normal. **Auscultation** is using a handheld ultrasound device to listen before, during, and at least 30 seconds after a contraction.

Ultrasound uses intermittent high-frequency sound waves to visualize the fetus, placenta, umbilical cord, and amniotic fluid. (See Figure 13-2). Gestational age, fetal growth, fetal structural abnormalities, number of fetuses, placental position, umbilical artery blood flow, and amniotic fluid volume can be assessed using this method. Abnormal findings will be explained by the physician and further testing may be done. Ultrasound is a common prenatal diagnostic tool in the United States.

> Ultrasound is a common prenatal diagnostic tool in the United States.

A **nonstress test (NST)** measures the response of the fetal heart rate to fetal movement, and is done if the pregnant woman has risk factors that may lead to diminished placental functioning. Using an electronic fetal monitor, fetal heart rate and fetal movement detected by the mother are recorded. Accelerations are increases in the fetal heart rate of 15 beats per minute or greater above the baseline, continuing for at least 15 seconds.

> Accelerations are increases in the fetal heart rate of 15 beats per minute or greater above the baseline, continuing for at least 15 seconds.

When accelerations occur two or more times in a 20-minute period, the NST is considered reactive, indicating adequate oxygenation to the fetus. If the test does not meet the criteria within 40 minutes, it is considered nonreactive and further evaluation is done.

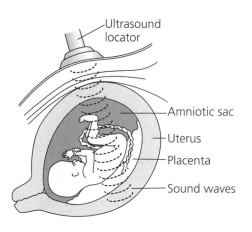

Ultrasound locator

Amniotic sac

Uterus

Placenta

Sound waves

Figure 13-2 Illustration of ultrasound.

A **biophysical profile (BPP)** is used to evaluate a fetus at risk for inadequate placental perfusion. Maternal conditions such as diabetes, hypertension, multiple gestation, or pregnancy past the due date often place a fetus at increased risk.

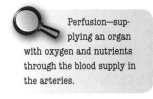

Perfusion—supplying an organ with oxygen and nutrients through the blood supply in the arteries.

BPP assesses five variables that reflect oxygenation of the fetus: fetal heart rate during an NST, body movement, muscle tone, breathing movements, and amniotic fluid volume during an ultrasound examination.

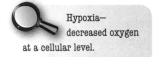

Hypoxia—decreased oxygen at a cellular level.

When there is fetal hypoxia, muscle tone, body, and breathing movements diminish; the heart rate pattern becomes nonreactive; and amniotic fluid volume decreases. Each of the five BPP parameters is scored with a 2 for a normal finding and a 0 for an abnormal finding. A score of 8 to 10 is considered normal; 6 is equivocal; 4 or less is abnormal, with interventions for birth indicated. With scores of 4 or less, the fetus must be delivered as soon as possible or it may be stillborn.

Invasive Techniques

In **chorionic villus sampling (CVS),** a small amount of chorionic villi from the edge of the developing placenta is obtained by inserting a needle through the vagina or abdominal wall of a pregnant woman. This is usually performed at weeks 10 to 12 of pregnancy to test for genetic abnormalities in the fetus.

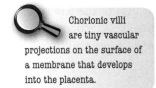

Chorionic villi are tiny vascular projections on the surface of a membrane that develops into the placenta.

Results can be obtained sooner than with amniocentesis and decisions about pregnancy continuation can be made earlier.

There is a slight increased risk of miscarriage associated with CVS.

Amniocentesis is the insertion of an ultrasound-guided needle through the mother's abdomen into the uterine cavity to obtain a sample of amniotic fluid. (See Figure 13-3.)

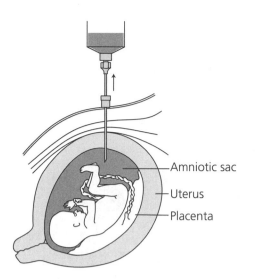

—Amniotic sac

—Uterus

—Placenta

Figure 13-3 Illustration of amniocentesis.

Amniocentesis is performed in early pregnancy at weeks 15 to 18, usually to detect chromosomal abnormalities. It may be done in late pregnancy at weeks 30 to 35, most often to determine fetal lung maturity.

The most common biochemical test done on amniotic fluid in late pregnancy is the lecithin/sphingomyelin (L/S) ratio to detect the amount of surfactant production in fetal lungs. An L/S ratio of at least 2:1 indicates fetal lung maturity.

Surfactant is a substance that reduces the surface tension of pulmonary fluids to allow gas exchange in the alveoli.

 Complications of the L/S test, although rare, include infection, pregnancy loss, or injury to the fetus.

Percutaneous umbilical blood sampling (PUBS) is the collection of fetal blood after 18 weeks of gestation for testing of blood disorders, infection, or genetic disorders. This procedure is done by inserting an ultrasound-guided needle through the mother's abdomen into the fetal umbilical vein.

 There is a slight increase in pregnancy loss following the PUBS procedure.

In a **contraction stress test (CST),** the response of the fetal heart rate to controlled uterine contractions is evaluated. This information helps to determine the ability of the fetus to tolerate the contractions of labor.

Using an electronic fetal monitor, uterine activity and fetal heart rate are recorded. Contractions are stimulated by either nipple stimulation or the use of intravenous oxytocin. Three contractions lasting 40 seconds or longer must occur in a 10-minute period.

The test is considered negative or reassuring when there are no decelerations of the fetal heart rate associated with contractions. This indicates circulation within the placenta and the uterus is adequate.

If late decelerations occur with 50% or more of the contractions, the test is interpreted as positive or nonreassuring. See Chapter 21 for a more detailed explanation of late decelerations.

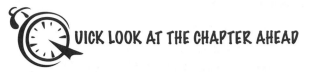

Nutrition prior to and during pregnancy is a major factor influencing the health of the infant.

Significant factors are nutritional needs during pregnancy, ways of managing nutrition-related discomforts of pregnancy, cultural influences on diet, and special needs. (See Table 14-1.)

The average recommended weight gain during pregnancy is 25 to 35 lb for a woman of normal weight.

Total calories consumed daily should increase by 300 during the second and third trimesters.

Daily protein intake should increase to 60 g to ensure adequate amino acids. Carbohydrate intake needs to be sufficient to prevent ketoacidosis.

Calories from fat should not exceed 30%. Low-fat dairy products and lean cuts of meat are recommended.

Daily calcium of 1200 mg is needed for development of fetal skeleton and teeth.

Daily iron requirements are 30 mg during pregnancy. All women of childbearing age should take 400 micrograms of folic acid daily to prevent neural tube defects in the first trimester.

Caffeine should be limited to 300 mg, or 10 oz, per day.

Women should avoid foods with additives, preservatives, or artificial sweeteners, and foods that might be contaminated with heavy metals such as mercury in fish.

14

Nutrition During Pregnancy

Pregnant women should never consume alcohol because of fetal alcohol syndrome.

Pica is the ingestion of nonfood substances with little or no nutritional value, such as clay, dirt, ice, and laundry or corn starch.

Nausea, vomiting, heartburn, and constipation are common discomforts of pregnancy. A low-fat, high-carbohydrate diet with frequent small meals is recommended.

Cultural beliefs and practices about nutrition during pregnancy may be difficult to change. However, the pregnant woman may be receptive to nutritional variations out of concern for the well-being of her baby.

 In most prenatal settings, nurses provide nutritional counseling and arrange for consults with a dietician when needed.

TERMS
- [ ] recommended weight gain
- [ ] protein
- [ ] carbohydrate
- [ ] fat
- [ ] calcium
- [ ] iron
- [ ] folic acid
- [ ] caffeine
- [ ] alcohol
- [ ] pica

Table 14-1 Special Nutritional Considerations During Pregnancy

Situation	Risks	Recommendations
Underweight: pre-pregnancy > 10% below ideal body weight	May tire easily, have iron deficiency anemia, reduced resistance to disease, higher incidence of low birth weight infant.	Determine if poverty, stress, depression, or eating disorder is contributing factor. Increase daily intake by 500–1000 calories. Recommend total weight gain of 25–35 lbs, plus enough to attain ideal weight.
Overweight: pre-pregnancy > 20% above ideal body weight	Increased incidence of gestational diabetes, pregnancy-induced hypertension, macrosomia with resulting cesarean birth, and postmaturity. Difficulty in auscultating fetal heart rate and palpating for fetal position and size.	Determine contributing factors such as stress, family or cultural preferences, or dietary habits. Dieting is not recommended during pregnancy. Recommend total weight gain of 15–25 lbs. Increase exercise and reduce intake of empty calories. Avoid excessive hunger to reduce the tendency to overeat.
Adolescent	Increased incidence of low birth weight infant, anemia, pregnancy-induced hypertension.	The younger the adolescent, the greater the need to meet own growth requirements. Determine dietary patterns, assess for eating disorders. Encourage a balanced, nutrient-dense diet with increased protein and calcium. Limit empty calories. Work with family member who purchases and prepares food.
Advanced maternal age (>40 yrs.)	More likely to have chronic diseases such as hypertension and type II diabetes. Increased incidence of gestational diabetes, superimposed pregnancy-induced hypertension, and multiple gestation.	Maintain a balanced diet and appropriate weight gain.
Vegetarian	Possible deficit in total calories, protein, and calcium. May not achieve optimum weight gain.	Determine what types of foods are consumed. Suggest energy-dense foods containing calcium and protein. Supplement B-12, iron, and calcium if necessary.
Lactose intolerance	Possible calcium deficiency.	Suggest substitution for dairy products such as tofu, soy milk, yogurt, or fortified orange juice.
Multiple gestation	Increased risk for maternal depletion of iron, calcium, and folic acid stores.	Recommended total weight gain of 40–45 lbs for twins and 45–50 lbs for triplets. Suggest nutrient-dense foods, with increased protein and calcium. Supplement with prenatal vitamins and iron.

MATERNAL WEIGHT GAIN

The average **recommended weight gain** during pregnancy is 25 to 35 lb for a woman of weight appropriate for her height and body type. The woman who is underweight should gain at least an additional 5 lb and an overweight woman should gain 5 to 10 lb less.

During the first trimester, a total weight gain of 3 to 5 lb is adequate. During the second and third trimesters a weight gain of 1 pound per week is typical.

Components of maternal weight gain are the fetus, placenta, amniotic fluid, increased uterine musculature, increased blood volume, increased breast tissue, and maternal fat stores.

NUTRITIONAL REQUIREMENTS

Having a balanced diet is essential for healthy fetal development. Total calories to meet daily energy requirements should increase by 300 cal during the second and third trimesters. To accomplish this, a woman could add two glasses of nonfat milk, two slices of bread, and one meat-equivalent serving to her daily consumption.

Daily **protein** needs increase by 10 g to 14 g to a total of 60 g. This ensures adequate amino acids for fetal growth and development, maternal tissue growth, and blood volume expansion.

Carbohydrate intake needs to be sufficient to prevent ketoacidosis from protein use for energy. Pregnancy is not the time for a woman to have a low-carbohydrate diet.

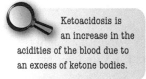
Ketoacidosis is an increase in the acidities of the blood due to an excess of ketone bodies.

Calories from **fat** should not exceed 30% of the daily intake. Low-fat dairy products and lean cuts of meat are recommended to achieve this proportion of fat in the diet.

Calcium is needed for development of fetal skeleton and teeth. If there is not adequate calcium intake, fetal needs will be met by decalcification of maternal bones. Daily calcium needs remain at 1200 mg. If the pregnant woman is not able to ingest dairy products, calcium supplements are recommended.

Iron requirements are greatly increased during pregnancy because of growth of the fetus and placenta, expansion of maternal blood volume, and iron stores in the fetal liver. Daily recommendations for iron intake increase from 15 mg before pregnancy to 30 mg during pregnancy.

> All women of childbearing age should take 400 micrograms of **folic acid** daily to prevent neural tube defects in the first trimester.

Although a balanced nutritious diet supplies most of the woman's needs, prenatal supplementation is often prescribed to ensure adequate intake of vitamin and mineral requirements.

 ## FOODS TO AVOID

Some substances added to foods should be avoided because of potential effects on the pregnancy. **Caffeine** should be limited to 300 mg/day. This is the amount found in 10 oz of coffee.

> Amounts of caffeine exceeding 300 mg/day may contribute to miscarriage, decreased placental blood flow from vasoconstriction, increased gastrointestinal motility which decreases absorption of nutrients, and increased hydrochloric acid production leading to increased nausea and vomiting.

Women should read product labels to identify foods with additives and preservatives or artificial sweeteners. The use of these substances is not recommended because the effects are not known.

Foods that might be contaminated with heavy metals such as mercury in fish should be avoided.

Women with a personal or family history of nut allergies should avoid foods containing peanuts.

Pregnant women should never consume **alcohol** because of the possibility of fetal alcohol syndrome.

 ## PICA

The ingestion of nonfood substances with little or no nutritional value is known as **pica**. Some common pica cravings include clay, dirt, ice, and laundry or corn starch. This behavior can interfere with the ingestion and absorption of essential nutrients. Pica is not linked to any particular race, creed, culture, geographical area, or socioeconomic status.

NUTRITION-RELATED DISCOMFORTS OF PREGNANCY

Nausea, vomiting, heartburn, and constipation are common discomforts of pregnancy that have nutritional implications. In most cases, nausea and vomiting, common in the first trimester, do not affect the nutritional status of the woman and fetus.

 If vomiting is severe and long lasting, loss of fluids, electrolytes, and nutrients may result.

CULTURE, SPECIAL NEEDS, AND NUTRITION

The nurse needs to determine cultural preferences and special needs as they relate to nutritional intake during pregnancy.

The pregnant woman may have special diet needs for such conditions as lactose intolerance or choices such as vegetarianism. Certain foods may be culturally prescribed or restricted during pregnancy. In many cultures, for example, beliefs about the balance between hot and cold determine the foods that may be eaten during pregnancy and after birth.

Cultural beliefs and practices about nutrition during pregnancy may be difficult to change. However, the pregnant women may be receptive to nutritional advice out of concern for the well-being of her baby.

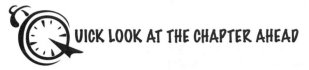

As a result of physiologic and anatomic changes, discomforts of pregnancy may occur. These discomforts may make the woman uncomfortable and anxious and have the potential to lead to more serious problems.

Nausea and/or vomiting, called "morning sickness," are common early symptoms of pregnancy. It is important to maintain adequate nutrition.

Urinary frequency occurs in early pregnancy because of pressure on the bladder from the growing uterus.

Breast tenderness occurs from increasing levels of estrogen and progesterone.

Increased metabolic demands are a major factor in early pregnancy fatigue.

Many women experience increased vaginal discharge, or leukorrhea, as a result of increased estrogen levels. Foul odor of discharge, irritation of the perineal area, and vaginal itching may indicate infection.

Late discomforts are heartburn, constipation, flatulence, hemorrhoids, ankle edema, varicose veins, and leg cramps. Avoiding gas-forming foods and chewing food thoroughly along with regular bowel habits can help.

Dyspnea, or shortness of breath, can increase in late pregnancy, with exertion, and/or when lying flat, and decreases when the fetus drops into the pelvis in preparation for labor.

15

Common Discomforts of Pregnancy

Posture change from the heavy uterus and relaxation of the pelvic joints can lead to backache. Round ligament pain from stretching may be felt as an intense, sharp sensation. Women can become anxious about its origin if they are not prepared to expect it.

Vena cava syndrome, or supine hypotension, occurs when the woman lies flat on her back. The symptoms are lightheadedness, dizziness, or feeling weak, all due to a drop in blood pressure.

 The nurse can educate the woman and her family to understand and manage these discomforts and promote overall health. (See Table 15-1.)

TERMS

- ☐ nausea
- ☐ vomiting
- ☐ "morning sickness"
- ☐ hyperemesis gravidarum
- ☐ urinary frequency
- ☐ breast tenderness
- ☐ fatigue
- ☐ leukorrhea
- ☐ heartburn
- ☐ constipation
- ☐ flatulence
- ☐ hemorrhoids
- ☐ dyspnea
- ☐ backache
- ☐ round ligament pain
- ☐ vena cava syndrome

Table 15-1 Management of Common Discomforts of Pregnancy

Discomfort	Nursing Recommendations
Nausea and vomiting	Eat dry crackers before getting out of bed. Eat small, frequent meals throughout the day. Drink fluids between rather than with meals. Avoid foods or odors that trigger nausea. Prevent fatigue.
Urinary frequency	Void when the urge is felt. Reduce caffeine intake since it is a bladder irritant. Increase daytime fluid intake while decreasing evening fluid intake.
Breast tenderness	Purchase and wear a supportive, well-fitting bra.
Fatigue	Increase amount of rest and sleep by planning a daily nap or quiet time. Go to bed earlier. Ask for help with household chores.
Increased vaginal discharge	Bathe daily. Wear cotton underwear. Avoid douching, nylon panties, and panty hose.
Heartburn	Eat small, frequent meals. Avoid fatty or fried foods. Sit upright after eating. Use low-sodium antacids as ordered by the health care provider.
Constipation	Drink at least 8 eight-ounce glasses of fluid daily. Increase fiber by eating more fruits and vegetables. Have adequate exercise to promote peristalsis. Laxatives, enemas, or herbal remedies are not recommended unless directed by health care provider.
Hemorrhoids	Avoid constipation. Lie with legs elevated or in knee-chest or left lateral positions. Use ice packs, topical ointments, astringent pads, warm soaks, or sitz baths to relieve discomfort.
Leg discomfort	Have regular exercise to promote venous return. Dorsiflex the foot frequently when standing or sitting. Avoid tight garters or restrictive bands in knee-high or thigh-high stockings. Do not cross legs at the knee. Elevate the legs and hips during rest periods. If leg cramps occur, extend the knee and dorsiflex the foot. Report persistent leg cramps to health care provider.
Dyspnea	Maintain proper posture when sitting or standing. Elevate head when lying down.
Backache	Wear shoes with low to moderate heels. Maintain proper posture. Use good body mechanics. Perform exercises to strengthen lower back muscles. Local heat, massage, or the pelvic rock exercise can be used to relieve backache.
Round ligament pain	Move slowly and carefully. Bring the knees to the abdomen for pain relief.
Difficulty sleeping	Drink a warm caffeine-free beverage before bedtime. Use back massage, pillows to provide support, and relaxation techniques. Over-the-counter medications or herbal remedies should not be used unless discussed with the health care provider.
Vena cava syndrome	Avoid lying flat on the back. Raise the head of the examination table, and place a pillow under the right hip when a woman needs to be in a back-lying position.

EARLY DISCOMFORTS

Nausea and/or **vomiting** are common early symptoms of pregnancy. The exact cause is unknown; however, elevated hCG and lowered blood sugar levels are thought to be major contributing factors.

Although it is called "**morning sickness**" because it frequently occurs in the morning, nausea and vomiting can appear throughout the day. For most women this gastrointestinal upset subsides by the end of the first trimester. It is important to maintain adequate nutrition while experiencing this early discomfort. A low-fat, high-carbohydrate diet with frequent, small meals is recommended during pregnancy.

> A low-fat, high-carbohydrate diet with frequent, small meals is recommended during pregnancy.

If nausea and vomiting are severe or extend beyond the first trimester, then the woman may be suffering from **hyperemesis gravidarum**.

Urinary frequency occurs in early pregnancy because of pressure of the growing uterus on the bladder, and subsides as the uterus rises out of the pelvis. The nurse should ask about signs of a urinary tract infection such as pain or burning on urination or blood in the urine.

Breast tenderness occurs from increasing levels of estrogen and progesterone, and may be one of the first symptoms noticed in pregnancy.

Increased metabolic demands are a major factor in the **fatigue** experienced in early pregnancy.

Many women experience increased vaginal discharge, or **leukorrhea**, as a result of increased estrogen levels. Increased acidity of the vaginal secretions makes the pregnant woman more susceptible to vaginal yeast infections.

 Women should be advised to report foul odor of discharge, irritation of the perineal area, and vaginal itching as these may indicate an infection.

LATE DISCOMFORTS

Most of the discomforts associated with the second and third trimesters are related to the growing fetus and enlarging uterus. Some gastrointestinal symptoms are heartburn, constipation, flatulence, and hemorrhoids.

Heartburn is caused by increased progesterone production leading to decreased GI mobility and relaxation of the cardiac sphincter of the stomach, as well as stomach displacement by the enlarging uterus.

Constipation results from the weight of the enlarging uterus pressing against the bowel, and slower peristalsis from increased progesterone levels. Some women experience flatulence with or without constipation. Avoiding gas-forming foods and chewing food thoroughly, along with regular bowel habits, can help with flatulence.

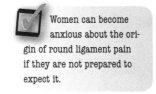
Avoiding gas-forming foods and chewing food thoroughly, along with regular bowel habits, can help with flatulence.

Hemorrhoids occur during pregnancy because of pressure on the rectal veins from the weight of the growing uterus. Constipation also contributes to the formation of hemorrhoids.

Late-pregnancy discomforts related to blood circulation in the legs are ankle edema, varicose veins, and leg cramps. These problems are the result of reduced circulation in the lower extremities from the pressure of the enlarging uterus on the blood vessels.

Dyspnea, or shortness of breath, occurs as the enlarging uterus exerts pressure on the diaphragm, causing lung compression. Dyspnea can increase in late pregnancy, with exertion, and/or when lying flat. It will decrease when the fetus drops into the pelvis in preparation for labor.

Change in posture from the heavy uterus and relaxation of the pelvic joints from increased progesterone levels can lead to **backache**.

Round ligament pain from stretching may be felt as an intense, sharp sensation in the lower abdomen and inguinal area usually associated with movement. Women can become anxious about the origin of round ligament pain if they are not prepared to expect it.

Women can become anxious about the origin of round ligament pain if they are not prepared to expect it.

Inability to find a comfortable position for sleep, dyspnea, fetal movements, urinary frequency, or leg cramps may contribute to difficulty sleeping.

Vena cava syndrome, or supine hypotension, occurs when the woman lies flat on her back and the uterus presses on the inferior vena cava, decreasing blood return to the heart. The symptoms experienced are light-headedness, dizziness, or feeling weak; all are due to a drop in blood pressure.

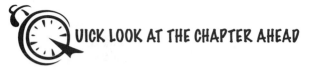

Preparing the couple for pregnancy, birth, post-partum, and beginning parenting is the major focus of perinatal education classes. An underlying principle in perinatal education is that knowledge empowers the family to make appropriate, informed decisions based upon their values and needs. Knowledge also helps to decrease anxiety, thereby enhancing ability to cope with a new situation.

Exercise during pregnancy should be maintained. Women need to practice exercises that strengthen abdominal, lower back, and perineal muscles.

Relaxation during labor conserves energy and permits more efficient use of the uterine muscles.

Controlled breathing during labor enhances the level of relaxation, maintains oxygen availability to the mother and fetus, and serves as a distraction.

Distraction or cutaneous stimulation may diminish the brain's ability to perceive pain. Distractions include imagery, music, and looking at a focal point.

Cutaneous stimulation during labor includes effleurage, massage, and sacral pressure, although, in late labor, the woman may not want to be touched.

Nurses have a vital role in providing information to families in office, home, and classroom settings. Classes are available for first-time or repeat parents, siblings, grandparents, and couples anticipating a cesarean birth.

16

Preparation for Childbirth

TERMS
- [ ] pelvic tilt
- [ ] kegel exercises
- [ ] progressive relaxation
- [ ] controlled breathing techniques
- [ ] cleansing breath
- [ ] focal point
- [ ] imagery
- [ ] visualization
- [ ] effleurage
- [ ] massage
- [ ] sacral pressure

PHYSICAL FITNESS

Exercise during pregnancy should be continued; however, it is not the time to learn a new or strenuous sport. The woman should take into consideration the effects of pregnancy, including the change in center of gravity and increased energy needs leading to fatigue. She should wear supportive shoes and clothing, avoid hyperthermia, and prevent dehydration.

Women need to practice exercises that strengthen abdominal, lower back, and perineal muscles. Exercises to increase abdominal muscle tone include tightening and relaxing of the abdominal muscles, along with deep breathing, and partial sit-ups, lifting head and shoulders off the floor with the knees bent.

Pelvic tilt or rocking increases flexibility of the lumbar spine and strengthens lower back muscles. In the **pelvic tilt**, the woman arches her lower spine while on her hands and knees, slowly rocking the pelvis back by tightening abdominal and buttocks muscles. Then she rocks the pelvis forward to hollow the spine. This can be done on hands and knees or standing.

Kegel exercises strengthen perineal muscles and involve contracting and relaxing the muscles around the vagina as if stopping and starting the flow of urine.

Kegel exercises should not be practiced during urination because they have been associated with increased risk of urinary stasis, leading to infection.

"Tailor sitting" or squatting are positions that stretch the perineal muscles.

LABOR AND BIRTH PREPARATION

There are many different approaches to management of labor pain, all based on education and preparation as important for coping with labor. Unfamiliar experiences can cause fear and anxiety, which increase muscle tension and exaggerate the perception of pain. Understanding the process of labor and birth decreases fear of the unknown. Learning specific coping strategies enhances a feeling of control and increases the self-confidence of the couple.

Relaxation during labor conserves energy and permits more efficient use of the uterine muscles. There are several relaxation techniques that can be taught: **Progressive relaxation** is the most common. In this technique, the woman is directed to tighten muscles of selected portions of the body, hold the tension for a few seconds, and then slowly release the tension.

In practicing progressive relaxation during pregnancy, the woman becomes familiar with the sensation of tension and develops the ability to relax muscles consciously. During labor she would be reminded to use this technique during a contraction.

Using **controlled breathing techniques** during labor enhances the level of relaxation, maintains oxygen flow to the mother and fetus, and serves as a distraction. (See Table 16-1.)

There are many different approaches to management of labor pain, all based on education and preparation as important for coping with labor. Unfamiliar experiences can cause fear and anxiety, which increase muscle tension and exaggerate the perception of pain. Understanding the process of labor and birth decreases fear of the unknown. Learning specific coping strategies enhances a feeling of control and increases the self-confidence of the couple.

- A deep, **cleansing breath** is taken at the beginning and end of each contraction.
- At the beginning of labor when contractions are less intense, a slow, deep abdominal breathing pattern is used.
- As the contractions increase in intensity, shallow, quick patterns of chest breathing are used.
- When the urge to push is felt and it is not yet time to push because of incomplete dilatation, blowing is combined with the breathing pattern to prevent pushing. Conscious blowing on each exhale counteracts the urge to bear down.
- Because some of the breathing patterns are complicated, the couple should practice together during pregnancy to use them during labor.

During the admission process for labor, the nurse should ask the couple what breathing techniques they have practiced so that their

During the admission process for labor, the nurse should ask the couple what breathing techniques they have practiced so that their efforts can be reinforced. If they have not learned breathing techniques, slow abdominal breathing and shallow chest breathing can be taught in labor.

Table 16-1 Breathing Patterns in Labor

Type of Breathing	Description	Illustration
Cleansing breath	Relaxed breathing in through the nose and out through the mouth. Use at the beginning and end of each contraction.	
Slow deep breathing	Slow-paced breathing about 6 to 12 breaths per minute, in through the nose and out through pursed lips. To maintain rhythm, counting may be done.	
Shallow breathing	Light, effortless breathing in and out through a relaxed mouth and jaw at a rate of 25 to 40 breaths per minute. The inhale should equal the exhale to avoid hyperventilation.	
Patterned breathing	Shallow, rhythmic breathing, and blowing in and out through a relaxed mouth in a varying pattern. Example of 3:1 pattern is IN-OUT/IN-OUT/IN-OUT/IN-BLOW.	
Breathing to prevent pushing	Blow on each exhale when the urge to push is felt and pushing should not be done. IN-BLOW/IN-BLOW/IN-BLOW/IN-BLOW.	
Breathing for pushing	Take deep breaths until the urge to push is strong, then bear down using open glottis method, grunting and exhaling with each push. Breath holding should be less than 6 seconds.	

efforts can be reinforced. If they have not learned breathing techniques, slow abdominal breathing and shallow chest breathing can be taught in labor.

In addition to patterned breathing techniques, activities such as distraction or cutaneous stimulation may diminish the brain's ability to perceive pain. This is based on gate-control theory, according to which only a limited number of sensations can move through nerve pathways at one time.

Distraction techniques include imagery, music, and use of a **focal point**. **Imagery**, or visualization of a mental image that is special to the woman, allows her to concentrate on something other than the pain of contractions.

Music promotes relaxation and can be used with other techniques to reduce pain sensation.

A picture or an object with special meaning can be used as a focal point. Looking at a focal point is an effective way of blocking pain sensation.

It is important for caregivers not to break the woman's concentration when she is using a distraction technique.

Cutaneous stimulation techniques during labor include effleurage, massage, and sacral pressure.

In **effleurage**, the woman slowly and gently traces a circular pattern over her abdomen with her fingertips.

Massage promotes relaxation in addition to decreasing perception of pain. Usually the support people provide massage of the arms, legs, back, shoulders, and forehead.

In late labor, the woman may not want to be touched.

Sacral pressure, which is firm counter-pressure applied with heel of the hand in the sacral area, can be used if the woman experiences lower back pain with contractions.

PART III · QUESTIONS

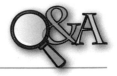

1. The nurse is answering questions during a woman's prenatal visit at week 24. What information would be most significant?
    a. At this time, the fetus is most sensitive to teratogens.
    b. Fetal lung maturity is complete at this gestation.
    c. Fetus weighs 2.5 lb and is about 14 in. long.
    d. Survival is possible if the fetus is born now.

2. What assessment data would the nurse expect to collect from a woman who is 13 weeks pregnant?
    a. Auscultation of fetal heart beat by Doppler.
    b. Counting fetal heart rate with a fetoscope.
    c. Fetal movement associated with fetal heart rate acceleration.
    d. Mother reports fetal movement.

3. What statement by the client would indicate understanding of the physiologic anemia of pregnancy?
    a. "All pregnant women are anemic, so I don't have to worry about it."
    b. "Because I am anemic, I am more likely to have high blood pressure."
    c. "I am a little anemic because my body is producing extra fluid in my blood."
    d. "I did not get enough iron in my diet before I became pregnant, so I am anemic now."

4. What change in the urinary system predisposes the pregnant woman to urinary tract infection?
    a. Decreased bladder capacity.
    b. Increased plasma volume flow.
    c. Pressure on the bladder from the enlarging uterus.
    d. Stasis of urine in the bladder and ureters.

5. A woman who comes to her health care provider for her first prenatal visit at 10 weeks of gestation says, "My husband says he doesn't know how we are going to pay for another baby; we already have two children. I am not sure how this is going to work out." What response to pregnancy does this indicate?

a. Attachment to the fetus has begun to occur.
b. Normal ambivalence about the pregnancy is being expressed.
c. Partner relationships are changing in anticipation of the birth.
d. The couple has accepted the fetus as an individual separate from the mother.

6. Which maternal behavior demonstrates the ensuring of safe passage through pregnancy, one of Rubin's tasks of pregnancy?
a. Arranges for prenatal care and education.
b. Looks for support from family and friends.
c. Prepares siblings for birth of the baby.
d. States feelings of attachment to the fetus.

7. A pregnant client comes to her first prenatal visit. She reports a pregnancy history of two babies born near the due date, twins born prematurely, and a miscarriage in the first trimester. Using the GTPAL notation, how would her pregnancy history be recorded?
a. Gravida 4 Para 2-1-1-4
b. Gravida 4 Para 2-2-1-4
c. Gravida 5 Para 2-1-1-4
d. Gravida 5 Para 2-2-1-4

8. A woman reports her last menstrual period began on January 10. Using Nagele's Rule, what is her expected date of delivery?
a. October 3
b. October 17
c. November 3
d. November 17

9. Which finding in a biophysical profile indicates diminished oxygenation to the fetus?
a. Frequent extension of fetal extremities.
b. Nonreactive fetal heart rate.
c. Normal amniotic fluid volume.
d. Well flexed arms and legs.

10. A pregnant woman asks the nurse, "My doctor told me some numbers about the baby's lungs. What does that mean?" In reviewing the medical record, the L/S ratio taken by amniocentesis is 1.5:1. What would be the best initial response by the nurse?
a. "Amniocentesis results indicate that your baby's lungs are not mature."

    b. "Delivery will be scheduled soon because the baby's lungs are mature."

    c. "I will arrange another appointment so your doctor can explain this to you."

    d. "This indicates there is a problem with your baby's lungs and needs further evaluation."

11. A client at 29 weeks of gestation weights 154 lb. She expresses concern about this weight gain. Her prepregnant weight of 125 lb is within her ideal body weight range. What would be the nurse's best response?

    a. "Let us talk about your diet. You are gaining too much weight."

    b. "Pregnancy is not the time to be concerned about your weight gain."

    c. "This weight gain is typical for this time in your pregnancy."

    d. "You are not gaining enough weight. Let us review your diet."

12. Which lunch menu would best meet the nutritional needs of a pregnant woman?

    a. Hamburger on a roll with tomato and lettuce, Jell-O, and iced tea.

    b. Fried chicken fingers, coleslaw, and milk.

    c. Macaroni and cheese, tossed green salad, and orange soda.

    d. Chicken salad sandwich with sliced tomatoes and milk.

13. Which statement by a client indicates that further teaching about nausea and vomiting of pregnancy needs to done by the nurse?

    a. "I hope that taking a nap when I get home from work makes me feel better."

    b. "I need to drink an extra glass of water with every meal."

    c. "I will ask my husband not to wear aftershave because it upsets my stomach."

    d. "I will try to eat five or six smaller meals during the day."

14. A woman at her 28-week prenatal visit complains of weakness and lightheadedness when lying on the examination table. What would be the primary nursing action?

    a. Assess the woman's blood pressure.

    b. Encourage the woman to take slow, deep breaths.

    c. Lower the head of the exam table.

    d. Turn the woman on her left side.

15. Which exercise would the nurse teach a pregnant woman in order to strengthen perineal muscles in preparation for labor?
    a. Kegel
    b. Partial sit-ups
    c. Pelvic tilt
    d. Sacral pressure

16. The patient in labor says that she feels like pushing. After doing a vaginal exam, the nurse tells the patient it is not yet time to push because she is not fully dilated. Which breathing technique would the nurse coach the patient to use?
    a. Light breathing, 25 to 40 times a minute.
    b. Rapid, shallow breathing, blowing on each exhale.
    c. Shallow, rhythmic breathing in a varying pattern.
    d. Slow-paced breathing, 6 to 12 times a minute.

PART III • ANSWERS AND RATIONALES

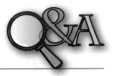

1. **The answer is d.** Viability or survival of the fetus outside the uterus is possible at approximately 24 weeks of gestation. Option a is incorrect because the period of most vulnerability to teratogens is 3 to 8 weeks. Option b is incorrect because lung maturity is not complete until 37 weeks. Option c is incorrect because fetal weight is about 1.5 lb and length is about 11 in. at 24 weeks of gestation.

2. **The answer is a.** Auscultation of the fetal heart rate by Doppler is possible by 8 weeks. Option b is incorrect because counting fetal heart rate by fetoscope can be done after 16 to 20 weeks of gestation. Option c is incorrect because accelerations of fetal heart with movement do not occur until 28 weeks. Option d is incorrect because fetal movement is usually not detected by mothers until 16 to 18 weeks of gestation.

3. **The answer is c.** Physiologic anemia of pregnancy is the result of hemodilution from increased plasma volume related to the amount of red blood cell production. For option a, although all pregnant women experience hemodilution, not all become anemic. However, anemia in a pregnant woman should be treated with diet and iron supplementation. Option b is incorrect because anemia may be associated with low blood pressure, not high blood pressure. Option d describes iron deficiency anemia.

4. **The answer is d.** Stasis of urine in the bladder, ureters, and renal pelves may lead to increased growth of organisms, resulting in increased risk for infection. Option a is incorrect because there is an increased bladder capacity during pregnancy. Options b and c are incorrect because increased plasma flow and pressure from the enlarging uterus encourage more frequent urination, thereby reducing urinary stasis.

5. **The answer is b.** In early pregnancy, both expectant mothers and fathers experience ambivalence, questioning the appropriateness of having a child at this time. The other options describe psychological responses during later trimesters of pregnancy.

6. **The answer is a.** Seeking prenatal care and knowledge are behaviors that ensure safe passage through pregnancy, labor, and birth, according to Rubin. The other options are behaviors demonstrating Rubin's other maternal tasks of pregnancy. Options b and c demonstrate the task of seeking acceptance of this child by others. Option d indicates the task of seeking commitment and acceptance of self as mother to the infant.

7. **The answer is c.** Gravida refers to the total number of pregnancies. In the GTPAL format, para refers to the number of pregnancies delivered at term, the number of pregnancies delivered prematurely, the number of miscarriages and abortions, and the number of living children. In the case described in the question, this is her fifth pregnancy, she has had two term births, the twins' birth is counted as one preterm pregnancy, she has had one miscarriage, and each twin is counted in the number of living children for a total of four living children.

8. **The answer is b.** According to Nagele's Rule, the due date is calculated by subtracting 3 months and adding 7 days to the first day of the last menstrual period. In the situation described in the question, October is 3 months before January 10. When 7 days are added, October 17 is the correct due date.

9. **The answer is b.** A nonreactive fetal heart rate in a nonstress test that is part of a biophysical profile indicates fetal hypoxia. All of the other options do not indicate diminished fetal oxygenation.

10. **The answer is a.** An L/S ratio of at least 2:1 indicates fetal lung maturity. Therefore, an L/S ratio of 1.5:1 would mean that the lungs are not yet mature. Option b is inaccurate because the lungs are not yet mature. Option c is incorrect because the nurse can give an explanation of the test results to the patient. Option d is not the best choice because there is not a problem with the lungs. Surfactant production indicated by the L/S ratio will increase with fetal lung maturation over time.

11. **The answer is a.** The recommended gain for women with normal prepregnant weight is 25–35 lb. The pattern of weight gain is 3 to 5 lb in the first trimester, and 1 lb per week in the second and third trimester. This woman has gained 29 lb at 29 weeks of gestation;

her expected weight gain at this time would be 19 to 21 lb. She is gaining too rapidly; her diet needs to be reviewed and contributing factors determined.

12. **The answer is d.** Option d meets the woman's needs for calcium, protein, vitamins, and carbohydrates without empty calories or too much fat. In option a, iced tea contains caffeine, and Jell-O has the empty calories of simple sugars. In option b, fats from fried foods and mayonnaise in the coleslaw would be excessive. In option c, the orange soda is not nutritious.

13. **The answer is b.** Option b indicates that the woman does not understand the need to drink fluids between meals instead of with meals. In the other options, understanding of the recommendations for managing nausea and vomiting of pregnancy is demonstrated.

14. **The answer is d.** Lightheadness and dizziness when lying flat indicate vena cava syndrome or supine hypotension. Option d is the only nursing action that addresses means of correcting this syndrome.

15. **The answer is a.** The Kegel exercise strengthens perineal muscles around the vagina. Option b is incorrect because partial sit-ups are done to increase abdominal muscle tone. Option c is incorrect because the pelvic tilt exercise strengthens lower back muscles. Option d is incorrect because sacral pressure is counter-pressure used to decrease back pain felt with contractions.

16. **The answer is b.** The most appropriate breathing to prevent pushing is to blow on each exhale. This conscious blowing on each exhale counteracts the urge to bear down. The other options describe breathing techniques used throughout labor.

IV

Intrapartum Period: The Client in Labor

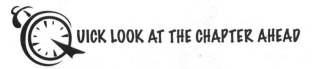

An understanding of the process of labor and birth is essential for the perinatal nurse in caring for women in labor and their families.

During labor, uterine contractions efface and dilate the cervix to allow the fetus to exit the mother's body through the vagina. After the birth of the fetus, the placenta and membranes are expelled.

Effacement is the thinning and shortening of the cervix and **dilation** is the widening of the cervical canal. (See Figure 17-1.)

The presenting part is the fetal body part entering the maternal pelvis first.

The first or dilation stage of labor is divided into three phases. In the latent phase the cervix dilates from 0 to 3 cm. The woman is talkative, excited, and apprehensive, able to answer questions and receptive to teaching.

In the active phase the cervix dilates from 4 to 7 cm. The woman experiences an increase in bloody show, nausea, a flushed face, and possible increases in blood pressure and pulse, and verbalizes her discomfort and fatigue.

In the transition phase the cervix dilates from 8 to 10 cm. There is copious bloody show, sweat on the upper lip, burping, hiccupping, vomiting, face very flushed, trembling extremities, and strong rectal pressure. Typical verbalizations are "I can't do this anymore!" and "I want to go home!"

17

The Process of Labor: The First Stage

The presenting fetal body part enters the maternal pelvis first. The head is called a cephalic presentation. The buttocks or feet is called a breech presentation. A shoulder presentation occurs when the fetus lies sideways in the uterus.

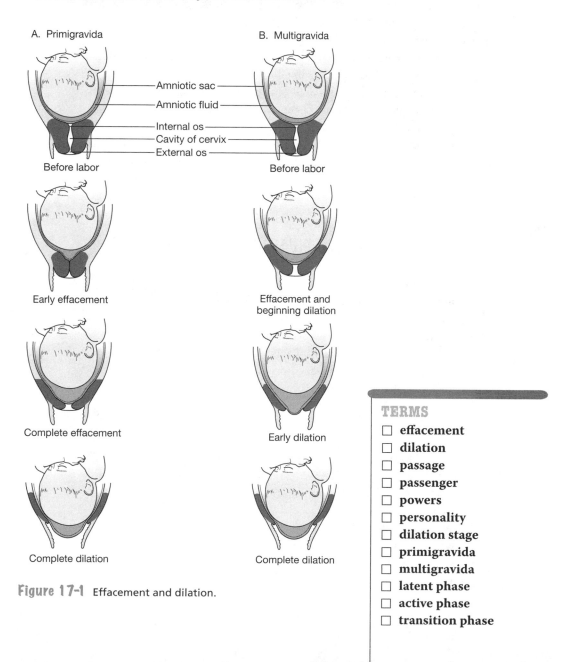

A. Primigravida   B. Multigravida

Amniotic sac
Amniotic fluid
Internal os
Cavity of cervix
External os

Before labor   Before labor

Early effacement   Effacement and beginning dilation

Complete effacement   Early dilation

Complete dilation   Complete dilation

Figure 17-1 Effacement and dilation.

TERMS
- ☐ **effacement**
- ☐ **dilation**
- ☐ **passage**
- ☐ **passenger**
- ☐ **powers**
- ☐ **personality**
- ☐ **dilation stage**
- ☐ **primigravida**
- ☐ **multigravida**
- ☐ **latent phase**
- ☐ **active phase**
- ☐ **transition phase**

THE FOUR Ps OF LABOR

The process of labor depends on the relationship among four factors: passage, passenger, powers, and personality.

The **passage** is composed of the pelvis, the bony canal through which the fetus must pass, as well as the soft tissues of the cervix, vagina, and perineum. The internal size and shape of the pelvis are crucial to a successful vaginal birth.

The fetus or **passenger** adjusts to the size and shape of the pelvis though the cardinal movements of labor (Chapter 18).

The **powers** may be positive or negative. The positive powers of labor, the uterine contractions and the use of abdominal muscles for the pushing stage, must overcome the negative powers, the resistance of the soft tissues.

The **personality** of the laboring woman influences her response to labor. Her knowledge of the labor process, her confidence in her ability to cope, and the support of the people around her will enable her to have a positive birth experience.

FIRST STAGE PHASES OF LABOR

Labor is divided into three stages. The first or **dilation stage** of labor lasts from the onset of contractions to complete dilation of the cervix. This stage may last for several hours,

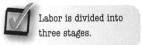

Labor is divided into three stages.

and is divided into three phases. Each phase is defined by the amount of cervical dilation, and has typical contraction patterns, physical signs, and maternal behaviors.

Latent Phase

The **latent phase** occurs as the cervix dilates from 0 to 3 cm. In the primigravida, the average length is 9 hours; in the multigravida, the average length is 5 hours.

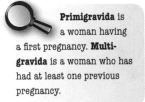

Primigravida is a woman having a first pregnancy. **Multigravida** is a woman who has had at least one previous pregnancy.

The typical contraction pattern is irregular, with mild to moderate intensity, 20 to 40 second duration, and 5 to 20 minute frequency. See Chapter 19 for an explanation of uterine contractions.

Physical signs usually associated with the latent phase include loss of mucus plug, presence of pink-tinged vaginal secretions known as "bloody show," and possible rupture of amniotic membranes. Maternal behaviors in this phase include being talkative, excited, and apprehensive. The woman is able to answer questions and is receptive to teaching.

 Maternal behaviors in this phase include being talkative, excited, and apprehensive. The woman is able to answer questions and is receptive to teaching.

Active Phase

The **active phase** is defined as the time when the cervix dilates from 4 to 7 cm. In the primipara, this phase averages 4 to 5 hours, with about 1 cm dilation per hour. In the multipara, this phase averages 2.5 hours with approximately 1.5 cm dilation per hour. The contraction pattern is regular, with moderate intensity, 40 to 60 second duration, and 2 to 5 minute frequency.

Maternal behaviors associated with this phase indicate an inward focus as labor becomes work. The woman verbalizes her discomfort, has increased dependency, and may question her ability to cope as she begins to tire.

The physical signs of the active phase include an increase in bloody show, nausea, flushed face, and possible increases in blood pressure and pulse. Maternal behaviors associated with this phase indicate an inward focus as labor becomes work. The woman verbalizes her discomfort, has increased dependency, and may question her ability to cope as she begins to tire.

Transition Phase

The **transition phase** lasts from 8 to 10 cm of cervical dilation. The average length is 1 to 2 hours for a primipara and up to 1 hour for a multipara. The contraction pattern is regular, with strong intensity, 60 to 90 second duration, and 2 to 3 minute frequency.

Maternal behaviors characteristic of this phase include irritability, fatigue, difficulty concentrating, feeling out of control, needing assistance controlling bearing down efforts, and feeling discouraged. Typical verbalizations during transition are "I can't do this anymore!" and "I want to go home!"

Physical signs include copious bloody show, sudden appearance of sweat on the upper lip, burping, hiccupping, vomiting, face very flushed, trembling extremities, and strong rectal pressure. Maternal behaviors characteristic of this phase include irritability, fatigue, difficulty concentrating, feeling out of control, needing assistance controlling bearing down efforts, and feeling discouraged. Typical verbalizations during transition are "I can't do this anymore!" and "I want to go home!"

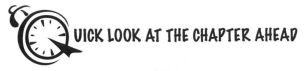

The second stage of labor is defined as the time from complete dilation to the birth of the infant. The average length is about 2 hours for a primigravida and about 15 minutes for a multigravida.

Contractions are regular, every 2 to 3 minutes, of strong intensity, and lasting 60 to 90 seconds. The woman sweats and feels the urge to push. The perineum bulges, the anus dilates, and the fetal head crowns at the vaginal opening.

The cardinal movements or mechanisms of labor are positional changes of the fetal head and body throughout birth.

The third or placental stage is the time from birth of the baby to delivery of the placenta and membranes.

The fourth stage is the immediate postpartum period, the first 4 hours after delivery. The new mother expresses joy and relief, eagerness to see and hold the infant, desire to share news of the birth, hunger, thirst, and fatigue.

Family bonding is encouraged by having the parents hold and interact with the infant. Breastfeeding is initiated as soon as possible after birth.

18

The Process of Labor: Second, Third, and Fourth Stages

TERMS

- [ ] pushing stage
- [ ] crowning
- [ ] cardinal movements
- [ ] mechanisms of labor
- [ ] engagement and descent
- [ ] station
- [ ] flexion
- [ ] internal rotation
- [ ] extension
- [ ] restitution and external rotation
- [ ] expulsion
- [ ] placental stage
- [ ] retained placenta
- [ ] signs of placental separation

SECOND STAGE

The second stage of labor, from complete dilation to birth, is called the **pushing stage**. It is characterized by strong urges to bear down as the presenting part presses on the stretch receptors of the pelvic floor muscles. Factors that affect pushing are position of the fetus, size of the fetus, maternal position, pelvic size and shape, use of epidural anesthesia, and the number of previous deliveries. Contractions during second-stage labor are regular, of strong intensity, with duration of 60 to 90 seconds and frequency of 2 to 3 minutes.

Physical signs exhibited by the woman include sweating, urge to push, bulging of the perineum, anal dilation, and appearance of the fetal head at the vaginal opening. When the largest diameter of the fetal head is circled by the vaginal opening, the head is said to be **crowning**.

> When the largest diameter of the fetal head is circled by the vaginal opening, the head is said to be **crowning**.

Maternal behaviors associated with second-stage labor include involuntary bearing down efforts, guttural sounds when pushing, increased focus on pushing efforts, sense of energy while still fatigued, burning or stretching sensations in the perineum, and a sense of accomplishment from finally being able to do something to help birth occur.

> Maternal behaviors associated with second-stage labor include involuntary bearing down efforts, guttural sounds when pushing, increased focus on pushing efforts, sense of energy while still fatigued, burning or stretching sensations in the perineum, and a sense of accomplishment from finally being able to do something to help birth occur.

If the woman has received epidural anesthesia, the length of the second stage may be significantly longer. Lack of sensation for bearing down efforts contributes to this delay. If there is no evidence of fetal or maternal compromise, and progress in descent is being made, there is no limit to a safe length for the second stage.

The **cardinal movements** or **mechanisms of labor** are positional changes of the fetal head and body throughout birth. (See Figure 18-1.)

> The **cardinal movements** or **mechanisms of labor** are positional changes of the fetal head and body throughout birth.

The mechanisms for birth of a fetus in cephalic presentation are described here.

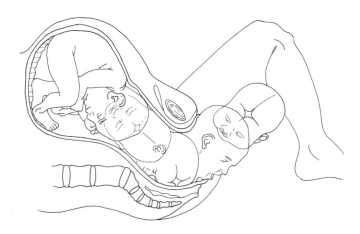

Figure 18-1   Cardinal movements or mechanisms of labor for a cephalic presentation birth.

- **Engagement and Descent:** The fetal head enters the pelvis and begins progressive movement through the pelvic cavity. Engagement of the fetal head usually indicates the pelvis is of adequate size for a vaginal birth.

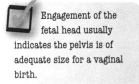

Engagement of the fetal head usually indicates the pelvis is of adequate size for a vaginal birth.

  Descent is measured by the **station** of the fetal presenting part in the pelvis. As the presenting part moves through the pelvis, it reaches the level of the ischial spines, which is the narrowest diameter of the pelvis. This is called the zero station. Negative numbers denote centimeters above zero station if the presenting part is higher than the ischial spines. Positive numbers denote a position of the presenting part lower than the ischial spines.

- **Flexion:** Resistance from the pelvic floor muscles causes the fetal chin to flex toward the chest.
- **Internal Rotation:** As the back of the fetal head meets resistance from pelvic floor muscles, the fetal head rotates to fit the diameter of the pelvic cavity.
- **Extension:** The fetal head emerges from under the symphysis pubis, first the occiput, then the face, and finally the chin.

- **Restitution and External Rotation:** After the head emerges, it resumes its original position. As the shoulders rotate to fit the outlet, the head is turned farther to one side.
- **Expulsion:** The anterior shoulder slips under the symphysis pubis, then the posterior shoulder. The rest of the body follows quickly.

THIRD STAGE

The third stage of labor, or the **placental stage**, is the time from birth of the baby to delivery of the placenta and membranes. The usual length of this stage is 2 to 15 minutes; a length more than 30 minutes is called **retained placenta**. After the infant is born, the uterus contracts firmly, decreasing the size and surface area of placental attachment.

The placenta separates from the wall of the uterus, drops into the lower uterine segment, and is delivered. **Signs of placental separation** include a gush of vaginal bleeding, lengthening of the cord protruding from the vagina, fundus rising in the abdomen, and the uterus becoming firm and globular. The woman may feel abdominal cramps and rectal pressure as the placenta separates. She bears down to deliver the placenta, or the health care provider lifts the placenta out of the vagina.

FOURTH STAGE

The immediate postpartum period is known as the fourth stage of labor, usually defined as the first 4 hours after delivery. Physical signs include a firm fundus near the umbilicus and in the midline, bright red vaginal bleeding, and shaking chills. Uterine cramps, perineal discomfort, leg cramps, or backache may occur. The perineum may begin to swell.

Physiological and psychological adjustments begin to occur immediately after delivery. Hemodynamic changes are most significant at this time. Because of blood loss and decreased pressure from the uterus on surrounding blood vessels, blood is redistributed. Contraction of the uterus controls bleeding from the placental site. In addition, the woman is recuperating from the effects of analgesia and anesthesia.

Maternal behaviors at this stage include a sense of joy and relief, eagerness to see and hold the infant, desire to share news of the birth, hunger, thirst, and fatigue. Family bonding is encouraged by having the parents hold and interact with the infant. Breastfeeding is initiated as soon as possible after birth.

Maternal behaviors at this stage include a sense of joy and relief, eagerness to see and hold the infant, desire to share news of the birth, hunger, thirst, and fatigue.

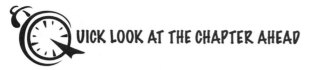
Assessment of the woman in labor is a major responsibility of the labor and delivery nurse. Assessments are performed and documented on a regular schedule.

Women are admitted into the health care setting if their membranes rupture or if they have signs of true labor. Upon admission, the nurse collects data about the client and takes baseline vital signs.

Uterine contractions are evaluated with manual palpation of the uterine fundus or by use of electronic monitoring.

Dilation, effacement, and fetal station are determined by vaginal examination.

Frequent blood pressure assessment is important because pregnancy-induced hypertension sometimes presents during labor.

Pain level and effectiveness of comfort measures are assessed throughout labor.

Hydration status and energy level are assessed throughout labor.

At least hourly, the bladder is assessed for distention.

Changes in behavior and physical signs characteristic of the different phases/stages of labor are assessed to determine labor progress.

The major reason for doing nursing assessments is to detect complications in labor: gestational hypertension, hemorrhage, intrauterine infection, dystocia (failure to progress in labor), or fetal distress.

19

Maternal Assessment During Labor

Although current technology affords increased accuracy in assessments, personal touch and "hands-on" assessment by the nurse are vitally important.

TERMS

- [ ] uterine contraction
- [ ] frequency
- [ ] duration
- [ ] intensity
- [ ] rupture of membranes
- [ ] gestational hypertension
- [ ] hemorrhage
- [ ] intrauterine infection
- [ ] failure to progress in labor
- [ ] fetal distress

> Frequent assessments are necessary to evaluate the progress in labor and to detect the development of complications.

Women are admitted into the health care setting if their membranes rupture or if they have signs of true labor. (See Table 19-1.)

Upon admission, the nurse should collect data about the client:

- age
- gravida and para, number of term pregnancies, preterm pregnancies, abortions, and living children
- date of last menstrual period (LMP)
- expected due date (EDD)
- weeks gestation
- time of onset of labor
- risk factors present; medications being taken
- allergies to medications, food, and other substances.

Prenatal labs including HIV, hepatitis B, rubella, VDRL, group beta strep, hemoglobin, and hematocrit are also reviewed. Baseline vital signs, blood pressure, fetal heart rate, contraction pattern, vaginal exam, and membrane status should be done.

Psychosocial assessment of the patient and family includes their existing knowledge of the birth process, use of childbirth preparation techniques, anesthesia preference, method of infant feeding, and desired amount of family involvement in the birth process.

Table 19-1   Comparison of True versus False Labor

	True Labor	**False Labor**
Contractions	Regular intervals	Irregular intervals
Intervals between contractions	Usually become shorter	Usually remain the same
Contraction intensity and duration	Increase in intensity and duration	Usually remain the same
Pain	Usually begins in the back and radiates to the abdomen, may increase with walking	Usually felt in the abdomen, walking has no effect or lessens contractions
Cervical effacement and dilation	Progressive increase	No change

UTERINE CONTRACTION PATTERN

Uterine contractions are evaluated with manual palpation of the uterine fundus or by use of electronic monitoring. **Frequency**, **duration**, and **intensity**, as well as uterine resting tone, are assessed. (See Figure 19-1.)

To evaluate contractions by palpation, a hand is placed gently on the fundus. Tightening and relaxation of the uterus can be felt with the fingertips. With experience, the nurse becomes proficient in judging contraction patterns by palpation.

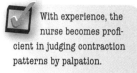

With experience, the nurse becomes proficient in judging contraction patterns by palpation.

Electronic monitoring of contractions is usually performed with an external transducer held in place at the fundus with a belt. Adjustments of the placement of the transducer are necessary with changes in maternal position and with fetal descent and internal rotation.

When more accurate information is needed, an intrauterine pressure catheter is inserted into the amniotic fluid to record pressures during the contraction cycle.

CERVICAL CHANGES

Dilation, effacement, and fetal station are determined by vaginal examination. (See Figure 19-2.) The amount of blood in vaginal secretions increases as dilation progresses. It is essential for the labor and delivery nurse to know the difference between heavy bloody show and overt hemorrhage.

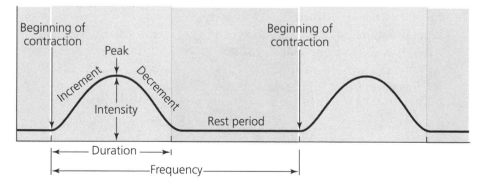

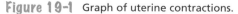

Figure 19-1 Graph of uterine contractions.

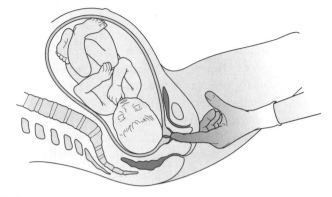

Figure 19-2 Vaginal examination to determine dilation, effacement, and fetal station.

 The nurse should use disposable gloves during vaginal exams as protection from exposure to vaginal secretions, bloody show, and amniotic fluid.

STATUS OF THE MEMBRANES

Amniotic membranes are either intact or ruptured. If membranes are ruptured, the alkaline amniotic fluid will turn Nitrazine paper blue, and will appear in a fern-like pattern when examined under the microscope.

Nitrazine paper is an absorbant strip of paper that changes color in response to acid or alkaline solutions. Also called pH paper.

The date and time of **rupture of the membranes** must be recorded. Once membranes rupture, ongoing assessments of fetal heart tone, color, odor, consistency, and amount of fluid are made.

 Ruptured membranes increase the risk of infection.

See Chapter 45 for a discussion of premature rupture of membranes. Assessment of the amniotic fluid during labor is discussed in Chapter 21.

VITAL SIGNS

Baseline vital signs are taken on admission. Temperature is evaluated every 4 hours during labor; if elevated or membranes rupture, temperature is taken every 2 hours.

Blood pressure, pulse, and respiration assessments differ with each phase of labor. In the latent and active phases they are taken every hour; in the transition phase they are taken every 30 minutes and in second stage they are taken every 5 to 15 minutes.

 Blood pressure assessment is important because pregnancy-induced hypertension sometimes presents during labor.

PAIN

Pain level and effectiveness of comfort measures are assessed throughout labor. Women are asked to rate their pain on a scale ranging from 0 denoting no pain to 10 denoting extreme pain. The intensity of the patient's pain is determined by her perception, not by an interpretation of the contraction pattern present on the monitor strip. Pain management techniques are addressed in Chapter 22.

NUTRITION AND ELIMINATION

Hydration status and energy level are assessed throughout labor. Signs of dehydration are dry lips and mucous membranes, expressions of thirst, and elevation of body temperature.

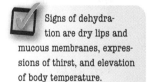
Signs of dehydration are dry lips and mucous membranes, expressions of thirst, and elevation of body temperature.

In most hospital settings intravenous fluids are administered and oral intake is limited to ice chips and/or clear liquids. In other birth settings, simple foods such as soup, crackers, or toast may be offered.

At least hourly, the bladder should be assessed for distention. A full bladder can impede fetal descent and increases patient discomfort. Patients who have had intravenous fluids or epidural anesthesia have higher risk for urinary retention. Measures to assist the patient to void should be initiated; if unsuccessful, catheterization will be necessary.

RESPONSES TO LABOR

Changes in behavior and physical signs indicate progress through the different phases/stages of labor. See Chapters 17 and 18 for descriptions of physical and behavioral changes during labor.

The nurse assesses the use of childbirth techniques, interactions with family members and health care providers, and the presence of fatigue or anxiety that may affect abilities to cope.

COMPLICATIONS

Detecting complications in labor is the major reason for doing nursing assessments. Significant problems and assessment findings during labor are listed here.

> Detecting complications in labor is the major reason for doing nursing assessments.

- **Gestational hypertension:** history of risk factors, elevated BP, decreased urinary output, proteinuria, hyperreflexia, presence of headaches, blurred vision, or other visual disturbances. (See Chapters 43 and 44.)
- **Hemorrhage,** especially placenta abruption: presence of risk factors, decreased blood pressure, increased pulse, elevated uterine resting tone, signs of fetal distress. (See Chapter 42.)
- **Intrauterine infection:** presence of risk factors, increased maternal temperature, fetal tachycardia, foul odor of amniotic fluid. (See Chapter 45.)
- **Failure to progress in labor** or dystocia: presence of risk factors, diminished uterine contractions, lack of cervical change.
- **Fetal distress:** fetal tachycardia, bradycardia, or decelerations, decreased fetal scalp pH, and decreased fetal oxygen saturation. (See Chapter 20.)

FREQUENCY OF ASSESSMENTS

Assessments are performed and documented on a regular schedule: at admission, every 30–60 minutes during the latent phase, every 30 minutes during the active phase, every 15–30 minutes during transition, and every 5 minutes during pushing. Nursing assessments during the fourth stage of labor are discussed in Chapter 25.

More frequent assessments are carried out if risk factors exist, if changes occur which warrant more frequent evaluation, or if the client is receiving analgesia, anesthesia, oxytocin, magnesium sulfate, or other medications that may affect labor. Nursing assessments during the administration of analgesia and anesthesia are discussed in Chapter 22. Nursing assessments during the administration of oxytocin are discussed in Chapter 51. Nursing assessments during the administration of magnesium sulfate are discussed in Chapter 44.

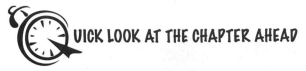
Fetal assessment is done to evaluate the fetal response to labor and to detect signs of fetal distress. Information about pertinent risk factors is gathered from the mother's medical record: gestational age, history of complications of pregnancy, status of the membranes, phase/stage of labor, administration of analgesia/anesthesia, and labor induction.

Fetal status during labor is determined by evaluating fetal heart rate patterns and assessing the amniotic fluid. If there are signs of fetal distress, fetal oxygenation can be further assessed by sampling fetal blood and monitoring fetal oxygen saturation.

An ongoing responsibility of the labor and delivery nurse is assessing the fetus during labor by checking fetal heart rate patterns and the amniotic fluid. The fetal heart rate reflects fetal oxygenation. Fetal heart rate (FHR) patterns are evaluated by auscultation or by electronic fetal monitoring.

Auscultation is using a handheld ultrasound device to listen before, during, and for at least 30 seconds immediately after a contraction.

Using electronic fetal monitoring for FHR pattern interpretation involves baseline rate, presence or absence of accelerations, variability, deceleration patterns, and changes over time.

The normal baseline rate is 110 to 160 bpm (beats per minute). A rate above 160 is called tachycardia. A rate less than 110 is bradycardia. Variability is fluctuation in the baseline.

20

Fetal Assessment in Labor

Accelerations are transient increases of 15 bpm or greater above baseline for at least 15 sec. Decelerations are transient decreases in the FHR. Late decelerations are an indication of fetal distress.

When membranes are ruptured, a normal amount of amniotic fluid is between 500 and 1200 ml. The fluid should be clear with no foul odor. A green or brown color indicates an episode of fetal distress and the FHR should be monitored closely. A foul odor means possible membrane infection increasing the risk of infection to the fetus.

When the FHR pattern indicates fetal distress, the physician may obtain a fetal scalp blood sample to test the pH. Normal fetal scalp blood pH is 7.25 or above. Normal fetal oxygen saturation is 30–70%.

In high-risk situations, continuous real-time recording of the fetal oxygen status is displayed on the uterine activity panel of the EFM tracing using a sensor inserted through the cervix into the uterus and resting against the fetal face.

 Assessment of the fetus during labor is an ongoing responsibility of the labor and delivery nurse.

TERMS
- [ ] auscultation
- [ ] electronic fetal monitoring
- [ ] baseline rate
- [ ] tachycardia
- [ ] bradycardia
- [ ] variability—marked, moderate, minimal
- [ ] accelerations
- [ ] decelerations—early, late, variable
- [ ] oligohydramnios
- [ ] hydramnios
- [ ] fetal scalp blood sample

EVALUATION OF FETAL HEART RATE PATTERNS

Fetal heart rate (FHR) patterns are evaluated by auscultation or by electronic fetal monitoring. Over the past three decades, electronic fetal monitoring has become in the United States and Canada the preferred method of fetal assessment during labor.

> Over the past three decades, electronic fetal monitoring has become in the United States and Canada the preferred method of fetal assessment during labor.

Auscultation

With **auscultation**, the nurse uses a handheld ultrasound device to listen before, during, and for at least 30 seconds immediately after a contraction. The fetal heart rate is heard most clearly at the fetal back. Maternal pulse should be compared to the fetal heart rate.

If no risk factors are present, auscultation every 30 minutes in the first stage and every 15 minutes in the second stage of labor is recommended. When risk factors are present, auscultation should be every 15 minutes in the first stage and every 5 minutes in the second stage.

Electronic Fetal Monitoring

Electronic fetal monitoring is an objective means of evaluating fetal well-being. The fetal heart rate reflects fetal oxygenation.

> The fetal heart rate reflects fetal oxygenation.

During a contraction, the tightening of the uterine muscles constricts blood flow through the placenta. If circulation within the placenta has been adequate, the fetus will have oxygen reserves and be able to tolerate temporary diminished blood flow, resulting in no change in the fetal heart rate. Signs of fetal distress can be detected by observing continuous fetal heart rate patterns and periodic changes during and after contractions.

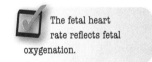

> Signs of fetal distress can be detected by observing continuous fetal heart rate patterns and periodic changes during and after contractions.

FHR pattern interpretation involves assessment of five components: baseline rate, variability, presence or absence of accelerations, deceleration patterns, and changes in these components over time.

Baseline Rate

Baseline rate refers to the upper and lower range of the FHR, observed between contractions during a 10-minute period of monitoring. The normal range is from 110 to 160 beats per minute.

Tachycardia is fetal heart rate above 160 beats per minute. The most common cause of fetal tachycardia is maternal fever. Fetal tachycardia also may be a compensatory mechanism for fetal hypoxia and an early sign of fetal distress.

Bradycardia is baseline rate less than 110 beats per minute. Common causes of fetal bradycardia are maternal hypotension, anesthesia/analgesia, and fetal hypoxia.

Variability

Variability is the fluctuation in the FHR baseline defined as marked, moderate, or minimal. **Marked** variability refers to a fluctuation above 25 beats per minute (bpm), **moderate** variability refers to fluctuations of 6 to 25 bpm, and **minimal** variability refers to fluctuations of 5 or less bpm.

Accelerations and Decelerations

Accelerations are transient increases of 15 bpm or greater above the FHR baseline, continuing for at least 15 seconds. Accelerations indicate adequate oxygenation to the fetal nervous system and occur with fetal movement or uterine contractions.

Decelerations are transient decreases in the FHR in relation to the contraction cycle. (See Figure 20-1.)

Early decelerations occur simultaneously with contractions, have uniform shape, and result from fetal head compression. This is considered a normal variation in FHR pattern.

Late decelerations begin after the contraction has started and reach their lowest point after the peak of the contraction. The FHR does not return to baseline rate until after the end of the contraction. They have uniform shape and indicate inadequate circulation within the placenta known as uteroplacental insufficiency.

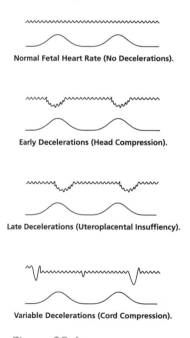

Normal Fetal Heart Rate (No Decelerations).

Early Decelerations (Head Compression).

Late Decelerations (Uteroplacental Insuffiency).

Variable Decelerations (Cord Compression).

Figure 20-1 Fetal heart rate patterns.

Late decelerations are an indication of fetal distress.

Variable decelerations occur abruptly, have irregular shape, and may not be related to the contraction cycle. They occur because of compression of the umbilical cord.

ASSESSMENT OF THE AMNIOTIC FLUID

When membranes are ruptured, amniotic fluid should be evaluated for color, odor, amount, and consistency. A normal amount of amniotic fluid is between 500 and 1200 ml. A decreased amount of amniotic fluid is called **oligohydramnios**; an increased amount is called **hydramnios**. Normal amniotic fluid has a thin, watery consistency. It should be clear with no foul odor.

If the fluid is green or brown in color, it is meconium-stained. This indicates there was an episode of fetal distress and the FHR should be monitored closely.

If there is a foul odor, infection of the membranes is suspected and there is increased risk of infection to the fetus. Maternal temperature should be checked.

Assessment of Fetal Oxygenation

When the FHR pattern indicates fetal distress, the physician may obtain a **fetal scalp blood sample** to test the pH. Normal fetal scalp blood pH is 7.25 or above. Normal fetal oxygen saturation is 30–70%. When hypoxia is present, blood pH falls because of acidosis. High-risk situations call for continuous real-time recording of fetal oxygen status, displayed on the uterine activity panel of the EFM tracing. This system uses a sensor that is inserted through the cervix into the uterus and rests against the fetal face.

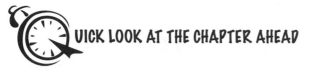

Nurses provide interventions during labor and birth for the patient and her family so that the woman is comfortable, safe, understands the birth events, participates in the labor process, and has the type of support she requests.

The nurse should help manage pain, detect and prevent complications, promote adequate hydration, provide ointment for dry mouth and lips, encourage the woman to urinate every 1 to 2 hr, promote safety, and encourage activity.

She should also teach the woman and her family what they should know and keep them informed during the birth process, encourage and assist the family to participate in the labor events to the extent they desire, and recognize how the culture of the patient and family can influence their responses to labor and birth.

She should assess the client for signs of hyperventilation—lightheadedness, dizziness, numbness and tingling of the face, lips, and fingers—and coach her on what to do about it.

The nurse should guide the woman through the various stages of labor, performing whatever exams, coaching, and activities that are needed, and keeping the family and health care provider aware of her progress in labor.

The primary goal of nursing care during labor and birth is for the woman to have a safe, empowering birth experience.

21

Nursing Care in Labor and Delivery

TERMS

- ☐ rupture of the membranes
- ☐ fetal distress
- ☐ vena cava syndrome
- ☐ hyperventilation

PAIN MANAGEMENT

- Observe response to contractions.
- Encourage the woman to rest between contractions.
- Provide comfort measures: ambulation, frequent position change, massage, soothing music, back rub, moist cloths to face, words of encouragement, changing pad under buttocks, shower, staying with woman and family, warmed blanket at back, sacral pressure.
- Assist with childbirth preparation techniques: patterned breathing, relaxation, use of focal point, visualization.
- If she has difficulty focusing, maintain eye contact and coach her through each contraction. Give very specific advice on breathing techniques with each contraction.
- Offer pain medication and give if requested.
- Assist with the administration of regional anesthesia.

DETECTION AND PREVENTION OF COMPLICATIONS

- Maintain ongoing assessments of mother and fetus. (See Chapters 20 and 21.)
- With **rupture of the membranes**, check fetal heart rate immediately to rule out prolapsed cord. See Chapter 20 for assessment of the amniotic fluid.
- Because there is an increased risk for infection after rupture, maternal temperature should be checked every 2 hours, underpads should be changed when wet, and vaginal exams should be limited.
- If there are signs of **fetal distress**, such as prolonged bradycardia, late or variable decelerations, or meconium-stained amniotic fluid, change maternal position, increase rate of IV flow, administer oxygen by face mask at 6 to 10 L/min, and notify health care provider.
- Observe for signs of other complications such as placental abruption, prolapsed cord, or prolonged labor.

HYDRATION

- Promote adequate hydration through IV fluids as ordered by physician, clear liquids, and ice chips. Monitor intake and output.
- Provide ointment for dry mouth and lips.

ELIMINATION

- Encourage the woman to urinate every 1 to 2 hours.
- If she is unable to void, perform catheterization if necessary.

SAFETY

- Promote safety by keeping siderails of the bed raised when the woman has been medicated with narcotics, or she is unable to maintain self-control in labor.
- Maintain bedrest immediately after adminstration of IV pain medication or after a regional block.

ACTIVITY

- Encourage ambulation unless contraindicated.
- Assist the woman into various positions at least every hour. Consider having her sit in a chair. Avoid the supine position, since this may cause **vena cava syndrome** (the weight of the uterus depresses the vena cava, reducing bloodflow, lowering maternal BP, and lowering FHR).

PATIENT/FAMILY TEACHING

- During admission, orient to the environment. Determine learning needs. Answer questions and provide information on labor process, procedures, and equipment.
- Teach relaxation, visualization, and breathing pattern if needed.
- Explain available comfort measures.
- During labor, keep patient and family informed of progress.

FAMILY INVOLVEMENT

- Determine patient's preference for family involvement.
- Assist family to provide comfort measures as requested by the laboring woman.
- Encourage patient and family to participate in the labor events to the extent they desire.

PSYCHOSOCIAL DIMENSIONS

- Recognize how the culture of the patient and family can influence their responses to labor and birth.
- Treat the woman and her family with respect.
- Accept nondisruptive behaviors during labor and birth without judgment.

COACHING

- Acknowledge that this is a special experience for the woman and her family.
- Reassure the client that she is doing a good job.
- Assist her with breathing, relaxation, and visualization techniques.
- Assess the client for signs of **hyperventilation**: lightheadedness; dizziness; numbness and tingling of the face, lips, and fingers. Remind her to slow her breathing rate, take shallow breaths, and breathe through her cupped hands or into a small paper bag.

TRANSITION PHASE

- Recognize behaviors that indicate the woman is in the transition phase of labor.
- Perform a vaginal exam if the laboring woman feels rectal pressure or an urge to push; determine if she is fully dilated and ready to begin the pushing stage.
- Encourage the woman to blow with short, forceful exhalations during a contraction to prevent pushing if she is not fully dilated and has the urge to push.

Short, forceful breathing increases the risk of hyperventilation.

If the woman bears down before the cervix is completely dilated, the cervix can swell or tear, prolonging the transition phase.

- Keep family and health care provider aware of her progress in labor.

SECOND STAGE: PUSHING

- Review breathing techniques for the pushing stage.
- Suggest that the woman rest until the urge to push is felt, allowing for the passive descent of fetus.
- Encourage active bearing down efforts when the fetal presenting part stimulates the woman's urge to push.
- Assist the woman to push and change position frequently. She could rotate from side to side, be semirecumbent, squat on a birthing ball, be on hands and knees, or lean over a birthing bar. (See Figure 21-1.)
- Encourage the woman to rest and extend her legs between contractions.

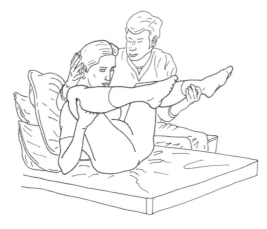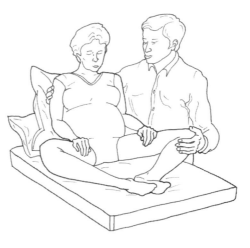

Figure 21-1 Positions for pushing.

- Praise the patient for her pushing efforts.
- Stay with the family.
- Continue to encourage drinking fluids and urination.
- Notify physician or midwife when presenting part is visible.

BIRTH

- Prepare birthing area as the time approaches.
- Notify the physician or midwife if he or she is not already present.
- Assist with pushing positions and breathing techniques.
- Prepare the instrument table, other equipment, and the infant assessment area.
- Prepare identification bracelets for mother and newborn.
- Note and record the time of birth.
- Acknowledge emotions the family expresses.

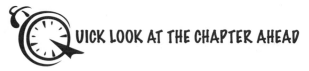

Normal physiological events cause most pain in labor. Labor pain is acute pain. Pain is perceived differently by each woman. Expression of pain is influenced by cultural expectations and norms.

Non-pharmacological techniques of pain management include relaxation techniques, patterned breathing techniques, cognitive distraction, and touch (if the woman is receptive).

Pharmacological techniques of pain management include barbiturates and antihistamines to sedate, and narcotics to decrease the perception of pain and allow the woman to rest between contractions. Narcotics for pain relief are usually administered intravenously.

Epidural anesthesia is most often administered to provide pain relief during active labor, birth, and episiotomy repair.

Spinal anesthesia is preferred over general anesthesia for cesarean birth. General anesthesia is used only in emergency situations or if spinal and epidural anesthesia are contraindicated.

When birth is imminent, the physician or midwife may inject a local anesthesia into the perineum before performing an episiotomy. This area may be reinjected after delivery of the placenta in preparation for a perineal repair.

 A high priority in the nursing care of the laboring woman is pain management, because labor pain is acute. Fear, anxiety, muscle tension, and fatigue decrease the ability to tolerate pain.

Nurses provide interventions to assist the woman to cope with the pain of labor, to have an active role in the labor process, and to experience a sense of accomplishment after birth.

22

Pain Management in Labor and Delivery

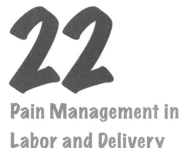

TERMS
- [ ] relaxation techniques
- [ ] patterned breathing techniques
- [ ] cognitive techniques
- [ ] touch
- [ ] barbiturates
- [ ] antihistamines
- [ ] narcotics
- [ ] side effects
- [ ] epidural anesthesia
- [ ] spinal anesthesia
- [ ] general anesthesia
- [ ] local anesthesia

135

PHYSIOLOGICAL BASIS FOR PAIN IN LABOR

Normal physiological events cause most pain in labor. In the first stage, uterine hypoxia; accumulation of lactic acid; stretching of the cervix and lower uterine segment; traction on the ovaries, fallopian tubes, and uterine ligaments; and pressure on the bony pelvis contribute to pain sensations.

In the second stage, distention of the pelvic floor muscles, vagina, perineum, and vulva, and pressure on the urethra, bladder, and rectum cause pain.

Pain is perceived differently by each woman, and her expression of pain is influenced by cultural expectations and norms.

Pain is perceived differently by each woman, and her expression of pain is influenced by cultural expectations and norms.

Factors influencing pain include intensity and duration of contractions, amount of cervical dilation, fetal position and size, length of labor, sleep deprivation, and past experiences.

NON-PHARMACOLOGICAL TECHNIQUES

Non-pharmacological techniques enhance a woman's sense of control and increase confidence in her ability to cope with the pain of labor. Non-pharmacological pain management provides a way for the nurse and family members to demonstrate support during the birth process.

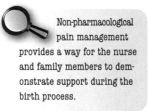
Non-pharmacological pain management provides a way for the nurse and family members to demonstrate support during the birth process.

With **relaxation techniques** the woman is taught to relax selected muscle groups while her uterus contracts. This decreases muscle tension, thereby decreasing uterine hypoxia.

Patterned breathing techniques can be used to control pain. See Chapter 16. The nurse needs to know what breathing techniques the couple has learned and teach simple techniques if needed.

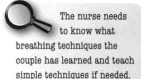
The nurse needs to know what breathing techniques the couple has learned and teach simple techniques if needed.

Cognitive techniques use the principle that the mind can focus on only one thing at a time. Thus, distracting the woman during labor decreases her perception of pain. Focusing on a picture, listening to music, counting during patterned breathing, concentrating on the voice of another person, having the presence of a support person, and hearing encouraging words about her efforts all assist the woman to cope with the discomfort of labor.

Touch helps the laboring woman to relax; it is both a distraction technique and tangible proof that she is not alone. Examples are massage, back rub, sacral counter pressure, acupressure, and light abdominal massage called effleurage.

> Touch must be used judiciously, as some women do not like to be touched during labor. Nurses should assess the woman's receptivity to touch.

PHARMACOLOGICAL TECHNIQUES

The goal of analgesia/anesthesia use in labor is to provide pain relief with minimal effects on the fetus or on labor progress.

> Most drugs used during labor affect either the mother's breathing or blood pressure, and have the potential to decrease the oxygenation to the fetus.

Two classes of drugs used in labor to produce sedative and hypnotic effects are **barbiturates**, such as secobarbital sodium, and **antihistamines**, such as promethazine hydrochloride. Barbiturates do not relieve pain; they induce sleep and decrease anxiety. These drugs may be used in early labor or to allow rest if a woman has a prolonged latent phase. Antihistamines are frequently given with narcotics to increase sedation and decrease nausea and vomiting.

Narcotics, such as meperidine or butorphanol, are the drugs most commonly given during labor. They are usually administered intravenously. Narcotics do not eliminate pain; instead, they decrease the perception of pain and allow the woman to rest between contractions. If the woman falls asleep, it is important to help her anticipate the beginning of a contraction rather than having her awaken at the most intense part. Narcotic use may decrease the frequency and duration of contractions in early labor; therefore, it is preferable to administer them after labor is well established.

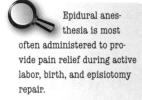

Narcotics will reduce fetal heart rate variability during labor.

Two major **side effects** of narcotics are maternal nausea and neonatal respiratory depression. To prevent nausea, IV push medications are given slowly over a period of 3 to 5 minutes. Sometimes antiemetics are given simultaneously.

Neonatal respiratory depression is most likely to occur if delivery happens during the peak effect of the narcotic. Optimally, birth should occur within 1 hour or after 4 hours following administration of a narcotic. If the newborn fails to breathe spontaneously, appears depressed, or requires prolonged resuscitation efforts, a narcotic antagonist, naloxone hydrochloride, is used.

 Epidural anesthesia is most often administered to provide pain relief during active labor, birth, and episiotomy repair.

Epidural anesthesia is most often administered to provide pain relief during active labor, birth, and episiotomy repair. **Epidural anesthesia** involves injection of a local anesthetic agent into the epidural space. (See Figure 22-1a.) When active labor is established, the epidural may be given.

The most common side effect of an epidural is maternal hypotension, which may lead to decreased oxygenation to the fetus. This is usually prevented by a rapid infusion of at least 1000 cc of intravenous fluids prior to epidural adminstration, then providing intravenous fluids continuously. Maternal blood pressure is checked every 2–5 minutes until there is effective anesthesia.

A Trendelenberg position is a position in which the head is lowered and the body and legs are elevated on an inclined plane.

If systolic BP falls below 100, corrective measures such as positioning the woman on her left side, increasing the IV rate, and placing the bed in a 10–20 degree Trendelenberg position are instituted. If maternal blood pressure does not increase within 1 to 2 minutes, vasoconstrictor drugs such as ephedrine may be administered by physician order.

Frequent assessment of the bladder to detect distention, measures to encourage voiding, and catheterization if necessary are nursing actions for inability to urinate.

Epidurals are associated with other side effects. The ability to urinate diminishes because of loss of sensation and motor control. Frequent assessment of the bladder to detect distention, measures to encourage voiding, and catheterization if necessary are nursing actions for inability to urinate.

Epidurals may be associated with increased length of the first and second stages of labor and with increased use of synthetic oxytocin medication. The woman should be assessed for progress in labor and will require assistance to push effectively. The use of forceps or vacuum extraction for delivery may be necessary.

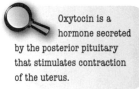

Oxytocin is a hormone secreted by the posterior pituitary that stimulates contraction of the uterus.

Spinal anesthesia is preferred for cesarean birth. Advantages over general anesthesia are that the woman is awake for birth, and neonatal respiratory depression is less likely to occur. The anesthetic agent is injected directly into the spinal fluid in the subarachnoid space. (See Figure 22-1b.)

The two major complications are immediate maternal hypotension and postpartum spinal headache. Prevention and treatment of hypotension are the same as with epidural anesthesia. In addition, positioning the woman with a wedge under the right side may prevent vena cava syndrome.

The postpartum spinal headache occurs because of leakage of spinal fluid at the puncture site in the dura. Hydration and keeping the woman flat in bed may be suggested to reduce the headache.

For cesarean birth, **general anesthesia** is used only in emergency situations, or if spinal and epidural anesthesia are contraindicated. Because general anesthesia leads to central nervous system depression of the mother and fetus, maternal and neonatal respiratory depression can be a serious problem. Most general anesthetic agents decrease the ability of the uterus to contract postpartum. Therefore, uterine assessments are important during the fourth stage of labor.

When birth is imminent, the physician or midwife may inject a **local anesthesia** into the perineum before performing an episiotomy. This area may be reinjected after delivery of the placenta in preparation for a perineal repair. This method provides the least effect on the progress of labor, mother's participation in labor, and the fetus.

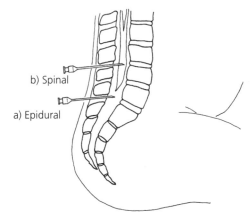

b) Spinal

a) Epidural

Figure 22-1 a) Epidural injection site. b) Spinal injection site.

PART IV · QUESTIONS

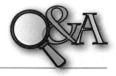

1. Which assessment indicates that a client is in true labor?
   a. Membranes ruptured.
   b. Presenting part is engaged.
   c. Cervix is at 4 cm dilation, 90% effaced.
   d. Contractions every 5–10 minutes, of 30-second duration.

2. A laboring patient pushes the nurse's hand away when the nurse tries to rub her back, saying "Leave me alone!" What would be the best nursing action?
   a. Ask another nurse to care for this client.
   b. Perform a vaginal exam to determine cervical dilation.
   c. Acknowledge this as normal behavior for the transition phase of labor.
   d. Continue to rub her back because the client does not mean what she says.

3. A client in labor received meperidine 2 hours before birth of a 7 lb, 3 oz girl. What drug should be available if needed?
   a. Butorphanol tartrate
   b. Naloxone hydrochloride
   c. Secobarbital sodium
   d. Promethazine hydrochloride

4. The nurse observes the fetal monitor tracing for a women who is 9 cm dilated and 100% effaced. The fetal heart rate begins to decrease when a contraction begins, and returns to the baseline as the contraction goes away. What is the most appropriate nursing action?
   a. Increase the IV flow rate.
   b. Change the mother's position.
   c. Administer oxygen by mask to the mother.
   d. Reassure the mother that the tracing reflects pressure on the baby's head.

5. Why should the mother in labor be encouraged to void every 2 hours?
   a. A full bladder may prevent the presenting part from descending.
   b. Several urine specimens are required during labor.

   c. There will be no need to catheterize the client at the time of delivery.

   d. Keeping the bladder empty will prevent postpartum cystitis.

6. What is the nurse's first action when an intrapartal woman's membranes rupture?
   a. Assess the fetal heart rate.
   b. Change the woman's bed linens.
   c. Document the time of rupture.
   d. Assess the amount and color of the fluid.

7. The nurse assesses variable decelerations on the fetal heart monitor of a woman in labor. What would be the first nursing action?
   a. Call the physician or midwife.
   b. Change the woman's position.
   c. Increase the IV flow rate.
   d. Administer oxygen by mask to the client.

8. A laboring woman is experiencing contractions of strong intensity. She complains of numbness and tingling of the lips and fingers and of dizziness. What would the nurse encourage her to do?
   a. Continue her breathing techniques.
   b. Hold her breath and bear down.
   c. Slow her breathing rate.
   d. Increase her breathing rate.

9. What observation would indicate that birth is immediate?
   a. Bulging of the perineum.
   b. Controlled urge to push.
   c. Decrease in bloody show.
   d. Sudden increase in fetal heart rate.

10. A woman has been admitted to the labor and delivery unit at 8 cm dilation. She is in which phase of the first stage of labor?
   a. Latent
   b. Active
   c. Transition
   d. Pushing

11. What nursing assessment is most important immediately after administration of epidural anesthesia for labor discomfort?
    a. Maternal respirations.
    b. Maternal blood pressure.
    c. Maternal pulse.
    d. Fetal heart rate.

12. A woman in labor begins to have difficulty maintaining her breathing pattern, expresses her discomfort by moaning softly, and asks for pain medication. Which statement is true about her behavior?
    a. It is appropriate for the latent phase of labor.
    b. It is indicative of the active phase of labor.
    c. It is indicative of complications in labor.
    d. It is appropriate for immediate birth.

13. A primipara in labor complains of a strong urge to push. She is examined and has reached 10 cm dilation. What is the most appropriate nursing action?
    a. Roll her on her side and tell her to breathe slowly during the contractions.
    b. Coach her to breathe out until the contraction is over.
    c. Explain that she is not yet ready to push and that doing so might harm the baby.
    d. Coach her to push with each contraction.

Using Figure Q-1, evaluate the contraction cycle and answer the next two questions.

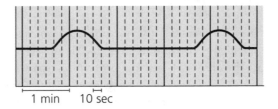

1 min   10 sec

Figure Q-1 The solid lines are at 1-minute intervals; the dashed lines are at 10-second intervals.

14. What is the duration of the contractions?
    a. 30 seconds
    b. 40 seconds
    c. 50 seconds
    d. 60 seconds

15. What is the frequency of the contractions?
    a. 2 minutes
    b. 3 minutes
    c. 4 minutes
    d. 5 minutes

PART IV • ANSWERS AND RATIONALES

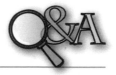

1. **The answer is c.** The essential ingredient of true labor is progressive dilatation and effacement of the cervix. Membranes may rupture before the onset of labor. The presenting part will reach 0 station when engagement occurs. Engagement can occur before the onset of labor. Contractions in true labor are regular and increase in frequency and duration. Women may have contractions; however, they may not be dilating.

2. **The answer is c.** The behaviors described in the question indicate the irritability experienced by the woman in the transition phase of labor. In a and d the nurse does not understand that this is normal behavior in the transition phase of labor. Vaginal exams are kept to a minimum in labor. A vaginal exam would be done if there are indications that the woman has reached complete dilation such as rectal pressure or an urge to push.

3. **The answer is b.** If the infant is delivered within 1 to 4 hours after the administration of meperidine, neonatal respiratory depression can occur. Naloxone hydrochloride is the narcotic antagonist used to reverse depressive effects. The other drugs are used for sedation or analgesia for the mother.

4. **The answer is d.** The question describes an early deceleration considered a normal variation of the fetal heart rate pattern. This is caused by head compression, and is not fetal distress. Reassuring the woman and her family that this is normal is an important nursing intervention. The other three choices list interventions performed when the fetal heart rate pattern indicates fetal distress.

5. **The answer is a.** The bladder should be kept empty in labor so that it does not interfere with the descent of the presenting fetal part. Voided urine specimens may not be accurate in labor because contamination from amniotic fluid and bloody show would alter the results. A clean catch urine specimen may be collected on admission to labor and delivery. There still may be a need to catheterize if the bladder is full and impeding the delivery. A full bladder in labor may be a contributing factor to postpartum cystitis; however, it is not the primary reason to keep the bladder empty.

6.   **The answer is a.** The first priority when membranes rupture in labor is to assess the fetal heart rate. The greatest concern is for a prolapsed cord. The other three choices describe nursing actions that would be done after determining the status of the fetus. Assessing the amount and color of the fluid is a second priority, followed by changing the linens and documenting the time of rupture.

7.   **The answer is b.** A variable deceleration occurs because of pressure on the umbilical cord. The first priority is to reduce the pressure on the umbilical cord by changing the mother's position. The other three choices are also nursing actions for fetal distress but would not relieve pressure on the cord.

8.   **The answer is c.** The question describes symptoms of hyperventilation. This occurs when clients breathe too fast or too deeply in labor. One action to correct this situation is to instruct the woman to slow her breathing rate. The other choices would not improve her symptoms and are not appropriate.

9.   **The answer is a.** Bulging of the perineum indicates that the fetal presenting part is at the vaginal opening and is a sign of late second stage labor. An uncontrolled urge to push is another sign of the second stage; however, birth may not be immediate. An increase in bloody show is a sign of transition. An acceleration of the fetal heart rate is not associated with impending birth.

10.   **The answer is c.** The laboring woman with cervical dilatation between 8 and 10 cm is in the transition phase of the first stage of labor.

11.   **The answer is b.** A major side effect of epidural anesthesia is maternal hypotension. Nursing assessments to detect a drop in blood pressure are imperative. Because blood pressure can drop suddenly, assessments every 2 to 5 minutes are necessary. While important, the other assessments do not take priority.

12.   **The answer is b.** The maternal behaviors indicative of the active phase of labor are described in the question. These behaviors are not typical of the latent phase, are normal behaviors not indicating complications, and are not indicative of immediate birth.

13. **The answer is d.** When the laboring woman is completely dilated and has the urge to push, she could be assisted to push with contractions. The other options would be appropriate if she is not ready to push or is not 10 cm dilated.

14. **The answer is d.** The solid lines are at 1-minute intervals. The dotted lines are at 10-second intervals. Duration is the length of the contraction from beginning to end. In the illustration, the contraction is 60 seconds in length.

15. **The answer is b.** The solid lines are at 1-minute intervals. The dotted lines are at 10-second intervals. Frequency is from the beginning of one contraction to the beginning of the next contraction. In the illustration, there are 3 minutes from the beginning of the first contraction to the beginning of the next contraction.

V

Postpartum Period: The Client After Birth

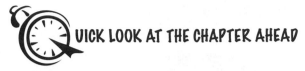
The postpartum period is the time between birth and the return of the mother's reproductive organs to their nonpregnant state. These changes usually take about 6 weeks to occur.

During involution, the uterus contracts, called involution, and the uterine muscles clamp off the blood vessels at the placental site. Muscle tone returns, but not fully, to the cervix, vagina, and perineum. Changes in lochia color and amount indicate healing of the placental site.

If breastfed, the infant's sucking efforts maintain prolactin production. If the infant is not breast-fed, the breasts return to the nonpregnant state within 2 weeks.

Immediately after delivery of the placenta, there is a rapid shift in blood flow in the maternal circulation, and blood volume returns to prepregnant levels.

Increased urination lasts for about a week. Urinary retention may require catheterization and can increase the risk of urinary tract infection.

A normal, balanced diet is encouraged for a woman without complications. Within 2 to 3 days normal bowel elimination usually returns, but other factors can cause constipation.

Weight is lost as the body returns to the nonpregnant state.

Chloasma and linea nigra fade, and striae take on their permanent coloration, white or silverish in Caucasian women, and brown in dark-skinned women.

23

Physical Adaptations to Postpartum

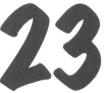

Assessments during the postpartum period focus on both physical and psychological responses to recovery from pregnancy and birth. The nurse must understand normal physical adaptations in order to interpret assessment findings and to teach the woman and her family what they need to make appropriate decisions about recuperation.

TERMS
- [ ] **involution**
- [ ] **lochia**
- [ ] **prolactin**
- [ ] **diaphoresis**
- [ ] **fibrinogen**
- [ ] **thromboembolus**
- [ ] **diuresis**
- [ ] **hypotonia**
- [ ] **edema**
- [ ] **meatus**

REPRODUCTIVE SYSTEM

The uterus returns to the nonpregnant state in a process called **involution**. Immediately following the delivery of the placenta, the uterus contracts to approximately the size of a grapefruit, weighs about 2 lb, and is located between the umbilicus and the symphysis.

> Throughout involution, the uterine muscles stay contracted, clamping off the blood vessels at the placental site, thereby preventing hemorrhage. The hormone oxytocin promotes these contractions.

By the end of the first week, the uterus weighs about 1 lb and is located just above the symphysis; by 6 weeks postpartum, it weighs about 2 oz and cannot be palpated through the abdominal wall.

Throughout involution, the uterine muscles stay contracted, clamping off the blood vessels at the placental site, thereby preventing hemorrhage. The hormone oxytocin promotes these contractions.

Healing of the placental site takes about 6 weeks.

The cervix, vagina, and perineum have been stretched and may be swollen or bruised. Muscle tone returns to these structures over the next 6 weeks but usually not to its prepregnant state.

Lochia is the postpartum discharge of blood, fragments of uterine lining, white blood cells, and mucus. Lochia is present usually up to 4 weeks after delivery. The changes in lochia color and amount indicate healing of the placental site. (See Table 23-1.)

Table 23-1 Types of Lochia

Type	Days Postpartum	Description
Rubra	Birth to day 2 to 4	Consists mainly of blood. Bright red changing to dark red or reddish brown. No more than the amount of a heavy menstrual period.
Serosa	Next 7 days	Amount of fresh blood diminishes. Serosanguineous,* lighter in color, turning pink or brownish.
Alba	Next 2 to 3 weeks	Yellow or white mucus. Scant amount.

*Serosanguineous refers to a thin, red discharge containing serum and blood.

Breast changes continue to occur after birth. Because of the reduction in estrogen and progesterone with the delivery of the placenta, **prolactin** levels increase and stimulate milk production. If breastfeeding is done, the sucking efforts of the infant

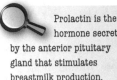

Prolactin is the hormone secreted by the anterior pituitary gland that stimulates breastmilk production.

maintain prolactin production. If the infant is not breastfed, prolactin levels diminish and the breasts return to the nonpregnant state within 2 weeks postpartum. See Chapter 33 on newborn nutrition for more detail on breastfeeding.

CARDIOVASCULAR SYSTEM

Immediately after delivery of the placenta, there is a rapid shift in blood flow in the maternal circulation. Blood volume from the placenta moves to the general circulation, and increases cardiac output and stroke volume. Cardiac output increases during labor, returns to prelabor values within 1 hour postpartum, and reaches prepregnancy levels within 3 weeks postpartum.

The additional blood volume gained during pregnancy is lost in the postpartum period through blood loss, increased urination, and **diaphoresis**. Within 2 to 4 weeks, the blood volume returns to prepregnant levels. The 30–50% increase in blood volume in pregnancy allows the woman to tolerate a normal blood loss during birth. In a vaginal birth, blood loss up to 500 cc is considered

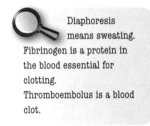

Diaphoresis means sweating. Fibrinogen is a protein in the blood essential for clotting. Thromboembolus is a blood clot.

normal. For cesarean birth, normal blood loss may be as much as 1000 cc.

Fibrinogen levels that have increased during pregnancy help protect the postpartum woman against hemorrhage, but increase her risk for **thromboembolus** formation. These fibrinogen levels gradually return to normal during the postpartum period.

URINARY SYSTEM

Within 12 hours of giving birth, excess tissue fluid is lost as **diuresis** begins. This increased urination lasts for about a week. The **hypotonia** and dilation of the ureters, renal pelves, and bladder that contribute to stasis may take up to 8 weeks to be reversed. **Edema** of the bladder, urethra, and urinary **meatus** from birth trauma, or diminished sensation from epidural or spinal anesthesia, may lead to urinary retention requiring catheterization.

 Diuresis means producing large amounts of urine. Hypotonia is decreased muscle tone. Edema is swelling. Meatus is an opening.

Stasis and retention increase the risk for urinary tract infection.

GASTROINTESTINAL SYSTEM

During the postpartum period, a normal balanced diet is encouraged for women without complications. Normal bowel elimination usually returns within 2 to 3 days after birth. Decreased motility of the gastrointestinal tract, discomfort from episiotomy or hemorrhoids, dehydration, or fear of having a bowel movement may lead to constipation.

WEIGHT CHANGES

Initial weight loss of 10 to 12 lb is due to delivery of the infant, placenta, and amniotic fluid. An additional 5 to 8 lb is lost in the first week from diuresis and lochia. Over the next 4 to 6 weeks, additional weight is lost as the body returns to the nonpregnant state. Nutrition, exercise, and breastfeeding influence the amount of weight lost by the end of the postpartum period.

SKIN CHANGES

Chloasma and linea nigra fade by the end of 6 weeks postpartum. In the next 3 to 6 months, the striae (stretch marks) that occurred during pregnancy will obtain their permanent coloration, white or silverish in Caucasian women and brown in dark-skinned women.

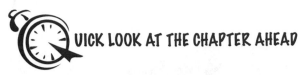
Intense maternal, parental, and family psychological changes begin during pregnancy and continue after the birth of the infant. (See Table 24-1.)

There are three maternal phases: taking-in, or dependency, taking-hold, or dependent-independent, and letting-go, or interdependent.

At first, many new mothers experience "baby blues," feelings of being overwhelmed and exhausted. This is normal, different from postpartum depression.

Both mothers and fathers experience attachment through eye contact, touch, verbalizations, and naming and nurturing of the infant.

Reciprocity is the interaction between the parent and the baby in response to cues. Synchrony is the correct interpretation of cues so that interaction between parent and infant is mutually rewarding.

Family dynamics change dramatically with the birth of an infant. Postpartum psychological adaptations also may vary according to culture.

The nurse has a unique opportunity to facilitate psychological adaptation, and thus family role development, during encounters with new parents. The nurse should be aware of normal postpartal psychological adaptations to make appropriate assessments, to recognize deviations from the normal, and to provide anticipatory guidance to the woman and her family.

24

Psychological Adaptations to Postpartum

TERMS
- [ ] **taking-in**
- [ ] **taking-hold**
- [ ] **letting-go**
- [ ] **"baby blues"**
- [ ] **attachment**
- [ ] **engrossment**
- [ ] **attachment behaviors**
- [ ] **reciprocity**
- [ ] **synchrony**

Table 24-1   Factors Influencing Psychological Adaptations

	Influencing Factors
Maternal	Length of labor; use of drugs, anesthesia; type of delivery; complications of pregnancy, labor, delivery, or postpartum; pain status; age; parity; past experience with mothering; role conflicts; relationship with partner; cognitive ability; level of education; culture; and ethnicity.
Paternal	Age, maturity, past experience with fathering, relationship with the mother, inclusion in the experiences, cognitive ability, level of education, culture, and ethnicity.
Infant	Gestational age, physical abnormalities, prolonged separation in special care, gender, appearance, and temperament.
Family	Socioeconomic factors, culture, ethnicity, demands of siblings, social support, family relationships, career demands, past experiences with own parents, and planned or unplanned pregnancy.

MATERNAL ADJUSTMENTS

In her classic work on the postpartum transition to being a mother, Rubin (1977) describes three separate phases. The successful outcome of these phases is attainment of the maternal role. In contemporary times, because of shorter hospital stays, less anesthesia, and earlier involvement in infant care, women experience these phases more quickly than originally described.

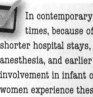

In contemporary times, because of shorter hospital stays, less anesthesia, and earlier involvement in infant care, women experience these phases more quickly than originally described.

The **taking-in** or dependent phase, in which the mother is passive and self-centered, focusing on her own needs and marveling about the baby, lasts from a few to 24 hours.

The second phase, which can last from one day to several weeks, is known as **taking-hold** or dependent-independent. In this phase, the new mother becomes more active in her own care and expresses interest in caring for her child. The mother is most receptive to teaching during this phase.

In the third phase, **letting-go** or interdependent, the woman redefines herself and becomes comfortable with taking on the role of mother in performing tasks and making decisions. Nurses can facilitate postpartum maternal adjustments. (See Table 24-2.)

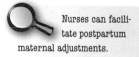

Nurses can facilitate postpartum maternal adjustments.

Table 24-2 Nursing Interventions to Enhance Postpartum Psychological Adaptations

Psychological Adaptation	Nursing Interventions
Taking-In Phase	"Mother the mother" by allowing her to be dependent. Assist mother in self-care activities. Focus explanations and teaching on immediate self-care. Encourage her to sleep, eat, drink, and talk about the birth experience. Allow opportunities for her to marvel at the baby by holding and observing, but not caring for the baby.
Taking-Hold Phase	Teach in more detail about self-care including normal lochial changes, normal involution pattern, breast care, and signs of infection. Teach infant-care skills; model attachment behaviors by talking to the baby, establishing eye contact, and cuddling. Provide positive reinforcement for mother's infant care activities.
Letting-Go Phase	Suggest options and resources for parental decision making. Reassure parents that it may take weeks or months to develop comfort in their new roles.
Attachment	Provide opportunities for parents to interact with the newborn. Observe for behaviors that indicate attachment. If attachment behaviors are not demonstrated, encourage verbalizations about their birth experience, model infant care skills and nurturing behaviors, and refer to social services as necessary.

In the first 2 to 3 weeks postpartum, many new mothers experience feelings of being overwhelmed and exhausted, and experience mood swings, irritability, anxiety, sadness, anorexia, insomnia, and fatigue. This cluster of symptoms is often called "**baby blues**" and is seen across all age, parity, socioeconomic, and ethnic groups. Although the exact cause is unknown, changes in hormonal levels, sleep deprivation, physical discomfort, and the emotions brought about by the assumption of the mothering role are contributing factors. "Baby blues" is considered normal, and is different from postpartum depression. See Chapter 55 for a discussion of postpartum depression.

> "Baby blues" is considered normal, and is different from postpartum depression.

PARENT-INFANT ATTACHMENT

Attachment is the emotional bond between a parent and an infant. Although it begins during pregnancy, the reality of having an infant encourages the development of this bond. Both mothers and fathers undergo the attachment process. Paternal attachment is sometimes called **engrossment**.

Attachment behaviors may be demonstrated in eye contact, touch, verbalizations, and naming and nurturing of the infant.

> Attachment behaviors may be demonstrated in eye contact, touch, verbalizations, and naming and nurturing of the infant.

Direct face-to-face and eye-to-eye contact is usually sought by parents when interacting with their infants. This position allows mutual gazing, another visual attachment behavior.

The typical touch sequence progresses from exploration of the newborn with fingertips, to using the fingers and palms to caress the baby, and finally enfolding the infant by cradling in the arms.

Verbalizations of what parents say and how they say it reflect attachment. Positive statements about the infant's appearance and behavior can be interpreted as signs of attachment. High-pitched, soft, and soothing tones provide comfort to the newborn and encourage the infant to look in the parent's direction. In most Western cultures naming a child is done soon after birth. Calling the baby by name indicates attachment. Other nurturing behaviors that may be demonstrated by the parents include performing infant care skills, soothing the crying infant, holding and rocking the baby, and expressing concern for the infant's well-being.

In developing attachment, both the parent and the infant respond to behavioral cues from the other. **Reciprocity** is the interaction between the parent and the baby in response to cues.

> In developing attachment, both the parent and the infant respond to behavioral cues from the other.

Synchrony refers to the correct interpretation of cues, so that the interaction between parent and infant is mutually rewarding. An example of synchrony would be recognizing that the infant's cry indicates sleepiness rather than hunger, soothing the infant, and having the infant fall asleep. Such positive responses stimulate continuing interactions to meet the infant's physical and emotional needs.

INTEGRATION OF THE INFANT INTO THE FAMILY

Family dynamics change dramatically with the birth of an infant. Families learn new skills, reorganize their time, assume new roles, reallocate family resources, and help one another adjust to changing family interactions. The newborn becomes a member of the family and is accepted by other family members as its needs and schedules are incorporated into daily activities. The nurse can assess the degree to which family integration of the infant has occurred by observing family members interact with the infant. Statements about similarity of family characteristics, continuation of usual family activities, and adaptations made by the family since the birth also indicate integration.

> The nurse can assess the degree to which family integration of the infant has occurred by observing family members interact with the infant. Statements about similarity of family characteristics, continuation of usual family activities, and adaptations made by the family since the birth also indicate integration.

CULTURAL IMPLICATIONS

Postpartum psychological adaptations may vary according to culture. The three phases of maternal adjustment may be expressed in different time frames:

- A mother may have a lengthened taking-in phase with family members assuming care of the newborn.
- A new mother may be expected to have a longer recuperation and remain dependent on others for a longer period of time.

In some cultures the father may not be expected to participate in care of the infant. Therefore, he may not be interested in the teaching about newborn care.

The dominant culture may be so different for new arrivals that these couples need additional understanding and support as they cope with the expectations now placed upon them.

Attachment behaviors as described in this chapter may not be as evident in a family of another culture. Restrictions in maternal activity and personal preferences may limit parental caretaking activities. When assessing for parent-infant attachment, the nurse should observe for interest in and awareness of the baby, concern for the crying newborn, and knowledge of where the infant is and what is happening to the infant.

> When assessing for parent-infant attachment, the nurse should observe for interest in and awareness of the baby, concern for the crying newborn, and knowledge of where the infant is and what is happening to the infant.

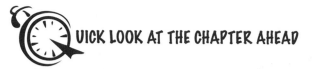

The first 4 hours after birth are known as the fourth stage of labor, and are a time of increased risk for hemorrhage. Because of this risk, the immediate postpartum physical assessments focus on hemodynamic changes and ability of the uterus to remain contracted.

Ongoing postpartum assessments focus more on changes that indicate return of body systems to the nonpregnant state. (See Table 25-1.)

Vital signs in the postpartum period reflect physiological adjustments made after birth.

Assessment of the uterus includes consistency, or firmness exhibited by the contracted uterine muscles; height, measured in fingerbreadths above or below the umbilicus; and position, in relation to the umbilicus.

Lochia is assessed for amount, presence of clots, color, and odor.

The bladder is assessed frequently for urinary retention.

The perineum is assessed for intactness, swelling, bruising, hemorrhoids, and the presence of a hematoma.

It is important that lacerations in the cervix, vaginal wall, or perineum be identified and repaired to prevent bleeding.

If an episiotomy was done, it should be assessed for REEDA: redness, edema, ecchymosis, drainage, and approximation of the edges.

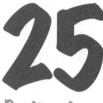

25

Postpartum Physical Assessment

TERMS
- [ ] uterus
  - [ ] consistency
  - [ ] height
  - [ ] position
- [ ] lochia
  - [ ] amount
  - [ ] color
  - [ ] odor
- [ ] lacerations
- [ ] sulcus tear
- [ ] episiotomy

Elimination patterns and presence of bowel sounds are assessed.

If a cesarean delivery or tubal ligation has been done, the abdominal incisions are assessed gently, using REEDA. The nurse modifies the position of hands during palpation to avoid direct pressure on the incision.

The breasts are assessed for signs of lactation, including engorgement, and evidence of trauma to the nipples from the infant's sucking.

Legs are assessed for edema and signs of phlebitis.

In addition, the nurse assesses for level of comfort, with special attention to breasts, abdomen, and perineum, and for psychological adaptations to the postpartum phase and attachment.

 Immediate and ongoing postpartum nursing assessments are important in identifying normal physical adaptations and the presence of complications.

Table 25-1 Guidelines for Postpartum Assessments

IMMEDIATE ASSESSMENTS IN FOURTH STAGE OF LABOR	
Frequency	**What is assessed**
q. 15 min x 4, q. 30 min x 2, then q. 1–2 hr x 2.	Vital signs, uterus, lochia, bladder, perineum, any incisions, and comfort status.
ONGOING ASSESSMENTS	
Frequency	**What is assessed**
After the first 4 hr, q. 4 hr for 24 hr, then q. 8 hr until discharge.	Vital signs, uterus, lochia, bladder, perineum, abdomen, incisions, breasts, legs, comfort, and psychological adaptations.

VITAL SIGNS

Vital signs in the postpartum period reflect physiological adjustments made after birth. Temperature may increase slightly during the first 24 hours due to dehydration during labor.

 If the temperature is above 100.4˚F or 38˚C after the first 24-hour period, the woman is considered febrile and further assessments for infection should be done.

Bradycardia is normal in the postpartum period; normal range for the pulse is 40 to 80 beats per minute.

 A rapid and thready pulse is abnormal and may indicate postpartum hemorrhage.

Respiration rate ranges from 16 to 24 breaths per minute.

Blood pressure should be stable and comparable to pregnancy and labor readings.

Elevated blood pressure should be evaluated for the presence of pregnancy-induced hypertension; decreased blood pressure may indicate orthostatic hypotension or postpartum hemorrhage.

UTERUS

Assessment of the **uterus** includes: consistency, height, and position. **Consistency** refers to the degree of firmness exhibited by the contracted uterine muscles. A well-contracted uterus feels hard to the touch; a non-contracted uterus may be difficult to palpate, feels soft to the touch, and is described as "boggy".

> A well-contracted uterus feels hard to the touch; a noncontracted uterus may be difficult to palpate, feels soft to the touch, and is described as "boggy."

The **height** of the uterus is measured in fingerbreadths above or below the umbilicus. In most situations, the uterus is located near the level of the umbilicus on the day of delivery and moves downward one fingerbreadth per day as involution progresses. By 10 to 14 days postpartum, the uterus can no longer be palpated through the abdomen. (See Figure 25-1.)

The usual **position** of the uterus is midline.

A full bladder displaces the uterus from the midline, usually to the right side, and may prevent the uterus from maintaining a contracted state.

LOCHIA

Lochia is assessed for amount, clots, color, and odor. In the first several hours following birth, the **amount** of lochia rubra may be heavy, saturating one pad an hour. After that, the volume will gradually diminish over the next several days. (See Figure 25-2.)

Clots may be present in lochia rubra, but should be less than the size of a plum. Clots occur due to pooling of blood in the uterine cavity or vagina.

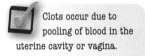
Clots occur due to pooling of blood in the uterine cavity or vagina.

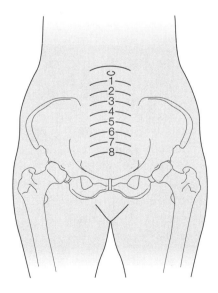

Figure 25-1 Involution of the uterus.

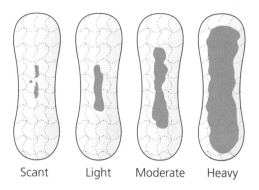

Scant   Light   Moderate   Heavy

Figure 25-2 Assessing amount of lochia.

 Excessive amount of bleeding, with or without clots, indicates postpartum hemorrhage.

Lab values of hemoglobin and hematocrit should be reviewed; for every 500 cc blood loss there is a 2% decrease in hematocrit.

Color of the lochia refers to the type of lochia: rubra, serosa, or alba. Refer to Chapter 23 for a description of types of lochia.

The normal **odor** of lochia is non-offensive, sometimes described as musty or fleshy, similar to that of menstrual flow.

 A foul or offensive odor lochia may indicate uterine infection.

BLADDER

The bladder is assessed frequently for indications of urinary retention. Urinary output should be at least 250 cc each voiding. As part of the assessment, the nurse asks about frequency and amount of voiding as well as any signs of urinary tract infection such as pain and burning on urination. The nurse also reviews the delivery record to determine if the woman had a periurethral laceration.

As part of the assessment, the nurse asks about frequency and amount of voiding as well as any signs of urinary tract infection such as pain and burning on urination. The nurse also reviews the delivery record to determine if the woman had a periurethral laceration.

Periurethral laceration may contribute to edema leading to urinary retention and cause burning on urination.

 ## PERINEUM

The perineum is assessed for intactness, swelling, bruising, hemorrhoids, and the presence of a hematoma. Some bruising, swelling, and mild discomfort are normal; small non-tender hemorrhoids may be present. Inflamed and painful hemorrhoids require specific comfort measures. Significant bruising, swelling, or pain in the rectal area may indicate the presence of a vaginal hematoma.

Lacerations can occur in the cervix, vaginal wall, or perineum during birth. A laceration of the vaginal wall is referred to as a **sulcus tear**.

 It is important that lacerations are identified and repaired to prevent bleeding.

Lacerations are classified by depth:

- A first-degree laceration involves mucus membrane and skin.
- A second-degree laceration goes deeper and includes the muscles of the perineum.
- A third-degree laceration involves the exterior sphincter of the rectum.
- A fourth-degree laceration extends through the entire perineum, the rectal sphincter, and into the anterior rectal wall.

Incisions involving these same structures are also classified as second, third, and fourth degree.

An **episiotomy**, or incision of the perineum, if done, is performed at the time of birth. This incision may be midline, down the center of the perineum, or mediolateral, angled to the right or left of the midline.

An episiotomy should be assessed for REEDA: redness, edema, ecchymosis, drainage, and approximation of the edges. Although most episotomies are second-degree incisions, sometimes they are extended to the third or fourth degree.

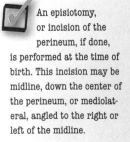
An episiotomy, or incision of the perineum, if done, is performed at the time of birth. This incision may be midline, down the center of the perineum, or mediolateral, angled to the right or left of the midline.

ABDOMEN

Elimination patterns and presence of bowel sounds are assessed. If a cesarean delivery or tubal ligation occurred, the abdominal incisions are assessed using REEDA—but the nurse performs the uterine assessment more gently, and modifies hand position during palpation to avoid putting direct pressure on the incision.

BREASTS

The breasts are assessed for signs of lactation, including engorgement, and evidence of trauma to the nipples from the infant's sucking. The signs of lactation begin about 36 to 72 hours after birth, and include progressive firmness of the breast tissue; sensations of fullness, tingling, or tenderness; enlarged veins visible on the surface of the breast; and leakage of fluid from the nipples. Engorgement often occurs with initial milk production. It is the term used to describe very firm, warm, throbbing breasts.

The nipples are assessed to determine if they become erect and protrude with stimulation. These conditions enhance the infant's ability to latch onto the nipple for breastfeeding. Signs of trauma to the nipple include redness, soreness, blistering, bruising, cracking, or bleeding.

LEGS

Legs are assessed for edema and signs of phlebitis. Ankle edema diminishes with postpartum diuresis and resolves in about a week. Thrombophlebitis is indicated by an area of warmth, redness, and tenderness in the calf, and a positive Homan's sign—pain in the calf muscle when the leg is sharply dorsiflexed.

OTHER ASSESSMENTS

In addition to the assessments described, the nurse assesses the postpartum woman for her level of comfort, with special attention to breasts, abdomen, and perineum. Assessment of postpartum psychological adaptations include observing for behaviors that indicate the postpartum phase and attachment.

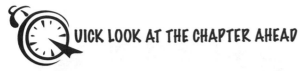

Hemorrhage and infection are the primary concerns of the nurse when providing postpartum care. After the immediate postpartum period, usually the new mother can assume responsibility for meeting most of her physical needs.

Hemorrhage from the inability of the uterus to contract is the primary nursing concern in the first 24 hours. Lacerations of the birth canal are suspected if heavy bleeding continues with a firm uterus. The usual postpartum infection sites are uterus, bladder, breast, and incision. Fever, chills, malaise, and body aches are general symptoms.

During the postpartum period, pain in the perineum from swelling, bruising, lacerations, incisions, and hemorrhoids may be relieved by use of an ice pack, perineal anesthetic sprays, sitz baths, and a side-lying position. In addition, astringent compresses can be used for hemorrhoids.

Comfort measures for afterpains from intermittent uterine contractions include massage of the uterus, emptying the bladder, ambulation, and lying on the abdomen.

In the breastfeeding mother, engorgement may be relieved by nursing the baby frequently, using warm compresses, and expressing milk to reduce pressure.

If bottlefeeding, a mother should not massage the breasts or express milk, avoid heat on the breasts, and use ice packs for discomfort.

Sore nipples may be prevented by ensuring correct latching of the infant, alternating the infant's position for breastfeeding, breaking the suction with a finger before detaching the infant, chang-

26

Postpartum Nursing Care

ing moist breast pads, air drying of the nipples for at least 20 minutes after nursing, and avoiding use of soap on the nipples.

If nipples are sore, the new mother can apply ice just before breastfeeding to numb the nipple, and have shorter, more frequent feedings.

After cesarean delivery, pain from the abdominal incision is relieved by adequate pain medication, prevention of abdominal distention from gas, encouragement of ambulation, promotion of urination, and recommendation for abdominal support during movement.

It is very important for postpartum women to empty the bladder frequently.

Postpartum women are at risk for developing constipation. Key nursing strategies are acknowledging the woman's fear, recommending increased intake of fluids and fiber, encouraging ambulation and regular bowel habits, teaching perineal comfort measures, and administering stool softeners.

Women who are not immune to rubella (German measles) should be given rubella vaccine before leaving the hospital.

The woman who is Rh negative with no evidence of antibody formation, and whose infant is Rh positive, is given Rh immune globulin (RhoGAM) within 72 hours after delivery.

Nursing strategies to help women assume the mothering role include providing opportunities for mother-infant interaction as early and as much as possible, teaching infant care procedures, and praising her efforts to care for her baby.

 The nursing care given during the postpartum period is in response to the findings from physical and psychological assessments. Ongoing nursing care focuses on developing the woman's ability to care for herself and her infant after discharge. The support and education she receives will facilitate a successful transition to the mothering role.

TERMS

☐ **fundal massage**
☐ **after pains**
☐ **engorgement**
☐ **sore nipples**

PREVENTION OF HEMORRHAGE

In the first 24 hours after birth, the most likely complication is hemorrhage from the inability of the uterus to contract. Oxytocin is given after delivery of the placenta to increase uterine contractility and prevent hemorrhage.

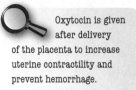

Oxytocin is given after delivery of the placenta to increase uterine contractility and prevent hemorrhage.

Frequent assessments of uterine muscle tone are done to make sure that the uterus is well contracted. If the uterus is not firm, the nurse performs **fundal massage** and expresses clots.

While supporting the lower uterine segment with one hand, the nurse gently massages the fundus with the other hand until the uterus is firm. To express clots, the nurse presses down on the fundus, giving firm counter pressure above the symphysis pubis. Additional nursing care includes promoting urination, encouraging breastfeeding, and administering oxytocin as ordered.

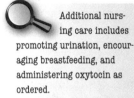

Additional nursing care includes promoting urination, encouraging breastfeeding, and administering oxytocin as ordered.

 Lacerations of the birth canal are suspected if heavy bleeding continues after the uterus becomes firm.

If excessive bleeding persists, the health care provider is notified. See Chapter 54 for discussion of postpartum hemorrhage.

PREVENTION OF INFECTION

Although infection can occur in the early postpartum period, most of the time infection is not evident for several days. The usual postpartum infection sites are uterus, bladder, breast, and incision. Fever, chills, malaise, and body aches are general symptoms.

Specific observations can be made to determine the exact location of infection. (See Table 26-1.)

Recommendations for prevention of postpartum infection include handwashing, daily bathing, frequent changing of sanitary pads, and use of warm water for cleansing the perineum after toileting.

Table 26-1 Assessment for Postpartum Infection

Site of Infection	Significant Assessments
Uterus	Lochia with foul odor; uterus large and tender to touch, excessive cramping.
Bladder	Pain and burning on urination, frequency and urgency of urination, blood in voided urine is most likely from lochia.
Breast	Localized redness, tenderness, and swelling around a palpable mass.
Incision	REEDA: redness, edema, ecchymosis, drainage, and edges not approximated.

To prevent bladder infections, frequent urination, perineal cleansing from front to back, and consumption of adequate fluids are encouraged. Suggestions for preventing breast infection include cleansing nipples with warm water only, and changing bra and breast pads frequently.

PROMOTION OF COMFORT

During the postpartum period, discomfort may result from trauma or normal physiological changes. The following interventions are suggested before administering pain medications:

- Pain in the perineum from swelling, bruising, lacerations, incisions, and hemorrhoids may be relieved by use of an ice pack, perineal anesthetic sprays, and sitz baths. In addition, astringent compresses can be used for hemorrhoids. A side-lying position may be more comfortable.
- Afterpains from intermittent uterine contractions are more common in multiparous women, after the birth of a large infant, or with multiple infants, and may increase while breastfeeding. Comfort measures include massage of the uterus, emptying the bladder, ambulation, and lying on the abdomen.

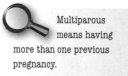
Multiparous means having more than one previous pregnancy.

Breast discomfort commonly occurs from engorgement or sore nipples. Wearing a supportive bra enhances comfort. In the breastfeeding mother, engorgement may be relieved by nursing the baby frequently, using warm compresses, and expressing milk to reduce pressure.

A bottlefeeding mother should not massage the breasts or express milk, should avoid heat on the breasts, and use ice packs for discomfort.

Sore nipples may be prevented by

- Ensuring correct latching of the infant
- Alternating the infant's position for breastfeeding
- Breaking the suction with a finger before detaching the infant
- Changing moist breast pads
- Air drying of nipples for at least 20 minutes after nursing
- Avoiding use of soap on the nipples.

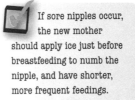

If sore nipples occur, the new mother should apply ice just before breastfeeding to numb the nipple, and have shorter, more frequent feedings.

If sore nipples occur, the new mother should apply ice just before breastfeeding to numb the nipple, and have shorter, more frequent feedings.

After a cesarean delivery, medication for pain from the abdominal incision is an appropriate first intervention because pain interferes with a mother's ability to interact with the baby, learn about self- and infant care, and begin to assume the mothering role. Other comfort measures are prevention of abdominal distention from gas, encouragement of ambulation, promotion of urination, and recommendation for abdominal support during movement.

PROMOTION OF ELIMINATION

A full bladder may contribute to postpartum hemorrhage, urinary tract infection, and discomfort. Also, the excess fluid gained during pregnancy is lost by diuresis in the early postpartum period. So it is very important for postpartum women to empty their bladders frequently.

Nursing strategies to promote urination include encouragement of ambulation and recommendation to void every two hours. If the woman is unable to void due to anesthesia or perineal trauma, she is instructed to run water in the sink, squirt or pour water over her perineum, dabble her fingers in warm water, or blow bubbles with a straw, all to relax the perineum.

Postpartum women are at risk for developing constipation. The woman may be hesitant to have a bowel movement because of

- perineal discomfort from birth trauma, episiotomy, lacerations, or hemorrhoids

- abdominal pain from a cesarean incision
- fear of pain during defecation.

When a woman is breastfeeding, she may not have adequate fluid intake for both milk production and prevention of constipation.
Key nursing strategies are

- acknowledging the woman's fear
- recommending increased intake of fluids and fiber
- encouraging ambulation and regular bowel habits
- teaching perineal comfort measures
- administering stool softeners.

> If there is a third- or a fourth-degree episiotomy or laceration, it is very important not to insert anything into the anus, such as a suppository or an enema tube.

PROMOTION OF MATERNAL ROLE ATTAINMENT

Experiences during the early postpartum period help women begin to assume the mothering role. Nursing strategies include providing opportunities for mother-infant interaction as early and as much as possible, teaching infant care procedures, and praising her efforts to care for her baby. Refer to Table 24-2.

RUBELLA VACCINE AND RHOGAM

Postpartum women may be candidates for two medications that prevent problems in future pregnancies. Women who are not immune to rubella (German measles) should be given rubella vaccine before leaving the hospital after birth.

The rubella vaccine is a live, attenuated virus; the woman is advised to prevent pregnancy for at least 3 months after receiving the injection.

If a pregnant woman develops a rubella infection in the first trimester, the fetus is at risk for congenital abnormalities such as deafness, cardiovascular defects, and cataracts.

The woman who is Rh negative with no evidence of antibody formation, and whose infant is Rh positive, is given Rh immune globulin (RhoGAM) within 72 hours after delivery. RhoGAM prevents the development of antibodies in the mother to Rh positive fetal red blood cells that could enter the mother's bloodstream when the placenta separates. Development of Rh-positive antibodies by the mother places a future fetus at risk for destruction of red blood cells known as erythroblastosis fetalis. Refer to Chapter 64 for a description of erythroblastosis fetalis.

Development of Rh-positive antibodies by the mother places a future fetus at risk for destruction of red blood cells known as erythroblastosis fetalis.

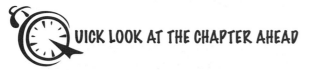
Topics important to cover when preparing the woman for discharge after a vaginal birth include:

- Dealing with normal physical changes in breasts, uterus, perineum, and lochia.

- What to do about and how to avoid heavy bleeding and signs of infection.

- Importance of proper personal hygiene.

- Signs of thrombophlebitis: warmth, redness, or tenderness in the affected leg; pain in calf when walking.

- Gradual resumption of physical activity, an activity schedule, and ways to conserve energy and promote rest.

- Importance and types of postpartum exercises.

- Proper nutrition and diet.

- Timing and nature of return to sexuality.

- Making emotional adjustments to having a child.

- Postpartum follow-up.

Nurses have an essential role in providing information to families about the woman's recovery from the birth process and care of the infant.

27

Discharge Teaching: Maternal Topics

TERMS
- [ ] subinvolution

Postpartum is a time when parents are very receptive to learning. But the nurse must evaluate the woman's ability to understand and retain information. Written instructions often need to accompany verbal explanations.

The following topics are important to cover when preparing the woman for discharge after a vaginal birth. Postpartum teaching after cesarean birth is discussed in Chapter 53.

Table 27-1 contains information about when to notify the health care provider.

NORMAL PHYSICAL CHANGES

- ◆ Review changes in breasts, uterus, perineum, and lochia.
- ◆ Describe how to assess for signs of lactation and engorgement, and teach comfort measures for engorgement.
- ◆ Demonstrate how to palpate the uterus through the abdomen and teach comfort measure for afterpains.
- ◆ Teach perineal hygiene and comfort measures.
- ◆ Explain expected lochial changes.

See Chapters 23 and 25 for details on this content.

Table 27-1   When to Call the Health Care Provider

Maternal Concerns

1. Temperature over 100.4°F (38°C) with or without chills.
2. Resumption of bright-red bleeding, passing clots.
3. Foul odor to lochia.
4. Uterine tenderness.
5. Pain or swelling of breast or leg.
6. Signs of urinary tract infection.
7. Signs of infection in perineal or abdominal incisions.
8. Severe mood swings or thoughts of harming self or baby.
9. Any other questions about self-care.

HEAVY BLEEDING

 Explain that reappearance of bright-red bleeding after lochia rubra has stopped is a danger sign, and the health care provider should be called.

- Explain that too much activity may increase bleeding, so rest is important.
- Describe how to assess uterus for signs of **subinvolution**: uterus is larger than expected, uterus does not remain firm, lochia may be excessive and does not progress to serosa or returns to rubra, backache and cramping may be present.

SIGNS OF INFECTION

- Teach signs and symptoms of breast infection: localized redness, tenderness, and swelling; palpation of a hard lump; flu-like symptoms.
- Teach signs and symptoms of bladder infection: urgency, frequency, or pain and burning on urination; suprapubic pain; blood in a voided urine specimen may be from lochia rather than infection.
- Teach signs and symptoms of intrauterine infection: chills and fever; tachycardia; headache; backache; malaise; anorexia; abdominal cramps; enlarged, boggy, and tender uterus; foul-smelling lochia; scant to profuse dark brown lochia.
- Teach signs and symptoms of infection in incision site: localized redness, swelling, bruising, pus drainage, separation of the incision, and pain to the touch.

 Explain the importance of notifying the health care provider if any signs and symptoms of infection occur.

PERSONAL HYGIENE

- Explain that the postpartum woman is vulnerable to intrauterine infection until the placental site is healed.

- Recommend showers rather than tub baths. If tub bath is preferred, the drain is kept open so that the woman is not sitting in dirty, soapy water.
- Advise no use of tampons or douching until after the postpartum check-up.
- Instruct wiping from vagina to anus when cleansing the perineum.

SIGNS OF THROMBOPHLEBITIS

- Explain that there is an increased risk in the postpartum patient.
- Teach signs and symptoms: warmth, redness, or tenderness in the affected leg; pain in calf when walking.
- Explain the importance of notifying the health care provider if these symptoms occur.

ACTIVITY AND REST

- Explain that physical activity is not contraindicated if vaginal delivery was uncomplicated. Fatigue is a common complaint of postpartum women; therefore, resumption of physical activity should be gradual.
- Suggest activity schedule: week 1 caring only for self and baby, week 2 doing light housework with no heavy lifting and carrying, week 3 performing usual housekeeping activities in the home, week 4 resuming errands and outside activity. Explain that postpartum recuperation is influenced by the amount of rest. Lack of rest can decrease milk supply, increase lochial flow, and negatively affect emotions.
- Suggest ways to conserve energy and promote rest such as napping when the baby naps, taking at least one nap during the day, accepting help from others, letting the housework go, and eating simple meals.

POSTPARTUM EXERCISES

- Explain that postpartum exercises can increase muscle tone, contribute to weight loss, promote urinary and bowel elimination, and improve self-image.
- Suggest to start with simple exercises and gradually increase in complexity and amount.
- The most common exercises that can be started in the early postpartum period are pelvic floor contractions (Kegel), abdominal tightening, chin to chest, bending the knees while lying flat, and circling and flexing the ankles. Exercises that can be added after the second week are pelvic rocking and abdominal crunch.
- Prepregnancy exercises or sports should be discussed with the health care provider before resuming them.

 NUTRITION

- Explain about expected weight loss. The non-breastfeeding woman should reduce her intake by 300 calories. The breastfeeding woman should increase her intake by 200 calories. The diet should be well balanced and contain adequate fluids. Prenatal vitamins and iron supplements are usually continued. Weight-loss programs should be discussed with a health care provider and started after the postpartum follow-up visit. See Chapter 23.
- Discuss dietary implications with the breastfeeding woman. The diet should contain adequate protein, carbohydrates, and calcium. Breastfeeding women should have at least 64 oz of fluid per day in the form of water, fruit juice, or milk. Avoid caffeine and alcohol. Adding an additional 12-oz glass of water with each meal will help meet the need for extra fluid intake.
- Suggest dietary restrictions of certain foods that may affect the breastfeeding infant. These foods include onions, turnips, cabbage, cauliflower, broccoli, chocolate, and some spices and seasonings.

RETURN OF MENSES

- Discuss the return of fertility and the resumption of menses. Ovulation usually occurs 2 weeks before menstruation; therefore, the woman may be fertile before her first menstrual flow.
- In the non-breastfeeding mother, the menstrual cycle returns within 6 to 12 weeks. In the breastfeeding woman, the return of the menstrual cycle is influenced by the amount of breastfeeding. Once formula or solid foods are introduced into the infant's diet, ovulation and menstruation may return.

RESUMPTION OF SEXUAL INTERCOURSE

- Advise to abstain from intercourse until the lochia has stopped and the perineum is healed and comfortable, which is usually about 3 weeks. Because of hormonal changes, vaginal dryness is common and water-soluble lubricants can be used.

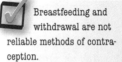

Breastfeeding and withdrawal are not reliable methods of contraception.

- Present information on contraception if the woman is receptive. (See Chapters 4 and 5.) Breastfeeding and withdrawal are not reliable methods of contraception.
- Mention that fatigue, discomfort, and the body's return to the nonpregnant state may interfere with the couple's sexual expression. There are ways to show affection and intimacy other than intercourse such as holding, kissing, caressing, and snuggling.
- Advise the breastfeeding woman that milk may leak during orgasm because of the release of oxytocin. Nursing the baby before intercourse may help prevent leaking, and a bra with nursing pads may be worn.

EMOTIONAL ADJUSTMENTS

- Explain the emotional adjustments that may occur during the postpartum period. See Chapter 24 for details on postpartum emotional adjustments.

- Explain the importance of caring for oneself in order to care for the baby and the need to maintain significant relationships.
- Suggest ways to set aside time for self, partner, other children, other family, and friends: arrange for child care, accept help from others, and prevent fatigue.
- Mention that "baby blues" are common. If these symptoms are prolonged or severe, the woman should contact her health care provider because this could indicate postpartum depression. See Chapter 55 for details on postpartum depression.

POSTPARTUM FOLLOW-UP

- Explain the need to schedule an appointment for a postpartum examination with her health care provider.
- Mention that she will be assessed for a successful return to the nonpregnant state, and her nutrition, immunizations, and ongoing health screening will be discussed.

PART V • QUESTIONS

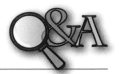

1. What findings would the nurse expect when assessing a client who had a vaginal birth 5 days earlier?
    a. Bright-red vaginal discharge; uterus at 4–5 fingerbreadths below the umbilicus.
    b. Light pink or brown vaginal discharge; uterus 4–5 fingerbreadths below the umbilicus.
    c. Pinkish, watery vaginal discharge; uterus 1–2 fingerbreadths below the umbilicus.
    d. Yellow, mucusy vaginal discharge; uterus at the umbilicus.

2. When assessing a client who gave birth 4 hours earlier, the nurse finds the uterus to be firm, 2 fingerbreadths above the umbilicus, and displaced to the right. Lochia rubra is moderate. What would be the first nursing action?
    a. Encourage the woman to urinate.
    b. Gently massage the fundus.
    c. Insert a foley catheter.
    d. Record these normal findings.

3. When teaching a client after a cesarean delivery, what would the nurse emphasize for the client to report to the health care provider about the incision?
    a. Edges are together.
    b. Fading bruises and slight swelling.
    c. Redness and drainage.
    d. Tenderness to touch during a shower.

4. When assessing the client 14 hours after birth, the following data are collected: Temperature 38.1°C (100.6°F), pulse 104, respirations 19, blood pressure 118/72. What would be the best nursing action?
    a. Assess for uterine tenderness and odor to lochia.
    b. Encourage the client to increase her fluid intake.
    c. Massage the uterus and express clots.
    d. Report these findings to the health care provider.

5. The nurse makes a postpartum home visit on day 5 to assess a first-time mother and her baby. The client states that she is beginning to care for her baby, has many questions about infant care, and indicates that she bathes the baby when her mother is there to help her. What nursing intervention is most appropriate?
   a. Give information about self-care.
   b. Identify resources for parental decision making.
   c. Make a referral for follow-up.
   d. Provide positive reinforcement for infant-care activities.

6. Which statement by a postpartum client indicates the need for further teaching about self-care after a fourth-degree episiotomy?
   a. "I can give myself a suppository if I become constipated."
   b. "Lying on my side will be more comfortable."
   c. "Salads and fruits in my diet will help keep me from getting constipated."
   d. "When my bottom is sore, I can use a sitz bath."

7. Thirty minutes after birth, the nurse has difficulty palpating the uterus because it is soft and boggy. There is heavy lochia rubra, with several small clots present. What would be the first nursing action?
   a. Assess for bladder distension.
   b. Increase the flow rate of intravenous fluids.
   c. Massage the uterus and express clots.
   d. Take the woman's pulse and blood pressure.

8. What behavior observed in the postpartum client indicates that the nurse needs to teach more about perineal self-care?
   a. Changes perineal pad with each voiding.
   b. Uses warm water to cleanse the perineum after toileting.
   c. Washes hands before and after perineal care.
   d. Wipes from back to front after toileting.

9. When teaching the woman after a vaginal birth about resumption of sexual activity, which statement by the nurse is most accurate?
   a. "After the bleeding has stopped and your perineum is comfortable, you can resume intercourse."
   b. "If you have no episiotomy, you can resume intercourse at any time."
   c. "The perineum will be healed in about a week and you can resume intercourse."
   d. "You should not resume intercourse until after your postpartum check-up."

10. A patient who is 5 days postpartum after a cesarean delivery reports a temperature of 38.9°C (102°F), muscle aches, a tender uterus, and increased cramping. What question would be most appropriate for the nurse to ask in order to collect more data?
    a. "Are there any lumps in your breasts?"
    b. "Do you have any pain when you urinate?"
    c. "How does your lochia smell?"
    d. "What does your incision look like?"

11. Which patient would be a candidate for postpartum administration of Rh immune globulin (RhoGAM)?
    a. Mother Rh negative with no antibody formation, infant Rh postive.
    b. Mother Rh negative with antibody formation, infant Rh postive.
    c. Mother Rh negative with no antibody formation, infant Rh negative.
    d. Mother Rh positive with no antibody formation, infant Rh negative.

12. When administering rubella vaccine, what information is essential for the nurse to explain to the client?
    a. Arrange for an antibody titer level to be done.
    b. Avoid becoming pregnant for at least 1 month after having the vaccine.
    c. Make an appointment for the administration of subsequent doses.
    d. Prevent pregnancy for at least 3 months after having the vaccine.

PART V · ANSWERS AND RATIONALES

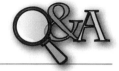

1. **The answer is b.** At 5 days postpartum, the vaginal discharge is lochia serosa, pink to brown in color and serosanguineous. Also, the uterus decreases in size 1 fingerbreath per day and would be about 4 to 5 fingerbreaths below the umbilicus. The other options do not reflect expected assessment findings at 5 days postpartum.

2. **The answer is a.** This assessment data indicates a full bladder. The first nursing action would be to have the woman empty her bladder. Option b is not the correct choice because massaging the uterus will not eliminate the underlying cause of the bogginess—the full bladder. Option c might be necessary if she is unable to urinate herself, but would not be the first nursing action. Option d is incorrect because these are not normal assessment findings of the newly delivered client.

3. **The answer is c.** Redness and swelling are signs of infection in the incision and should be reported to the health care provider. The other options indicate normal findings of a cesarean incision.

4. **The answer is b.** An increase in temperature in the first 24 hours postpartum usually indicates dehydration rather than infection. The data given does not indicate an increased risk for infection. Therefore, fluids would be encouraged. Option a would be appropriate interventions to assess for intrauterine infection. Option c gives interventions appropriate for increased uterine bleeding. Because a slightly increased temperature is normal during the first 24 hours, this does not need to be reported to the health care provider.

5. **The answer is d.** The data indicates the woman is in the taking-hold postpartum phase. Nursing interventions to enhance adaptation include positive reinforcement of infant care-taking activities. Option a is incorrect because the woman did not ask questions about self-care. Option b is more appropriate for the letting-go phase when the woman is more comfortable in the mothering role and ready to make decisions. Option c is incorrect because this is normal behavior for a new mother and there is no need for follow-up.

6. **The answer is a.** After a third- or fourth-degree episiotomy or laceration, it is important not to insert anything into the anus such as a suppository or enema tube. The other three options indicate that the client understands key concepts for self-care after a fourth-degree episiotomy.

7. **The answer is c.** A well-contracted uterus prevents hemorrhage. Massage stimulates the uterus to contract. Clots will usually be expressed during this procedure. The nurse needs to do the massage first in order to get the uterus to contract. Although the other options would be performed, massage of the uterus is the first priority.

8. **The answer is d.** Perineal cleansing from front to back prevents contamination that could lead to infection. The other options indicate that the woman understood recommendations for prevention of postpartum infection.

9. **The answer is a.** Abstaining from intercourse should be advised until the lochia has stopped and the perineum is healed and comfortable, which is usually about 3 weeks. In option b, if there is no episiotomy, the couple should abstain from intercourse until bleeding has stopped. In option c, it will take longer than 1 week for the perineum to heal. In option d, abstaining until after the postpartum check-up is no longer routinely advised.

10. **The answer is c.** The information the woman reported indicates symptoms of uterine infection. Another significant finding would be foul-smelling lochia. Therefore, the nurse would want to ask about the odor of the lochia. The other options would be asked to gather information about other sites of infection.

11. **The answer is a.** Postpartum women are candidates for RhoGAM within 72 hours after delivery if they are Rh negative with no evidence of antibody formation and their infant is Rh positive. The other options do not fit these criteria.

12. **The answer is d.** The rubella vaccine is a live attenuated virus that would put the fetus at risk for congenital abnormalities in the first trimester. The woman should be advised to prevent pregnancy for at least 3 months after receiving the injection. Option a is incorrect because antibody titers are done to determine if the vaccine is necessary. They do not need to be repeated after the vaccine. Option b is inaccurate because prevention of pregnancy for only one month would be an inadequate length of time. Option c is incorrect because only one dose of rubella vaccine is necessary.

VI
The Normal Newborn

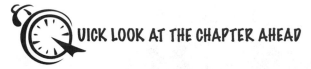

QUICK LOOK AT THE CHAPTER AHEAD

Numerous physiologic alterations occur within the newborn immediately after birth. The respiratory, cardiovascular, and thermoregulatory systems undergo profound changes within minutes of birth to ensure successful transition from the fetal to extrauterine environment. Breathing is initiated by four types of stimuli: mechanical (fetal chest compression during birth and chest wall recoil after birth), chemical (elevated peripheral carbon dioxide and decreased peripheral oxygen and pH stimulating the respiratory center of the brain), thermal (temperature change from uterus to outside environment), and a crying response to tactile, auditory, and visual stimuli at birth that expands the lungs.

Three structures within the fetal circulation allow the blood to bypass the liver and lungs: ductus venosus, foramen ovale, and ductus arteriosus. After birth, they constrict and close to allow normal blood circulation.

The mechanisms of a newborn's heat loss are evaporation, conduction, convection, and radiation.

The infant conserves heat by assuming a curled or flexed position that decreases the body surface area, and by peripheral vasoconstriction, resulting in a mottled appearance of the skin.

The infant produces heat by metabolizing brown fat and increasing its basal metabolic rate.

The newborn who loses heat faster than it can produce it experiences cold stress, which may lead to respiratory distress, metabolic acidosis, and hypoglycemia.

28
Transition to Extrauterine Life

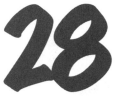
The nurse plays a major role in promoting the well-being of the newborn by assessing physiologic alterations, evaluating for problems, and providing appropriate interventions.

TERMS
- [ ] **surfactant**
- [ ] **initiation of breathing**
- [ ] **ductus venosus**
- [ ] **foramen ovale**
- [ ] **ductus arteriosus**
- [ ] **heat loss**
- [ ] **heat conservation**
- [ ] **heat production**
- [ ] **brown fat metabolism**
- [ ] **cold stress**

RESPIRATORY SYSTEM

Usually, by 37 weeks of gestation, the fetal lungs are developed and can maintain breathing and adequate exchange of gases. Sufficient amounts of **surfactant** are necessary to lower the surface tension within the alveoli so they remain open during expiration. **Initiation of breathing** in the newborn is triggered by four types of stimuli: mechanical, chemical, thermal, and sensory.

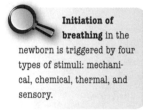

Initiation of **breathing** in the newborn is triggered by four types of stimuli: mechanical, chemical, thermal, and sensory.

Mechanical events that initiate breathing are compression of the fetal chest during passage through the birth canal and chest wall recoil after birth. Both bring about passive inspiration of air.

Chemical stimuli to the respiratory center of the brain that contribute to the onset of breathing are elevated peripheral carbon dioxide and decreased peripheral oxygen and pH. The change in temperature from inside the uterus to the extrauterine environment also stimulates the newborn to breathe.

The newborn responds to tactile, auditory, and visual stimuli at the time of birth with crying, which maintains expansion of the lungs.

Amniotic fluid within the respiratory tract is absorbed by the pulmonary capillaries and lymphatic vessels, as blood flow increases and pulmonary vascular resistance decreases.

CARDIOVASCULAR SYSTEM

Three structures within the fetal circulation allow blood to bypass the liver and lungs: ductus venosus, foramen ovale, and ductus arteriosus. (See Figure 28-1.)

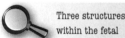

Three structures within the fetal circulation allow blood to bypass the liver and lungs: ductus venosus, foramen ovale, and ductus arteriosus.

When these three fetal structures close, blood flow assumes the circulation pattern that will be followed throughout the rest of life. In fetal circulation, the **ductus venosus** brings blood from the umbilical vein directly into the vena cava bypassing the liver. This structure will constrict after birth when the umbilical cord is severed and blood flow ceases through the umbilical vessels.

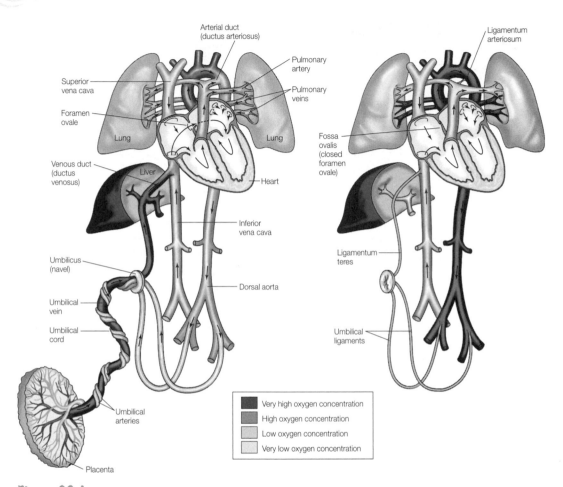

Figure 28-1 Fetal circulation.

In the fetus, the **foramen ovale**, an opening between the right and left atria, allows blood to move directly to the left side of the heart, where it enters the left ventricle and is pumped into the aorta. This shunting results in blood bypassing the vasculature of the lungs.

When breathing begins after birth, pressure in the left side of the heart increases and the foramen ovale is held closed. Blood now circulates from the right atria to the right ventricle and then to the lungs.

During fetal circulation, most blood that enters the right atrium passes through the foramen ovale; the rest is pumped to the right ventricle. It then enters the pulmonary artery going toward the lungs. Before reaching the lungs, most of this blood is shunted to the aorta through the **ductus arteriosus**.

After birth, changes of pressure within the heart and pulmonary vasculature occur with breathing, and the ductus arteriosus constricts and closes within hours. After constriction of the ductus arteriosus, blood flows from the right ventricle directly to the lungs.

THERMOREGULATION

At birth the infant moves from a very warm intrauterine environment to a much colder extrauterine environment. The newborn must now balance heat loss and heat generation by regulating body temperature. This is done by changing the rate of metabolism and the amount of oxygen consumption.

Because of a large body surface-to-weight ratio, and the limited amount of subcutaneous fat for insulation, the newborn tends to lose heat without assistance. For example, the head is large in proportion to the rest of the body, and significant amounts of heat can be lost if the head is not covered.

The mechanisms of **heat loss** after birth are evaporation, conduction, convection, and radiation. The newborn is at risk for heat loss from evaporation immediately after birth and during baths because of the moisture on the skin. Heat is also lost through conduction, when the infant has direct contact with cooler surfaces such as unheated mattresses or blankets, scales, and caregivers' hands.

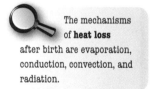

The mechanisms of **heat loss** after birth are evaporation, conduction, convection, and radiation.

Convection is the loss of heat to cooler air around the body from air drafts, air conditioning, or air outside an incubator.

With radiation, heat is lost to cooler solid objects around but not touching the infant, such as the walls of the room or windows not covered by drapery.

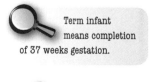

Term infant means completion of 37 weeks gestation.

Heat conservation occurs when the term infant assumes a curled or flexed position that decreases body surface area. Another mechanism for heat conservation is peripheral vasoconstriction, resulting in a mottled appearance of the skin. Shivering is rarely seen in newborns.

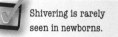

Shivering is rarely seen in newborns.

Heat production or thermogenesis is accomplished through **brown fat metabolism** and increased basal metabolic rate. Unique to the newborn, production of brown fat begins around 26 weeks gestation and continues for the first 4 weeks of life. Brown fat is deposited primarily in the midscapular area, mediastinum, around the neck, and in the axilla.

What should the nurse do in response to signs of new born distress from heat loss?

When heat production is needed, brown fat stores are metabolized. If these stores are depleted, the newborn's ability to respond to cold by increasing metabolic rate is limited. When the basal metabolic rate increases as a result of low body temperature, oxygen and glucose consumption increases.

Cold stress may lead to respiratory distress, metabolic acidosis, and hypoglycemia in the newborn. **Cold stress** occurs when the newborn loses heat faster than it can be produced. The compensatory mechanisms of metabolism of brown fat and increased basal metabolic rate are not effective to maintain core body temperature.

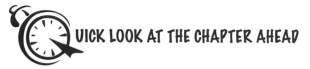

QUICK LOOK AT THE CHAPTER AHEAD

Once the infant's head it born, the health care provider suctions the nose and mouth of the infant to clear the oral respiratory passages. Then the nurse assists the infant to begin regular respiration, and continues to assess the newborn's breathing.

The Apgar score rates the condition of the newborn at 1 minute and 5 minutes after birth. It is the total of scores of five criteria: heart rate, respiratory effort, muscle tone, reflex irritability, and skin color.

To prevent significant heat loss, the infant is dried, covered with a warm, clean blanket, and its head covered by a hat. For assessments and immediate newborn care, the infant is placed under a radiant heater.

A brief head-to-toe assessment is done to determine general appearance, normal newborn characteristics, vital signs, and reflexes, along with gestational age, birth trauma, and abnormalities such as spina bifida, cleft lip/palate, or extra digits.

Identification bracelets with matching numbers should be placed on the infant and the mother before they are separated.

Within one hour of birth, vitamin K and prophylactic eye medication are routinely administered to the newborn.

The parents and other family members when appropriate should be encouraged to interact with the infant as soon as possible after birth.

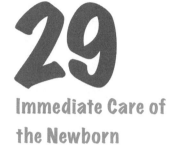

29

Immediate Care of the Newborn

The newborn is most receptive to begin breast-feeding in the first hour after birth.

 During the time immediately after birth, the nurse is responsible for providing care that assists the newborn in its transition to extrauterine life. The first priority is establishing and maintaining breathing; the second priority is providing and maintaining warmth. Throughout these interventions, many assessments are being done simultaneously.

 The time immediately after birth is a period of heightened attachment between the parents and the infant, and is the beginning of the incorporation of the infant into the family.

TERMS

- ☐ **establish respirations**
- ☐ **Apgar score**
- ☐ **maintain body temperature**
- ☐ **head-to-toe assessment**
- ☐ **infant identification**
- ☐ **vitamin K**
- ☐ **prophylactic eye medication**

ESTABLISHING AND MAINTAINING RESPIRATION

- Once the infant's head emerges, the health care provider suctions the nose and mouth of the infant to clear the oral respiratory passages for the first breath.
- Interventions that assist the infant to begin regular respiration are placing the infant on the mother's abdomen, massaging the infant while drying, putting the infant in a position that allows drainage of the nasopharynx and trachea, and continued suctioning of the nose and mouth as needed.
- Interventions that encourage the infant to cry promote expansion of the lungs and movement of fluid out of the lungs.
- The most common activities to make the infant cry are rubbing the back and tapping the feet.

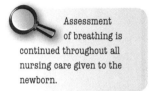

Assessment of breathing is continued throughout all nursing care given to the newborn.

Assessment of breathing is continued throughout all nursing care given to the newborn.

DETERMINING APGAR SCORE

The **Apgar score**, usually determined by the nurse, evaluates the condition of the newborn at 1 minute and 5 minutes after birth.

There are five criteria for the Apgar score: heart rate, respiratory effort, muscle tone, reflex irritability, and skin color.

Reflex irritability is the infant's response to stimulation such as rubbing or tapping the sole of the foot or rubbing the back.

The infant may receive a score from 0 to 2 for each criterion with a maximum score of 10. A score of 8 or above indicates the infant has dealt well with the transition to extrauterine life. A score between 4 and 7 indicates the need for stimulation, and a score under 4 indicates the need for resuscitation. (See Table 29-1 for a description of the Apgar scoring system.)

Table 29-1 Apgar Scoring System

SIGN	SCORE		
	0	1	2
Heart rate	Absent	Slow – below 100	Above 100
Respiratory effort	Absent	Slow – irregular	Good crying
Muscle tone	Flaccid	Some flexion of extremities	Active motion
Reflex irritability	None	Grimace	Vigorous cry
Color	Pale, blue	Body pink, blue extremities	Completely pink

Apgar, V. (1966). The newborn (Apgar) scoring system, reflections and advice. *Pediatric Clinics of North America, 13*, 645.

PROVIDING AND MAINTAINING WARMTH

Assisting the newborn to **maintain body temperature** is a major focus of initial nursing interventions.

> Assisting the newborn to **maintain body temperature** is a major focus of initial nursing interventions.

In order to prevent significant heat loss, the infant needs to be dried, covered with a warm, clean blanket, and have a hat placed on the head. For assessments and immediate newborn care, the infant is placed under a radiant heater to maintain temperature as monitored by a skin probe.

If the infant has spontaneous breathing and there are no signs of complications, the infant may be placed skin-to-skin on the mother's abdomen or chest immediately after birth to promote attachment.

PERFORMING INITIAL PHYSICAL ASSESSMENT

A brief **head-to-toe assessment** is done to determine gestational age, detect birth trauma, and observe general appearance, normal newborn characteristics, vital signs, and reflexes. This assessment includes observation for obvious abnormalities such as spina bifida, cleft lip/palate, or **extra digits**. The details of this assessment are in Chapter 32.

Conducting this physical assessment may be incorporated into other aspects of immediate newborn care.

IDENTIFYING THE NEWBORN

Infant identification is done as part of the initial care. Identification bracelets with matching numbers are placed on the infant and the mother. These bracelets are to be checked each time the infant is brought to the mother. The footprints of the infant and a fingerprint of the mother are taken as an additional identification measure and are part of the permanent hospital record.

 It is very important for identification procedures to be completed before the infant is separated from the mother.

ADMINISTERING MEDICATIONS

Within 1 hour of birth, **vitamin K** and **prophylactic eye medication** are routinely administered to the newborn. An intramuscular injection of vitamin K is given because the newborn is at risk for bleeding. The gastrointestinal tract of the newborn does not contain the bacteria necessary for vitamin K production and the newborn has low prothrombin levels. Usually erythromycin ointment is placed in the eyes as prophylaxsis against gonorrhea and chlamydia infections. If possible the parents should have eye-to-eye contact with the infant before eye ointment is administered.

> If possible the parents should have eye-to-eye contact with the infant before eye ointment is administered.

PROMOTING ATTACHMENT

The nurse plays a vital role in providing opportunities for initiating attachment. Encouraging the parents to interact with the infant as soon as possible after birth,

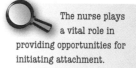 The nurse plays a vital role in providing opportunities for initiating attachment.

completing nursing interventions in the presence of the parents, and providing privacy for parent-infant contact are ways that nurses can support parents as they begin the attachment process. Other family members such as siblings or grandparents may need to be included during this time. The nurse should also be aware of cultural considerations when planning times for interaction.

INITIATING BREASTFEEDING

The time the newborn is most receptive to begin breastfeeding is in the first hour after birth. The newborn is awake, active, appears hungry, and has a strong sucking reflex. Nursing interventions to assist the mother with breastfeeding should be undertaken. See Chapter 33 for information on breastfeeding.

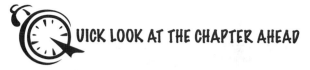

In addition to the immediate respiratory, circulatory, and temperature transitions after birth, more gradual adaptations occur within the gastrointestinal, renal, hepatic, immune, and neurological systems. These contribute to the infant's ability to function during the neonatal period. The gastrointestinal tract of the newborn has the ability to digest most fats, protein, and simple carbohydrates, but not complex starches.

Meconium, the first stool, is thick, tarry, sticky, greenish-black material that accumulated in the large intestine before birth. Transitional stools consisting of part meconium and part fecal material are thinner, less sticky, and brown to green in color. Within one week milk stools appear, characteristic of the type of feeding.

The newborn is less able to concentrate urine and can become dehydrated if fluid intake is inadequate.

Glycogen reserves in the liver provide energy and may be depleted if metabolic needs of the infant increase.

Because of immaturity of the liver in the newborn, there is decreased ability to conjugate bilirubin and increased risk for jaundice.

During the last trimester of pregnancy, the newborn receives passive immunity against bacterial and viral diseases until its own antibody production begins with vaccinations. But the newborn is vulnerable to systemic infections.

The neurological system continues to mature after birth. Progression through periods of reactivity indicates normal neurological status.

30

System Adaptations in the Newborn

An understanding of system adaptations occurring after birth is necessary for the nurse to accurately assess the newborn.

TERMS
- [ ] meconium
- [ ] transitional stools
- [ ] milk stools
- [ ] conjugation of bilirubin
- [ ] physiologic jaundice
- [ ] passive immunity
- [ ] active immunity
- [ ] periods of "reactivity"

GASTROINTESTINAL SYSTEM

In the term newborn, the suck, rooting, and swallowing reflexes are well developed. The gastrointestinal tract has the ability to digest most fats, protein, and simple carbohydrates.

Pancreatic amylase, needed to digest more complex starches, is the only enzyme not being produced at birth; therefore, starches should not be introduced into the diet for several months. The stomach of the term newborn has a capacity of about 2 oz with an emptying time of 2 to 4 hours.

An immature cardiac sphincter of the stomach contributes to regurgitation in the neonatal period. Peristalsis begins and bowel sounds are present within the first hour of life.

It is normal for the newborn to lose 5 to 10% of birth weight because of minimal caloric and fluid intake in the first few days while a feeding pattern is being established. However, the infant should regain its birth weight by two weeks of age.

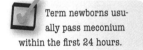
Term newborns usually pass meconium within the first 24 hours.

Term newborns usually pass meconium within the first 24 hours. **Meconium**, the first stool, is thick, tarry, sticky, greenish-black material that accumulated in the large intestine before birth.

As breastmilk or formula is ingested, **transitional stools** consisting of part meconium and part fecal material are produced. They are thinner, less sticky, and brown to green in color.

Within one week, **milk stools** characteristic of the type of feeding are present. The stool of the breastfed infant is small, semi-liquid, golden yellow, and more frequent. Formula-fed infants have less frequent stools that are more formed and pale yellow.

RENAL SYSTEM

The newborn is less able to concentrate urine; therefore, the infant could become dehydrated if fluid intake is inadequate.

Concentrating urine means the ability of the kidney to conserve fluid by moving water back into the circulation.

Most newborns urinate within 24 hours of birth, then 2 to 6 times daily for the first 2 days, then at least 6 to 8 times daily.

Rusty-colored stains from urates may appear on the diaper during the first few days of life.

HEPATIC SYSTEM

The newborn's liver is large and may extend below the costal margin. If the mother's iron intake is adequate during pregnancy, sufficient iron has been stored in the newborn's liver for use during the first 6 months of life. Glycogen reserves in the liver provide energy and may be depleted if metabolic needs of the infant increase, as during cold stress or respiratory distress.

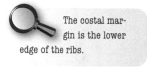

The costal margin is the lower edge of the ribs.

The liver plays an important role in the **conjugation of bilirubin**. Normally there is an increased number of red blood cells (RBCs) in the fetus for oxygen transport. After birth, this amount of RBCs is not needed and begins to break down. Bilirubin is a by-product of RBC destruction.

High levels of circulating bilirubin in the blood produce jaundice. Conjugated bilirubin can be excreted by the intestines. Because of immaturity of the liver in the newborn, there is decreased ability to conjugate bilirubin and increased risk for jaundice. In the first few days of life, about 50% of babies exhibit **physiologic jaundice.**

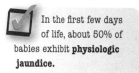

In the first few days of life, about 50% of babies exhibit **physiologic jaundice.**

IMMUNE SYSTEM

The infant is at greater risk for infection in the first 2 months of life. During the last trimester of pregnancy, the newborn receives **passive immunity** against bacterial and viral diseases to which the mother was exposed or vaccinated. This passive immunity protects the newborn from these diseases until its own antibody production begins with vaccinations.

Passive immunity does not protect the newborn if exposed to other bacteria or

During the last trimester of pregnancy, the newborn receives passive immunity against bacterial and viral diseases to which the mother was exposed or vaccinated. This passive immunity protects the newborn from these diseases until its own antibody production begins with vaccinations.

viruses like *E. coli*, group B streptococcus (GBS), staphylococcus, listeria, or herpes simplex virus. The newborn has limited inflammatory response and is vulnerable to systemic infection such as pneumonia, septicemia, and meningitis. *Active immunity* begins to develop when immunizations are given.

NEUROLOGICAL SYSTEM

The neurological system continues to mature after birth. The term newborn is in flexed position, resists extension of extremities, cries vigorously when disturbed, and exhibits typical reflexes such as sucking, palmar grasp, and Moro. See Chapter 32 for assessment of reflexes.

In the first hours after birth, the newborn has a predictable pattern of behavior called **periods of "reactivity."** In the first period of reactivity, lasting approximately 30 minutes, the newborn is awake, alert, has a strong sucking reflex, and may appear hungry. Heart and respiratory rates increase.

The newborn then enters a resting phase lasting from a few minutes to about 2 hours. During the resting phase the infant is in a deep sleep, has no interest in feeding, and the heart and respiratory rates slow down.

In the second period of reactivity, usually lasting 4 to 6 hours, the newborn is again awake, alert, and shows readiness for feeding. Periods of apnea may occur at this time, as well as gagging and regurgitation of mucus. The first meconium stool and first voiding often occur.

The progression through periods of reactivity indicates normal neurological status. See Tables 30-1 and 30-2 for descriptions of behavioral states and sensory capabilities of the newborn.

Table 30-1 Behavioral States of the Newborn

State	Description
Deep sleep	Eyes closed with no eye movement, breathing regular and even, heart rate as slow as 100, responses to stimuli often delayed, difficult to arouse.
Active REM sleep	Eyes closed with rapid eye movement, irregular respirations, irregular sucking motions, some motor activity, stimuli may cause a startle reflex and a change of state.
Drowsy	Open or closed eyes, fluttering eyelids, slow regular movements of the extremities, change of state results from sensory stimulus.
Wide wake	Alert, eyes open, fixates on faces or sounds, minimal body movement, delayed response to stimuli, optimal state for interaction with the newborn.
Active awake	Alert, eyes open, intense body movements with thrusting of the extremities, stimuli increase motor activity.
Crying	Intense crying, vigorous body movements, agitation, diminished response to stimuli.

Table 30-2 Sensory Capabilities of the Newborn

Sense	Description
Vision	Sees most clearly at 8 to10 in., sensitive to light, prefers human face and bright-colored objects, more attracted by black and white patterns, follows objects, and maintains eye-to-eye contact.
Hearing	Similar to adults when no amniotic fluid or vernix in ears, responds readily to parents' voices, startle reflex response to loud noise, soothed by low-frequency sound like calm voice or lullaby.
Touch	Well-developed response over the entire body, specific reflexes elicited when stroked in certain areas, soothed by swaddling or holding.
Taste	Well-developed, sweet elicits vigorous sucking, sour causes puckering of the lips, bitter causes a grimace.
Smell	Well-developed, able to differentiate mother's odor, influences attachment between mother and newborn.

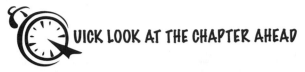
Assessment of gestational age characteristics identifies the preterm, term, or postterm infant. (See Table 31-1.) Heart rate, respiratory rate, and temperature are routinely assessed. However, blood pressure is usually measured only when indicated by prematurity or suspected cardiac abnormality.

Measurements are taken of birth weight, head-to-heel length, head circumference, and chest circumference.

The general appearance and behavioral state of the newborn are surveyed to assess the overall condition of the infant.

Some features, primarily skin characteristics, are unique to the newborn:

- Milia are tiny white spots on the nose, forehead, and chin.

- Newborn rash appears as a small white or pale yellow papule surrounded by a reddened area.

- Lanugo are the fine downy hairs found on shoulders, back, forehead, and ears.

- Vernix caseosa is a white cheesy substance that covers the fetus in utero.

- In a post-term infant, the skin may be wrinkled, leathery, and cracked, with significant desquamation or peeling.

- Skin turgor is assessed for hydration.

31

Newborn Assessment: Physical Characteristics

- Acrocyanosis is a bluish discoloration of the hands and feet.

- Mottling is a bluish, lacy pattern on the skin often associated with chilling.

- Stork bites are deep pink or reddish spots found on the eyelids, bridge of the nose, or back of the neck.

- Mongolian spots are irregular areas of dark pigmentation on the sacrum and gluteus.

- Jaundice, a yellowing of the skin or sclera of the eyes, may occur from high levels of bilirubin.

- Molding of the infant's head occurs when the cranial bones overlap to accommodate the shape of the mother's pelvis during descent through the birth canal.

- Caput succedaneum is edema of the scalp at the presenting part.

- Cephalhematoma is a collection of blood between the periosteum and the bone.

- Forceps marks on the cheeks or bruising of the scalp may occur when delivery was assisted.

The assessment of physical and behavioral characteristics of the newborn provides information needed to plan nursing care.

TERMS

- [ ] **periodic breathing**
- [ ] **small for gestational age (SGA)**
- [ ] **appropriate for gestational age (AGA)**
- [ ] **large for gestational age (LGA)**
- [ ] **milia**
- [ ] **newborn rash, or erythema toxicum**
- [ ] **lanugo**
- [ ] **vernix caseosa**
- [ ] **desquamation**
- [ ] **skin turgor**
- [ ] **tenting**
- [ ] **acrocyanosis**
- [ ] **mottling**
- [ ] **stork bites**
- [ ] **mongolian spots**
- [ ] **jaundice**
- [ ] **molding**
- [ ] **caput succedaneum**
- [ ] **cephalhematoma**
- [ ] **forceps marks**

VITAL SIGNS

Heart rate, respiratory rate, and temperature are routinely assessed. However, blood pressure is usually measured only when indicated by infant condition such as prematurity or suspected cardiac abnormality.

The normal heart rate is 120 to 160 beats per minute. The heart rate may fluctuate with activity. During crying the rate may rise to 180 and during sleep may decrease to 100. Because of this variation, heart rate should be counted for 60 seconds.

Respiratory rate in the newborn should be 30 to 60 breaths per minute at rest. It may increase with crying. The respiratory rhythm is irregular with short periods of apnea known as **periodic breathing**. For this reason, the respiratory rate should be counted for 60 seconds. In the first few hours after birth, breath sounds may be coarse due to amniotic fluid in the respiratory tract.

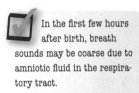

In the first few hours after birth, breath sounds may be coarse due to amniotic fluid in the respiratory tract.

Temperature is usually taken by the axillary method. The normal range is 36.5° to 37.2°C (97.9–99°F). The infant may have difficulty maintaining a stable body temperature in the first 12 hours of life.

Normal blood pressure ranges from 60 to 80 mm Hg systolic and from 40 to 60 mm Hg diastolic. Variations occur with activity.

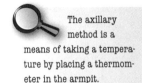

The axillary method is a means of taking a temperature by placing a thermometer in the armpit.

GENERAL MEASUREMENTS

Normal birth weight at term may vary from 5 lb 8 oz to 8 lb 14 oz (2500–4000 g). Infants weighing less than 2500 g may be premature or **small for gestational age** (**SGA**). Infants between 2500 and 4000 g are considered to be **appropriate for gestational age** (**AGA**). Infants more than 4000 g are considered **large for gestational age** (**LGA**).

Usual head-to-heel length is 18 to 22 in. (46–56 cm). Head circumference usually measures 13 to 14 in. (33–35 cm) and is about 1 in. (2–3 cm) larger than the chest circumference. Chest circumference usually measures 12 to 13 in. (30.5–33 cm).

GENERAL SURVEY

The general appearance of the newborn conveys information about the overall condition of the infant. The head is large and the extremities are short in proportion to the body. The behavioral state of the infant influences the general appearance. The flexed position is typical, with resistance when the extremities are straightened. Hands are tightly clenched; the abdomen is rounded and prominent. Skin color is consistent with genetic background, although healthy newborns should have pink undertones. The cry should be vigorous and lusty. Activity of the newborn is demonstrated by active motion of all extremities, especially when crying.

NEWBORN CHARACTERISTICS

Some features, primarily skin characteristics, are unique to the newborn. **Milia** are immature sebaceous glands that appear as tiny white spots on the nose, forehead, and chin. They disappear spontaneously within 4 weeks.

Newborn rash, or **erythema toxicum**, appears as a small white or pale yellow papule surrounded by a reddened area. They are found all over the body, may appear suddenly, are transient, require no treatment, and usually disappear completely by 2 weeks of age.

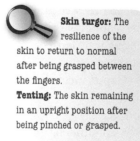

Skin turgor: The resilience of the skin to return to normal after being grasped between the fingers.
Tenting: The skin remaining in an upright position after being pinched or grasped.

Lanugo are the fine downy hairs found on shoulders, back, forehead, and ears. The amount of lanugo decreases as the fetus reaches term. By two weeks after birth, lanugo has been rubbed away.

Vernix caseosa is a white cheesy substance that covers the fetus in utero. It lubricates and protects the skin in the amniotic fluid environment. The amount of vernix decreases as the fetus matures. In the term newborn, vernix may appear only in the skin folds.

After birth, the skin of the newborn becomes dry, and **desquamation,** or peeling, may occur. The skin of the postterm newborn may be wrinkled, leathery, and cracked with significant peeling. **Skin turgor** is assessed for hydration status. Elastic skin turgor with no **tenting** is normal.

There are additional skin characteristics indicated by color. **Acrocyanosis**, a bluish discoloration of the hands and feet, is present for up to 48 hours after birth and is due to immature peripheral circulation.

Circumoral or central cyanosis is an abnormal finding and the primary health care provider should be notified for further evaluation.

Mottling is a bluish, lacy pattern on the skin as a result of general circulation fluctuations often associated with chilling.

Stork bites, also called telangiectatic nevi, are deep pink or reddish spots found on the eyelids, bridge of the nose, or back of the neck. They are more common in newborns of light complexion and usually fade by two years of age.

Mongolian spots are irregular areas of dark pigmentation on the sacrum and gluteus. They are common in infants of dark complexion and usually fade by age 4. The size and location of mongolian spots should be documented since they may be mistaken for bruises.

The size and location of mongolian spots should be documented since they may be mistaken for bruises.

Jaundice, a yellowing of the skin or sclera of the eyes, may occur from high levels of bilirubin.

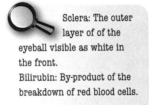

Sclera: The outer layer of of the eyeball visible as white in the front.
Bilirubin: By-product of the breakdown of red blood cells.

Molding of the infant's head occurs when the cranial bones overlap to accommodate to the shape of the mother's pelvis during descent through the birth canal. The normal shape of the head returns within a few days of birth.

Caput succedaneum is edema of the scalp at the presenting part. This soft, diffuse swelling crosses suture lines and disappears within three to four days.

Cephalhematoma is a collection of blood between the periosteum and the bone. This does not cross suture lines, is firm to touch, and is reabsorbed over the next 4 to 6 weeks.

Forceps marks on the cheeks or bruising of the scalp may occur when delivery was assisted with forceps or a vacuum extractor.

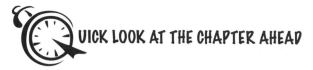

The nurse performs a systematic head-to-toe assessment of the newborn to detect abnormalities.

- The size and shape of the head are noted.

- The face is assessed for placement of facial features and symmetry of movement.

- Respiratory and cardiac assessments and measurements of chest circumference are done.

- The abdomen, bowel sounds, and umbilical cord are asssessed.

- Extremities are assessed for symmetry, range of motion, and the presence of deformities, extra digits, or webbing.

- Palmar and plantar creases are assessed. One palmar crease is suggestive of Down syndrome. Plantar creases are part of the gestational age assessment.

- Legs should be equal in length, with symmetrical thigh, popliteal, and gluteal skin folds.

- Hips are evaluated by observing for equal leg length, equal knee height, symmetrical gluteal folds, and the ability to abduct the thighs.

- The spine should be straight, flat, and intact. The base of the spine is examined carefully for openings, masses, dimples, or hairy tufts which may indicate spina bifida.

- The anus should be patent.

32

Newborn Assessment: Head-to-Toe Examination

- The passage of the first meconium stool indicates an intact gastrointestinal tract.

- Genitals are assessed for signs of gestational age and abnormalities in structure.

- Reflexes are evaluated.

 Head-to-toe examination is sometimes done in the presence of the parents and provides teaching opportunities about newborn characteristics and care.

 The gestational age, the behavioral state, time since last feeding, and maternal medications in labor may influence assessment findings.

TERMS
- ☐ fontanelles
- ☐ clavicles
- ☐ umbilical cord
- ☐ congenital hip dysplasia
- ☐ newborn reflexes

The assessment is done in a warm, well-lit area, free of drafts. The nurse performs a systematic head-to-toe assessment of the newborn to detect abnormalities. The gestational age, the behavioral state, time since last feeding, and maternal medications in labor may influence assessment findings.

HEAD

The size and shape of the head are noted. Palpation for molding, caput succedaneum, and cephqlhematoma is done.

Cranial sutures and fontanelles are assessed. **Fontanelles** are spaces at the intersection of the six cranial bones. The anterior fontanelle is diamond-shaped, 3 to 4 cm long by 2 to 3 cm wide, and the posterior fontanelle is triangle-shaped, 1 to 2 cm wide.

The posterior fontanelle may be difficult to palpate because of overlapping bones. The fontanelles should feel soft and flat. They may pulsate, and when the infant is crying may bulge slightly.

Caput succedaneum: Edema of the scalp at the presenting part; it crosses the suture line, is soft, and resolves in 3–4 days.
Cephalhematoma: The collection of blood between the skull bones and the membranes covering the bones. It does cross the suture line, is firm to touch, and is reabsorbed over 4 to 6 weeks.

A bulging fontanelle in a quiet infant is a sign of increased intercranial pressure; a depressed fontanelle is a sign of dehydration. Abnormal fontanelles should be reported to the primary health care provider.

FACE

The face is assessed for placement of facial features and symmetry of movement. Eyes should be level, move in all directions, blink in response to light, and have clear cornea and white sclera. Pupils should be equal, round, and reactive to light. Edema of the eyelids and subconjunctival hemorrhage may be present from the birth process. The top of the ear should be level with the outer canthus of

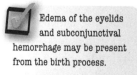

Edema of the eyelids and subconjunctival hemorrhage may be present from the birth process.

the eye. The nose may appear flattened and needs to be assessed for patency because newborns are nose breathers. Sneezing is a common newborn mechanism for clearing the nasal passages. The mouth should be assessed for an intact palate, presence of the sucking reflex, a freely moving tongue, and symmetrical movements when crying, sucking, and swallowing.

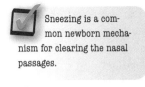

Sneezing is a common newborn mechanism for clearing the nasal passages.

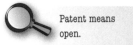

Patent means open.

CHEST

During the assessment of the chest, respiratory and cardiac assessments and measurements of chest circumference are done. (See Chapter 31.) **Clavicles** are palpated for intactness. Breast tissue is palpated for breast bud development as part of gestational age assessment.

ABDOMEN

The abdomen should be soft and cylindrical, protrude slightly, appear large in relation to the hips, and move with respiration. Bowel sounds can be heard shortly after birth. The **umbilical cord** is bluish white in color, gelatinous, with two arteries and one vein.

EXTREMITIES

Extremities appear short, remain flexed, move symmetrically, and have full range of motion. They are assessed for symmetry, range of motion, and the presence of deformities, extra digits, or webbing. Peripheral pulses are palpated at the radial, brachial, and femoral sites for equality and symmetry.

Hands are assessed for the presence of more than one palmar crease. A single palmar crease is frequently seen in children with Down syndrome. Plantar creases are part of gestational age assessment.

A single palmar crease is frequently seen in children with Down syndrome.

Legs should be equal in length with symmetrical thigh, popliteal, and gluteal skin folds.

Hips are evaluated for **congenital hip dysplasia** by observing for equal leg length, equal knee height, symmetrical gluteal folds, and the ability to abduct the thighs. Ortolani's and Barlow's maneuvers may be carried out to determine the presence of hip dysplasia.

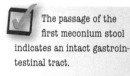 **Ortolani's and Barlow's maneuvers** are movements of the hips that determine if they are dislocated.

BACK

The spine should be straight, flat, and intact. The base of the spine is examined carefully for openings, masses, dimples, or hairy tufts which may indicate spina bifida.

The anus should be patent. The passage of the first meconium stool indicates an intact gastrointestinal tract.

The passage of the first meconium stool indicates an intact gastrointestinal tract.

GENITALS

Genitals are assessed for signs of gestational age and abnormalities in structure. Male genitals are inspected for position of the urinary meatus at the tip of the penis, pigmentation of the scrotum, and amount and depth of scrotal rugae. Palpation of the testes in both scrotal sacs should be done. In the female, the labia may be **edematous**, a hymenal tag may be present, and a vaginal discharge of thick, white or blood-tinged mucus is common.

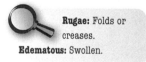 **Rugae:** Folds or creases. **Edematous:** Swollen.

REFLEXES

Newborn reflexes are evaluated as part of the head-to-toe assessment. (See Table 32-1.)

Table 32-1 Newborn Reflexes

Reflex	Stimulus	Response	Implications*
Moro or startle	A loud noise, jarring of the crib, or allowing the supported head to suddenly drop back an inch or two.	Abduction and extension of the arms and legs with the fingers in the C position, then flex arms and legs, often cry.	Symmetrical arm movement indicates intact clavicles and brachial plexus, should disappear by 6 months.
Rooting	Touch of cheeks, mouth, or lips.	Head turns toward side that is touched and mouth opens.	Indicates readiness for feeding, should disappear by 4 months.
Sucking and swallowing	When lips are touched or object placed in the mouth.	Coordinated sucking and swallowing.	A strong suck is essential for adequate feeding, non-nutritive sucking important as quieting behavior.
Palmar grasp	Object placed in hand.	Closing of fingers in strong grasp.	Should disappear by 6 months.
Plantar grasp	Pressure on the ball of the foot.	Flexion of all toes on stimulated foot.	Disappears in preparation for walking.
Babinski	Sole of foot stroked upward from heel to little toe then across to big toe.	Fanning and extension of the toes.	Normal in newborn infants, after 3 months toes should flex instead of extend upon stimulation.
Step	Infant held upright with feet touching a hard surface.	Rhythmic, stepping movements.	Should disappear by 3 months.
Tonic neck	With infant lying on back, head is turned to one side.	The arm and leg on the side the infant is facing extend while opposite arm and leg flex.	Should disappear by 3 months.
Trunk incurvation	With the infant lying prone, trunk is stroked upward lateral to the vertebrae.	Flexion of trunk in the direction of the touch.	Should disappear by 1 month.

*Absence of a reflex or persistence of a reflex beyond the expected time frame may indicate central nervous system damage and should be evaluated by the primary care provider.

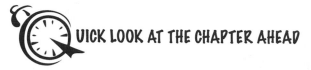

QUICK LOOK AT THE CHAPTER AHEAD

For the newborn to grow and develop adequately, nutritional needs must be met by either formula or breastmilk. Human breastmilk is the standard for determining nutritional requirements of the newborn. Breastmilk or formulas should be used for the first year.

The newborn should regain the birth weight by 2 weeks, double it between 4 and 5 months, and triple it by 1 year. Birth length increases about 1 in. per month for the first 6 months, one half inch per month in the second 6 months, and by 50% at 1 year.

Breastmilk changes in appearance, consistency, and content during postpartum and during a feeding. The hormone oxytocin stimulates milk ejection through the let-down reflex.

There are major benefits to breastfeeding, shown in Table 33-1. In the first 2 weeks, the infant should be fed every 1.5 to 3 hours. Once the milk supply is established, the infant can be fed on demand. The infant should nurse for up to 15 minutes on each breast to get the foremilk and the hindmilk. The infant should be in an alert state and demonstrate the rooting reflex before breastfeeding.

Typical positions for breastfeeding are the cradle hold, the football hold, and side-lying. It is essential to have proper latch-on to prevent sore, cracked, or bleeding nipples. To detach the infant from the breast, the mother should break the suction by placing a finger in the corner of the infant's mouth and pulling down on the lower jaw. The mother can determine whether her infant is getting a sufficient amount of breastmilk by observing the infant's fecal output.

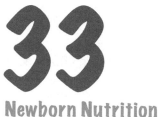

33
Newborn Nutrition

Common problems during breastfeeding are engorgement and sore nipples. The mother should discuss any medications she is taking while breastfeeding with her primary health care provider. With education and support, women who have given birth to a premature or sick infant are able to breastfeed successfully. Breastfeeding is contraindicated when the mother has breast cancer or HIV/AIDS.

Bottlefeeding allows both the mother and father to participate. The frequency of bottlefeeding is usually on demand or at least every 4 hours. Parents should be encouraged to soothe a crying infant if it is not yet time to feed. Bottle milk stools are pale yellow, formed, and pasty and may occur only once a day. A fresh bottle should be used for each feeding. The infant should be burped at least halfway through and at the end of the feeding. Proper instructions should be followed in preparing, storing, and heating bottle milk. Use nipples with the correct size of holes.

To assist new parents in meeting the nutritional needs of their newborn, the nurse must know the composition of human milk and formula, the physiology of breastfeeding, the advantages and disadvantages to both feeding methods, and feeding techniques.

TERMS
- [ ] **prolactin**
- [ ] **colostrum**
- [ ] **mature breastmilk**
- [ ] **foremilk**
- [ ] **hindmilk**
- [ ] **oxytocin**
- [ ] **let-down reflext**
- [ ] **latch-on**

NUTRITION FACTS

Commercially prepared formulas are modified to approximate the nutritional content of breastmilk, providing 20 kcal/oz and a comparable balance of carbohydrates, proteins, and fats.

Vitamin C, calcium, and phosphorus are important for infant growth and are present in both breastmilk and formulas.

Iron in breastmilk is well absorbed; a formula-fed infant may be given an iron-fortified formula.

Breastmilk or commercially prepared formulas should be used for the first year. Whole milk should not be given during the first year and skim milk should not be given until age 2, because they do not contain the appropriate nutrients.

The newborn should regain birth weight by 2 weeks and should gain between one half to 1 ounce per day for the first 6 months. Birth weight usually doubles between 4 and 5 months of age, and should triple by 1 year of age.

Birth length increases about 1 in. per month for the first 6 months and by one half inch per month in the second 6 months. Birth length usually increases by 50% at 1 year of age.

PHYSIOLOGY OF LACTATION

Regardless of whether or not the mother plans to breastfeed, there will be breast changes preparing for lactation. See Chapter 25 for signs of lactation and engorgement.

During pregnancy, the effect of **prolactin**, a hormone that stimulates milk production, is suppressed by high levels of estrogen and progesterone. After delivery of the placenta, these levels drop, triggering milk production.

Prolactin secretion continues in response to the infant's sucking, and repeated breastfeeding facilitates ongoing milk production. The amount of breastmilk produced is related to duration and frequency of breastfeeding — a supply and demand phenomenon.

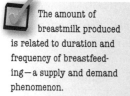

The amount of breastmilk produced is related to duration and frequency of breastfeeding—a supply and demand phenomenon.

Colostrum is produced by the breasts from week 16 of pregnancy, and is present for up to 5 days postpartum.

This thick, yellow fluid contains high levels of immunoglobulins, proteins, fat-soluble vitamins, and minerals.

Within 2 weeks, white or blue-tinged and watery **mature breastmilk** is being produced. During the first 10 minutes of feeding, **foremilk** is high in water content, vitamins, and protein. **Hindmilk**, released after 10 minutes of nursing, has a fat content four times higher than foremilk, satisfies hunger, and promotes weight gain.

The hormone **oxytocin** stimulates milk ejection through the **let-down reflex**. When the alveoli of the breast contract, milk moves into the ducts, the sinuses, and out through the nipple. Some signs of let-down are a tingling sensation, a warm feeling deep in the breast, and leakage of milk from the nipples.

> Some signs of let-down are a tingling sensation, a warm feeling deep in the breast, and leakage of milk from the nipples.

Until involution of the uterus is complete, the release of oxytocin with let-down produces uterine contractions, and for the first week this is felt as increased afterbirth pains.

BREASTFEEDING

Breastfeeding is often initiated within the first hour.

There are major benefits to breastfeeding for both mother and newborn. (See Table 33-1.) The frequency and duration of breastfeeding help establish an adequate milk supply. In the first 2 weeks, the infant should be fed every 1.5 to 3 hours.

> There are major benefits to breastfeeding for both mother and newborn. (See Table 33-1.)

Once the milk supply is established, the infant can be fed on demand. The infant should nurse for up to 15 minutes on each breast to get the foremilk and the hindmilk.

The newborn should be in an alert state and demonstrate the rooting reflex before attempting to breastfeed. If the infant is sleepy, the mother can arouse the baby by loosening blankets, massaging the back and limbs, or touching the face around the mouth to stimulate the rooting reflex.

The mother should be in a comfortable position, with pillows to support her back. The infant's head and spine should be in alignment, with the head well-supported. Typical positions for breastfeeding are the cradle hold, the football hold, and side-lying.

Table 33-1 Benefits of Breastfeeding

Nutrition	Ideally suited for newborn's digestive system: balanced composition of carbohydrates, fats, proteins, vitamins, and minerals; easily digested; readily absorbed.
Immunologic	Contains immunoglobulins, enzymes, and leukocytes to protect against infections; these proteins are not present in formula.
Anti-allergic	Eliminates exposure to potential allergens in cow's milk or soy-based formulas.
Cost	Less expensive to increase mother's daily caloric intake and buy nursing bras and breast pads than to buy bottles, nipples, and formula for one year.
Convenience	No time required for preparation or warming.
Psychosocial	Enhances maternal attachment, increases sense of maternal well-being; although only mother can breastfeed, other family members can give expressed breastmilk in a bottle.
Maternal	Faster uterine involution, faster weight loss, reduced risk for breast cancer.

When the infant's mouth is wide open and the tongue is down, the infant can be brought to the breast for correct **latch-on**.

 It is essential to have proper latch-on to prevent sore, cracked, or bleeding nipples.

Signs of correct latch-on are that the infant has as much of the areola in its mouth as possible, smooth jaw motion with suck and swallow, no clicking or smacking sounds indicating the infant is sucking on its tongue, and a firm tug on the nipple with no pain.

To detach the infant from the breast, the mother should break the suction by placing a finger in the corner of the infant's mouth and pulling down on the lower jaw.

 ## DETERMINING SUFFICIENCY

The mother can be reassured that her infant is getting a sufficient amount of breastmilk by observing the infant's output. During the first week, the stool becomes golden yellow, soft, and loose, and is excreted at least 3 to 4 times per day. Also, the infant should urinate at least 6 to 8 times per day.

Special Circumstances

- Common problems during adjustment to breastfeeding are engorgement and sore nipples. Nursing care to relieve breast-feeding discomforts is discussed in Chapter 26.
- The mother should discuss the safety of taking any medications while breastfeeding with her primary health care provider.
- With education and support, women who have given birth to a premature or sick infant are able to breastfeed successfully. They may have to pump their breasts until the infant is able to nurse at the breast.
- Mothers who have multiple births can produce adequate milk supply for more than one baby.

Breastfeeding is contraindicated when the mother has breast cancer or HIV/AIDS.

BOTTLEFEEDING

Bottlefeeding is begun when the infant shows signs of hunger or by 4 hours after birth. The frequency of bottlefeeding is usually on demand or at least every 4 hours. The newborn usually takes 1–2 oz at a feeding and increases to 4 oz by 2 months. Over-feeding should be avoided; parents should be encouraged to use techniques to soothe a crying infant if it is not yet time to feed. Stools of the bottle-fed infant change as the intake of formula increases. Bottle-milk stools are pale yellow, formed, and pasty, and may be excreted only once a day.

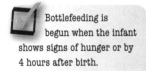
Bottlefeeding is begun when the infant shows signs of hunger or by 4 hours after birth.

Bottlefeeding is a safe choice for infant nutrition when a fresh bottle is used for each feeding. It allows both the mother and father to participate in infant feeding.

The caregiver should be sitting in a comfortable position to cradle the infant closely. The nipple should be placed in the infant's mouth and the bottle tilted so formula fills the nipple to avoid ingestion of excessive air.

The infant should be burped at least halfway through and at the end of the feeding. For the first few days, burping should be done after every one half ounce.

Formula preparation should follow the directions on the container. Bottles and nipples should be very clean. Refrigeration is necessary for bottles made in advance of feeding. Refrigerated bottles are usually warmed before feeding.

Do not use a microwave to warm a bottle because there could be "hot spots" in the milk.

The nipple hole should be large enough for milk to drip slowly.

Too large an opening in the nipple of a bottle may cause choking or regurgitation.

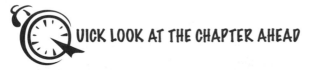
While the infant is in the hospital, the nurse continues to assist the newborn in its transition to extrauterine life. Vital signs of the infant are usually done every 4 hours and a physical assessment is performed every shift. The nurse observes color, character of cry, muscle tone, signs of excess mucus, nasal flaring, grunting, and chest retractions. The infant is positioned on the back for sleeping, and a bulb syringe placed in the crib for oral-nasal suctioning.

The nurse attempts to maintain a neutral thermal environment to minimize heat loss in the infant.

Breastfeeding is initiated in the first hour. Bottle feeding is begun when the infant shows signs of hunger or by 4 hours after birth. Frequency and duration or amount of formula, strength of suck, and each stool and voiding are recorded to monitor intake and output. The newborn is weighed daily to measure hydration and nutrition.

Because the newborn is at increased risk for infection, special antiseptic precautions are part of nursing care: handwashing, clean gloves, equipment cleaned before use. No one with illness or infections should care for mothers or newborns.

The umbilical cord site is observed for signs of infection such as redness, purulent drainage, or odor, and exposed to air to prevent infection.

Infants whose mothers are hepatitis B positive are given the first dose of vaccine within 12 hours of birth.

34

Nursing Care of the Newborn

Parent-infant attachment can be encouraged while the nurse provides care for the newborn.

The nurse detects complications by frequent assessment for hypothermia, respiratory distress, hypoglycemia, jaundice, and infection.

Blood for newborn metabolic screening tests is collected by the nurse before discharge. Parents are instructed to bring the child to a laboratory for a repeat test after discharge.

 In the hospital, the nurse monitors the infant's status, observes for complications, and prepares the parents for their new roles and responsibilities.

TERMS

- [ ] **signs of respiratory distress**
- [ ] **neutral thermal environment**
- [ ] **antiseptic precautions**
- [ ] **parent-infant attachment**
- [ ] **newborn metabolic screening tests**

MONITORING CARDIOPULMONARY STATUS

In all interactions with the infant, the nurse evaluates the cardiopulmonary status of the newborn by observing color, character of cry, muscle tone, signs of excess mucus, and **signs of respiratory distress** such as nasal flaring, grunting, and retractions of the sternum.

 Special attention is given to infants who might have increased amounts of fluid or mucus in the lungs: infants delivered by cesarean or infants with meconium-stained amniotic fluid.

All infants should be positioned on the back for sleeping, and a bulb syringe may be placed in the crib for use if oral-nasal suctioning is needed due to increased mucus or regurgitation.

MONITORING TEMPERATURE

The nurse attempts to maintain a **neutral thermal environment** to minimize heat loss by the infant. The infant is dressed, wrapped in at least two blankets, and wears a hat.

When bathing or other procedures are done, the infant is left exposed to the air for as short a time as possible. The initial bath is delayed until the temperature is stable for 1 to 2 hours; usually this is several hours after birth.

When bathing or other procedures are done, the infant is left exposed to the air for as short a time as possible. The initial bath is delayed until the temperature is stable for 1 to 2 hours; usually this is several hours after birth.

Temperatures are closely monitored for infants who have difficulty maintaining body temperature, have low birth weight, have signs of respiratory distress, or are under phototherapy for jaundice.

MONITORING HYDRATION AND NUTRITION

The frequency and duration of breastfeeding or the amount of bottle-fed formula ingested and the strength of the suck are recorded. See Chapter 33 for more information on the frequency of feeding and infant nutrition.

The first voiding and the first stool usually occur within 24 hours of birth. Recording of each stool and voiding is important to monitor intake and output.

The newborn is weighed daily at approximately the same time, and the expected weight loss is explained to the parents. See Chapter 30 for norms for weight loss.

PREVENTING INFECTION

Because the newborn is at increased risk for infection, **antiseptic precautions** are part of nursing care:

- Handwashing before and after contact with every newborn is standard practice.
- Clean gloves are worn when handling the newborn until the first bath is given.
- Equipment such as stethoscopes or thermometers is cleaned before use.
- Health care personnel with respiratory or gastrointestinal illness or eye or skin infections should not care for mothers or newborns.

The umbilical cord site is observed for signs of infection such as redness, purulent drainage, or odor, and exposed to air to prevent infection. Application of antiseptics such as alcohol, dyes, or ointments to the umbilical cord site is no longer recommended.

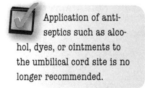
Application of antiseptics such as alcohol, dyes, or ointments to the umbilical cord site is no longer recommended.

Infants whose mothers are hepatitis B positive should be given the first dose of hepatitis B vaccine within 12 hours of birth.

ENHANCING ATTACHMENT

Parent-infant attachment can be encouraged while the nurse provides care for the newborn. Assessments and procedures can be done in the presence of the parents. Explanations of newborn characteristics and behaviors provide opportunities for parents to learn about their infant.

Participation in demonstrations of infant care such as bathing, dressing, and feeding enable the parents to develop caretaking skills.

MONITORING FOR COMPLICATIONS

An important role of the nurse is detecting complications. (See Table 34-1.) The infant's status can change quickly; therefore, frequent assessment alerts the nurse to developing problems. In addition to hypothermia or respiratory distress, complications for which the nurse should be alert are hypoglycemia, jaundice, and infection.

METABOLIC SCREENING

According to most state laws, blood for **newborn metabolic screening tests** is collected by the nurse before discharge. Parents are instructed to bring the child to a laboratory for a repeat test after discharge. Phenylketonuria, hypothyroidism, galactosemia, and maple syrup urine disease are the usual metabolic conditions detected in this screening.

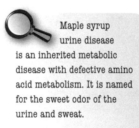

Maple syrup urine disease is an inherited metabolic disease with defective amino acid metabolism. It is named for the sweet odor of the urine and sweat.

Table 34-1 Monitoring for Selected Complications

Complication	Infants at Risk	Assessment	Action
Tachypnea	Preterm infant, post-term infant, meconium-stained amniotic fluid, infant of diabetic mother, cesarean birth.	Observations for nasal flaring, circumoral cyanosis, expiratory grunt, sternal retractions.	Stimulate infant to cry, perform chest physical therapy. If not resolved with intervention, report to health care provider.
Hypoglycemia	Small for gestational age (SGA), large for gestational age (LGA), infant of diabetic mother, preterm infant, postterm infant.	Blood glucose levels below 40 mg/dL. Jitteriness, tremors, lethargy, high-pitched cry, tachypnea, sweating.	Offer breastmilk, infant formula, or glucose water. Avoid cold stress.

Table 34-1 Monitoring for Selected Complications (continued)

Complication	Infants at Risk	Assessment	Action
Hyperbilirubinemia	O blood type mother, Rh negative mother, small for gestational age (SGA), large for gestational age (LGA), infant of diabetic mother, preterm infant, postterm infant, cephalhematoma, bruising.	Observations for jaundice in skin or sclera. Transcutaneous bilirubinometry readings above established norms for age and birth weight.	Report abnormal readings to health care provider. Encourage frequent feedings.
Infection	Amniotic membranes ruptured more than 24 hours before birth, history of maternal infection.	Unstable temperature, tachypnea without other signs of respiratory distress, pale or dusky color, feeding problems, lethargy, irritability.	Report signs of infection to health care provider.
Circumcision	Circumcised male infants.	Observations for excessive bleeding or excessive swelling every 15 minutes for 1 hour. Observe for first voiding of urine within 6 hours.	Apply petroleum jelly to the site except with Plastibell. If bleeding does occur, apply light pressure. If bleeding does not subside, report to health care provider.

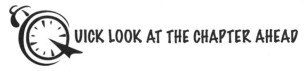

Topics to assist the parents to meet both physical and emotional needs of the newborn are as follows.

- For safety: place baby on the back for sleep; use tummy time to strengthen head, neck, and shoulder muscles; support head and neck during care; keep crib rails up; use firm crib mattress with no pillows; do not leave the infant alone on a couch, table, or bed; avoid shaken baby syndrome.

- Demonstrate taking axillary temperature with a digital thermometer; advise to take temperature before contacting the health care provider; remind parents of normal temperature range.

- Review signs of infection in umbilical cord, circumcision sites, the eye; advise to contact health care provider if signs occur.

- Review essentials for infant feeding; recommend that nursing continue for at least 6 months but preferably for the first year; advise to contact health care provider with any concerns.

- Demonstrate bathing, diapering, and dressing. Review umbilical cord care. Explain circumcision care and observations.

- Explain normal newborn characteristics and reflexes seen in their infant.

- Describe behavioral states and sensory capabilities of the newborn, and advise on suitable parental responses.

35

Discharge Teaching: Infant Topics

- Explain and describe interactions for enhancing the infant's development.

- Discuss integration of the infant into the family.

- Discuss mother's return to work and selection and safety issues of child care, if appropriate. If breastfeeding, discuss options for maintaining milk supply.

- Tell parents to discuss with their pediatric health care provider the schedule for examinations and immunizations, and to contact the provider with any questions or concerns about their infant.

 Before the infant is discharged, the nurse evaluates the ability of the parents to care for their infant. Taking into account cultural variations, the nurse instructs the mother and other family about newborn needs and care.

Topics to assist the parents to meet both physical and emotional needs of the newborn are as follows.

 SAFETY

- Advise placing baby on the back for sleep, to reduce the risk of SIDS (Sudden Infant Death Syndrome). Provide **"tummy time"** by placing the baby on its abdomen for a short time each day under supervision to strengthen head, neck, and shoulder muscles.
- Demonstrate how to support the head and neck when providing care to the newborn, since the neck muscles are not well developed.
- Discuss general safety measures such as keeping crib rails up; firm crib mattress with no pillows; not leaving the infant on a couch, table, or bed; and supervising the infant at all times.

 Describe **shaken baby syndrome** and the importance of prevention. Advise never to shake a baby during play or in anger or frustration.

 TAKING THE BABY'S TEMPERATURE

- Demonstrate how to take an axillary temperature with a digital thermometer.
- Advise to take the temperature before contacting the health care provider with a concern about the infant's condition.
- Remind parents of normal temperature range for infants — 97.8 to 99.5˚F or 36.5 to 37.5˚C.

 SIGNS OF INFECTION

- Review signs of infection in umbilical cord or circumcision sites: redness, purulent discharge, or odor.
- Review signs of infection in the eye: yellowish or greenish discharge, redness, or swelling.

 Advise to contact health care provider if any signs of infection occur.

FEEDING

- Review the essentials for infant feeding. Refer to Chapter 33 for information on newborn nutrition.
- If breastfeeding, recommend that nursing continue for at least 6 months but preferably for the first full year.
- Advise to contact health care provider with any concerns about infant's feeding behavior.

HYGIENE

- Demonstrate bathing, diapering, and dressing.
- Advise that daily bath is not necessary; however, face and diaper area should be cleaned every day. For infant girls, genitals should be cleaned from front to back. A sponge bath is given until the umbilical cord detaches and site is healed. After that, a tub bath may be given. The use of lotions, creams, or oils in bathing an infant is not recommended.

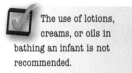
The use of lotions, creams, or oils in bathing an infant is not recommended.

- Review umbilical cord care, demonstrating folding diaper away from cord. See Chapter 34 for more information.
- Explain circumcision care and observations. See Table 34-1 in Chapter 34 for details on circumcision care.
- Inform parents that during the healing process, a yellow granulation tissue may form at the circumcision site. This is not a sign of infection and they should not attempt to remove it.

NEWBORN CHARACTERISTICS

- Explain normal newborn characteristics and reflexes seen in their infant.
- Inform parents that it is safe to touch the fontanelles and that milia are normal and do not need to scrubbed or squeezed.

INFANT BEHAVIORS

- Describe behavioral states and sensory capabilities of the newborn. See tables on newborn characteristics in Chapter 30.
- Inform parents that infants can block out sensory stimuli and it is not necessary to be quiet, whisper, or tip-toe around the infant.
- Advise parents to allow the infant to attempt self-quieting behavior such as sucking the fist before responding to infant's cries. If fussiness persists for several minutes, then parents should intervene. Discuss that the parents will learn to differentiate among types of cries.
- Describe sleep patterns and "fussy" periods common in newborns. Each infant has its own pattern for sleep and wake periods. Usually there is one longer sleep cycle in a 24-hour period. Infants may be more fussy in the evening. Reassure parents that they will learn their own infant's patterns.

INFANT STIMULATION

- Explain the need for interactions to enhance the infant's development, often called **infant stimulation**. Infants can see best at a distance of 8 to10 in., prefer contrasting primary colors, especially black and white, like geometric shapes rather than straight lines; and respond most readily to the human face and voice.
- Advise parents to interact with the infant in a developmentally appropriate manner by providing mobiles and toys, talking to the infant, and exposing the infant to a variety of sights, sounds, odors, and textures.

INCORPORATION INTO FAMILY

- Discuss integration of the infant into the family. See Chapter 24 for details on family integration.
- Recommend techniques for sibling introduction: supervising interactions between young children and the newborn, providing gifts for the older siblings from the new baby, encouraging age-appropriate assistance with infant care, and spending time with the older siblings without the newborn.

RETURNING TO WORK

- Discuss the mother's return to work and selection of child care, if appropriate. See Chapter 7.
- Many parents are concerned about leaving the infant with child care and need reassurance that the infant will thrive. Safety issues surrounding day-care selection can be discussed.
- Suggest contacting community resources, if they are needed to assist the family with child care.
- If the mother is breastfeeding, discuss options for maintaining milk supply, pumping and storing breastmilk, or partial weaning.

FOLLOW-UP

- Explain the need for well-baby health care. Parents should discuss with the pediatric health care provider the schedule for examinations and immunizations.
- Encourage parents to contact the pediatric health care provider with any questions or concerns they have about their infant. (See Table 35-1.)

Table 35-1 When to Call the Health Care Provider

Infant Concerns

1. Difficulty breathing: continuous sighing, grunting, or excess mucus.
2. Cyanosis: blue or blotchy skin.
3. Jaundice: yellow color to skin or eyes.
4. Axillary temperature above 100.4°F (38.0°C) or below 97.5°F (36.4°C).
5. Vomiting: frequent or forceful.
6. Refusal of two feedings in a row.
7. Loose, green, watery bowel movements.
8. No bowel movement for more than 24 hours.
9. No urination for 12 hours.
10. Signs of infection in eyes, umbilical cord, or circumcision.
11. Pustules, blisters, or rashes on skin.
12. Difficulty in waking baby.
13. More that usual fussiness.
14. Any unusual changes in the infant's behavior or appearance.
15. Any other questions about infant care.

PART VI • QUESTIONS

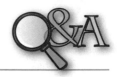

1. Drying the infant immediately after birth helps prevent heat loss from what mechanism?
   a. Conduction
   b. Convection
   c. Evaporation
   d. Radiation

2. Which chemical stimulus contributes to the initiation of breathing immediately after birth?
   a. Chest wall compression with recoil.
   b. Decreased peripheral oxygen levels.
   c. Rubbing the infant's back with a blanket.
   d. Temperature change in extrauterine environment.

3. Nursing assessment data of a term newborn includes temperature 36.1°C (97°F), pulse rate 148, respiration rate 52, color pink, and strong cry. Rank the nursing actions from 1 to 4 in order of priority.
   _____Assess for tremors.
   _____Place the infant under a radiant warmer.
   _____Recheck the temperature in 30 minutes.
   _____Verify the temperature.

4. The nurse observes a new mother applying a dressing or belly band over the umbilical cord site when getting the baby ready to go home. Although she states she understands reasons why a belly band is not necessary, the mother insists on using it. What is the best response by the nurse to this situation?
   a. "I will explain again why you don't need to use the belly band."
   b. "If you use a belly band, the baby will get a cord infection."
   c. "Let us discuss the signs of infection of the cord."
   d. "When you are at home, you do what you think is best."

5. What behavioral state of the newborn would be an optimal time for breastfeeding?
   a. Active REM sleep
   b. Crying

c. Drowsy

d. Wide awake

6. The nurse makes a home visit to a mother and her newborn. The infant weighed 7 lb and 9 oz (3430 g) at birth and now weighs 6 lb and 15 oz (3147 g) at 4 days of age. What nursing action would be most appropriate?

a. Notify the health care provider of the infant's condition.

b. Reassure the mother that the weight loss is in the appropriate range.

c. Recommend the mother stop breastfeeding and put the baby on formula.

d. Suggest the mother supplement with formula after each breastfeeding.

7. One minute after an infant's birth, the nurse assesses the newborn for an Apgar score. Assessment findings are heart rate of 110 beats per minute, breathing slow and irregular, active motion of the extremities, grimace when sole of foot is tapped, and blue body and extremities. What would be the Apgar score for this infant?

a. 4

b. 5

c. 6

e. 7

8. What would be the priority nursing action immediately after the birth of an infant?

a. Assess infant for Apgar score.

b. Dry infant with blanket.

c. Give infant vitamin K injection.

d. Put identification bracelets on infant.

9. A newborn male infant at 39 weeks of gestation is born. What gestational age characteristic would the nurse expect to observe during the initial assessment?

a. Creases over the entire sole.

b. Dry, leathery skin with deep creases.

c. Smooth scrotal sac with undescended testicles.

d. Thick lanugo on face, shoulders, and back.

10. The newborn medical record indicates the presence of a cephalhe-matoma. What assessment data would support this finding?
    a. Circular area of bruising on the back of the head.
    b. Cranial bones overlap with palpable sutures.
    c. Edema over the entire back of the scalp.
    d. Firm swelling on the left side of the head.

11. Which data from the nursing assessment should be reported to the primary care provider?
    a. Anterior fontenelle bulges slightly when infant cries.
    b. Positive Babinski sign.
    c. Subconjuctival hemorrhage present in right eye.
    d. Tuft of hair at base of spine.

12. The mother observes the nurse holding her infant's head and letting it to drop back suddenly. She expresses concern that this is too rough and would hurt the baby. What would be the best response by the nurse?
    a. "Sometimes it appears that we are rough with the baby, but it is the only way we can evaluate the spinal cord."
    b. "This is a way to evaluate the nervous system through the Moro response. I am very careful to support your baby's head and neck."
    c. "The tonic neck reflex is tested this way. You will notice that I am supporting the baby's head and neck."
    d. "Your baby won't be hurt by what I am doing. I need to do this to test for the Babinski reflex."

13. Upon entering the room of a postpartum client, the nurse can hear the breastfeeding infant make smacking sounds as it nurses. What is the appropriate nursing intervention?
    a. Assist the mother to detach the infant from the breast and have the infant latch on again.
    b. Detach the infant and have the mother nurse the infant on the opposite breast.
    c. Encourage the mother to continue breastfeeding because correct technique is being demonstrated.
    d. Observe the mother's technique when she has the infant latch on the opposite breast.

14. A pregnant woman tells the nurse she is undecided about infant feeding and requests information to make a choice. Which statement by the nurse would be most helpful?
    a. Allergies are less common in formula-fed infants.
    b. Bottle feeding is less expensive than breastfeeding.
    c. Breastmilk contains properties that protect the infant from infection.
    d. Mothers who breastfeed have an increased risk for breast cancer.

15. During assessment of a term newborn, the nurse observes temperature 36.5°C (97.7°F), pulse rate 158, respiration rate 82. The infant is demonstrating nasal flaring and occasional grunting. What nursing action would be most appropriate?
    a. Assess infant for jitteriness.
    b. Evaluate blood sugar level.
    c. Observe infant for jaundice.
    d. Perform chest physical therapy.

16. Which statement by the new mother indicates that further infant discharge teaching by the nurse needs to be done?
    a. "Baby's bowel movements are often green and watery."
    b. "I will call the doctor if the baby doesn't look or act right."
    c. "If my baby's eyes look yellow, I should call the doctor."
    d. "The newborn should urinate at least 6 to 8 times a day."

PART VI • ANSWERS AND RATIONALES

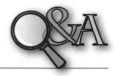

1. **The answer is c.** Immediately after birth, the infant is covered with amniotic fluid. Therefore, drying the infant will remove the fluid and decrease the risk of heat loss through evaporation. Drying the infant would not affect heat loss by the other mechanisms described in options a, b, and d.

2. **The answer is b.** Option b is correct because it describes a chemical stimulus to breathe. Options a, c, and d describe the other types of stimuli for initiation of breathing.

3. **The ranking of these nursing actions would be 3, 2, 4, 1.** Verifying temperature would be the first priority. If the temperature is low, the nurse needs to take action to increase the infant's temperature. Often this is done by placing the infant under a radiant warmer. Because low body temperature can lead to hypoglycemia, the infant needs to be assessed for signs of hypoglycemia, including tremors. To determine if thermogenesis is accomplished, the body temperature would be rechecked after the infant is under the radiant warmer for 30 minutes.

4. **The answer is c.** Cultural beliefs and practices should be respected. The nurse would inform the family of possible infection when the cord is not exposed to air, and teach the signs of infection. The family would then be able to detect signs of infection in the umbilical cord and seek appropriate health care. Options a and d do not reflect sensitivity to cultural practices, and option b is inaccurate.

5. **The answer is d.** During the wide-awake state, the infant is alert and ready for interaction with the environment. The infant would be most receptive to stimulation of the rooting and sucking reflexes necessary for breastfeeding. In the active REM sleep or drowsy states, the newborn would be less likely to open its mouth and latch on to the nipple. In the crying state, the newborn would be agitated and have difficulty latching.

6. **The answer is b.** A weight loss of 10 oz in this baby is within the 10% limit for expected weight loss after birth. Since the weight loss

falls within the expected range, the primary care provider does not need to be notified. The mother should be reassured, encouraged to continued breastfeeding, and taught signs that indicate that the baby is receiving adequate nourishment. Supplementation with formula is not necessary; more frequent and longer feedings could be suggested to increase the infant's intake.

7. **The answer is c.** A heart rate of 110 is rated 2. Respiratory effort that is slow and irregular is rated 1. Muscle tone as demonstrated by active motion of the extremities is rated 2. A grimace when the sole of the foot is stroked gives a reflex irritability rating of 1. Color is rated 0 when body and extremities are blue. The total Apgar score for this infant is 6.

8. **The answer is b.** Establishing and maintaining breathing is the first priority in the immediate care of the newborn. Providing and maintaining warmth is the second priority. Drying the infant with a blanket will implement both of these priorities. Apgar scoring is done at 1 minute and 5 minutes after birth. Assessment occurs simultaneously with other activities. The other options describe nursing care given after the infant's condition is assessed and stabilized.

9. **The answer is a.** An infant at 39 weeks of gestation is a term infant. Plantar creases would be seen over the entire sole of the foot. Option b is a characteristic of the postterm infant and options c and d are characteristics of the preterm infant.

10. **The answer is d.** Cephalhematoma presents as a firm swelling that does not cross suture lines. Option a describes bruising most likely from the use of a vacuum extractor. Option b describes molding. Option c describes caput succedaneum.

11. **The answer is d.** A tuft of hair at the base of the spine needs further evaluation to determine if spina bifida is present. The other options describe normal newborn assessment findings.

12. **The answer is b.** The description of the nurse activity suggests the Moro reflex is being tested. This response informs the mother of the purpose of the examination and reassures her about techniques that make it a safe procedure. The other options are incorrect because they refer to other reflexes or do not adequately address the mother's concern for her infant's safety.

13. **The answer is a.** Smacking sounds when the infant nurses indicate incorrect latch-on, which increases nipple discomfort. The nurse should assist the mother to use the proper technique. Option b is incorrect because the infant needs to continue to empty the same breast using correct latch-on. Option c is incorrect because correct technique is not being used when smacking sounds occur. Option d is incorrect because the nurse would not wait until the infant latches on the opposite breast to assist the mother in her breast-feeding technique.

14. **The answer is c.** Breastmilk contains immunologic properties that protect against infection; these are not present in formula. Option a is incorrect because allergies to cow or soy protein are more common in formula-fed infants. Option b is incorrect because cost of formula, bottles, and nipples is more than the cost of increased maternal nutrition and breastfeeding supplies. Option d is incorrect because women who breastfeed have a *decreased* risk of breast cancer.

15. **The answer is d.** A breathing rate of 82, nasal flaring, and grunting indicate newborn tachypnea. Nursing actions to remove secretions from the respiratory tract include doing chest physical therapy and stimulating the baby to cry. The other options do not address tachypnea.

16. **The answer is a.** Bowel movements that are loose, green, and watery should be reported to the health care provider. The other options indicate understanding of when to call the health care provider.

VII

The High-Risk Perinatal Client

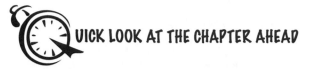

The majority, though not all, of high-risk pregnancies are identified during the first prenatal visit. Areas to be assessed are obstetrical history, medical history, current obstetric status, and social-personal characteristics.

Circumstances that can lead to increased risk of complications include:

* Pre-existing medical conditions.

* Risk factors identified during the course of pregnancy.

* Inadequate prenatal care.

* A maternal age less than 16 and over 35.

* Primagravidas (first-time pregnancies).

* A history of more than 3 previous births.

* Low education, low income, unmarried, and nonwhite.

* Underweight at conception.

* Smoking.

* Family violence.

The nurse plays an important role in caring for the high-risk perinatal client by helping in the early identification of high-risk factors, collaborating with other health team members to monitor the woman's condition, implementing interventions that minimize complications, and promoting a healthy response by the woman and her family to the situation.

36

Identification of High-Risk Factors

TERMS
- [ ] **high-risk pregnancy**
- [ ] **pre-existing medical conditions**
- [ ] **inadequate prenatal care**
- [ ] **socioeconomic factors**

A pregnancy is considered to be high risk when there is significantly increased risk for problems or complications in mother, fetus, or newborn.

The majority of **high-risk pregnancies** are identified during the first prenatal visit through careful history taking, complete physical examination, and laboratory studies. Areas to be assessed for high-risk factors include obstetrical history, medical history, current obstetric status, and social-personal characteristics.

A significant number of problems occur in women who have not been identified as being at high risk. (See Table 36-1.)

> A significant number of problems occur in women who have not been identified as being at high risk. (See Table 36-1.)

In the remaining chapters, selected high-risk complications will be discussed in more detail.

OBSTETRICAL HISTORY

Although a history of problems with a previous pregnancy does not make it certain that a current pregnancy will be high risk, in some situations there may be increased risk. For example, there is increased risk for ectopic pregnancy and for multiple gestation in women who have been treated for infertility.

A history of cervical insufficiency or anomalies of the uterus or cervix can predispose a woman to a second-trimester loss.

A woman who has had a previous history of gestational hypertension, preterm labor or birth, two or more spontaneous abortions, ectopic pregnancy, stillbirth, or neonatal death has an increased risk of experiencing the same complication again.

Pregnancies spaced less than one year apart do not give the woman's body time to recover.

Diabetes mellitus is often associated with large-for-gestational-age infants over 4000 g.

MEDICAL HISTORY

Pre-existing medical conditions can predispose a pregnant woman to have complications. There is an increased risk of gestational hypertension associated with chronic hypertension, diabetes mellitus, and renal or vascular disease.

Table 36-1 High-Risk Factors

Obstetric History	Current Obstetrical Status
Infertility	Total weight gain < 10 lb
Cervical insufficiency or incompetent cervix	Weight loss > 5 lb
Uterine or cervical anomaly	Excessive weight gain
Previous preterm labor/birth	Intrauterine-growth-restricted fetus
Previous cesarean birth	Large-for-gestational-age fetus
Previous gestational hypertension	Abnormal fetal surveillance tests
Previous infant over 4000 g	Abnormal presentation
2 or more spontaneous or elective abortions	Hydramnios
Previous ectopic pregnancy	Oligohydramnios
Previous stillbirth/neonatal death	Maternal anemia
Previous multiple gestation	Hypermesis gravidarum
Previous pregnancy less than 1 year ago	Gestational hypertension
	Placenta previa
	Placental abruption
	Fetal or placental malformation
	Rh sensitization
	Preterm labor
	Multiple gestation
	Premature rupture of membranes
	Postdate pregnancy
	Sexually transmitted infections
	Maternal infections

Medical History	Social-Personal Characteristics
Chronic hypertension	Inadequate prenatal care
Diabetes mellitus	Maternal age < 16
Major organ system disease: cardiac, pulmonary,	Maternal age > 35
renal, GI, thyroid, neurological,	Primigravida
hemaglobinopathies	Multiparity > 3
Sexually transmitted infections	Education under 11 years
Previous surgery, especially reproductive	Low socioeconomic status
Emotional or cognitive disorders	Minority status
	Single marital status
	Over/underweight at conception
	Smoking > 10 cigarettes/day
	Drug or alcohol abuse
	Family violence

Diabetes mellitus can worsen during pregnancy with increased risk of deteriorating vascular changes. Diabetes mellitus also increases a pregnant woman's risk for fetal congenital anomalies, stillbirth, cesarean delivery related to macrosomia and fetal distress, and neonatal complications.

The physiologic stresses on major organ systems during pregnancy can exaggerate problems of cardiac, pulmonary, renal, gastrointestinal, thyroid, neurological, or hematological functioning.

Infections during pregnancy can increase the risk of congenital anomalies, may require a cesarean delivery, and can increase the risk for preterm labor.

A history of depression or bipolar disorder is a risk factor for postpartum depression.

Previous surgery of the reproductive organs can affect fertility, the ability to carry a pregnancy to term, and method of delivery.

CURRENT OBSTETRICAL STATUS

Many times risk factors are identified during the course of pregnancy. A total weight gain of 10 lb or a weight loss of more than 5 lb has serious implications for fetal growth, and indicates the need for dietary intervention. Excessive weight gain can result from edema associated with gestational hypertension or caloric intake above the recommended amount.

Indications of intrauterine fetal growth restriction (IUGR) should be evaluated for limited circulation to the placenta.

A fetus that is large for gestational age is often associated with gestational diabetes and increases maternal risk for instrument-assisted birth or cesarean delivery and fetal risk for birth injury.

When fetal surveillance tests are abnormal, additional assessments for chromosomal abnormalities, congenital defects, and placental functioning are performed at the physician's direction.

An abnormal fetal presentation such as breech or transverse lie requires a cesarean delivery.

Hydramnios or increased amount of amniotic fluid is associated with certain conditions such as Rh sensitization, diabetes, and fetal neurological or gastrointestinal defects.

Oligohydramnios or a diminished amount of amniotic fluid is found with postmaturity, IUGR, and fetal renal abnormalities.

Maternal anemia can be an indication of inadequate iron intake or of a hemaglobinopathy such as sickle cell anemia.

Obstetrical complications during a pregnancy place the woman at significant risk. Vomiting associated with hyperemesis gravidarum has an impact on nutritional status.

Gestational hypertension results in constriction of maternal blood vessels that can cause decreased placental perfusion, leading to low birth weight and fetal distress.

Maternal risks from gestational hypertension include cerebral, renal, cardiovascular, or hepatic problems.

Placental problems such as previa or abruption can interfere with circulation to the fetus, lead to maternal hemorrhage, and require cesarean delivery.

Rh sensitization causes destruction of fetal red blood cells that can lead to fetal or neonatal complications.

Preterm labor affects maternal physical and emotional well-being, and if it progresses to preterm birth, can affect the newborn. Contributing factors to preterm labor are premature rupture of membranes, multiple gestation, and maternal infection.

Postdate pregnancy, a pregnancy continuing more than 2 weeks after the due date, can lead to complications in the fetus or newborn.

SOCIAL-PERSONAL CHARACTERISTICS

Inadequate prenatal care is care begun after the first trimester, or inconsistent attendance at appointments. This contributes to late recognition of problems.

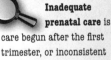

Inadequate prenatal care is care begun after the first trimester, or inconsistent attendance at appointments. This contributes to late recognition of problems.

A maternal age less than 16 increases the risk for premature labor, maternal anemia, PIH, prolonged labor, cesarean delivery, and IUGR. The adolescent woman is also more likely to have less education and income.

With maternal age over 35, there is an increased likelihood of chronic disease and an increased risk of congenital or chromosomal abnormalities, PIH, premature labor, and cesarean delivery.

Primagravidas (first-time pregnancies) have an increased risk of PIH, prolonged labor, and cesarean delivery. A history of more than 3 previous births is a multiparity greater than 3 and increases the risk for antepartum or postpartum hemorrhage.

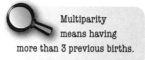

Multiparity means having more than 3 previous births.

Socioeconomic factors such as low education, low income, being unmarried, and being nonwhite are associated with increased incidence of gestational hypertension, inadequate prenatal care, preterm birth, and IUGR.

Being underweight at conception increases the risk for anemia, prolonged labor, and IUGR; being overweight at conception increases the risk for gestational hypertension, diabetes, cesarean delivery, and macrosomia.

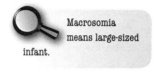

Macrosomia means large-sized infant.

Smoking contributes to IUGR and preterm labor or birth. Drug addiction or alcohol abuse increases the risk of preterm labor, IUGR, inadequate maternal nutrition, and abnormal fetal development.

Family violence leading to physical abuse increases the rate of spontaneous abortion, preterm birth, and stillbirths. The woman who experiences violence is more prone to anxiety, depression, alcohol or drug use, and is more likely to have inadequate prenatal care.

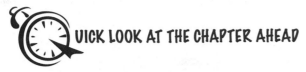

With a high-risk pregnancy, the perinatal experience is different from what was expected.

- The life and health of the mother and fetus may be at risk.

- The unpredictable nature of the situation and the uncertainty of the outcome can lead to a sense of loss of control.

- The management of the high-risk condition produces additional sources of stress.

- Sometimes there are restrictions in the woman's activity that may require changes in family roles.

- Additional necessary testing can require time that interferes with work or family responsibilities.

- Hospitalization can cause a significant increase in stress to the woman and her family.

Responses to the uncertainty of a high-risk pregnancy include fear, anxiety, frustration, anger, denial, threat to self-esteem, blaming of self and others, noncompliance, and an increased risk of postpartum depression. Many of these responses are part of the grieving process for the loss of a normal pregnancy.

Complications in the first trimester can heighten the feelings of ambivalence, as well as delay validation and acceptance of the pregnancy.

37

Psychological Adaptations to High Risk

It is difficult for the couple to develop an identity as parents, and the attachment process can be delayed because of fear, which can lead to rejection.

In addition, one of Rubin's maternal tasks, ensuring safe passage, is difficult to achieve when complications threaten the health of the mother or the fetus.

Nurses play a vital role in helping a family develop appropriate coping strategies. In collaboration with primary health care providers, the nurse clarifies information about the high-risk condition, treatment options, test results, and possible outcomes to help the family have a realistic perception of the situation. Whenever possible, the nurse encourages the woman to participate in her care and decision making.

Many women in high-risk situations have activity restrictions; feelings of isolation, boredom, and loss of control can result. Diversions become important.

Nursing interventions help maintain family cohesiveness in this time of crisis. The entire family can be included in the care of the hospitalized woman, and referrals made to a social worker, pastoral care provider, nutritionist, or a support group.

 The nurse needs to understand high-risk stressors, assess the responses of the woman and her family, and provide nursing interventions to facilitate coping. Table 37-1 lists questions the nurse may ask. Assessing the impact of high-risk factors on the family will assist the nurse in determining specific teaching or referrals needed.

With a high-risk pregnancy, a woman and her family experience variations in the usual psychological adaptations to pregnancy. There is a disruption in the typical adjustments because the perinatal experience takes an unexpected course, and medical management becomes more complex.

Table 37-1 Assessing the Impact of High-Risk Conditions

Topic	Nursing Assessment Questions
Nutrition	Are there dietary changes you have been told to make? How do you plan to make these changes? Do you anticipate any problems?
Elimination	Have there been any changes in your urination or bowel habits? What are you doing to maintain your usual habits?
Activity/Exercise	What changes in exercise and activity do you need to make? How are you going to do this? Do you expect any problems?
Sleep/Rest	Have there been changes in your usual sleep patterns? Do you feel rested after sleeping? Are you having dreams? What kind?
Sexuality	Has your condition required changes in your sexual activity? How do you and your partner feel about this? What do you plan to do to make these changes?
Understanding of situation	What do you know about your condition, the treatment plan, and possible effects on yourself and the baby? Do you have any other questions?
Coping	What are you most concerned about? What feelings are you experiencing? Are there other things happening to cause you stress? Have you had past experiences to help you cope with the stress you are feeling now? What things have you done in the past to manage stress? How supportive are your partner, family, and friends? What support do you have to help you?
Roles/Relationships	How has this high-risk condition affected you and your family? What changes in family roles do you need to make? Do you expect any problems? How has this condition affected your work responsibilities? Will there be any problems?
Cultural/Spiritual issues	Has this high-risk condition affected your cultural or spiritual practices? How do you feel about this?
Finances	Are there financial concerns about medical bills, child care expenses, or additional expenses such as family meals, lodging, and transportation? What resources do you have?

HIGH-RISK STRESSORS

In a high-risk situation, the perinatal experience is different from what was expected. The life and health of the mother and fetus may be at risk. The unpredictable nature of the situation and the uncertainty of the outcome can lead to a sense of loss of control. The management of the high-risk condition produces additional sources of stress.

Sometimes there are restrictions in the woman's activity that may require changes in family roles. For example, the father of the baby may assume housekeeping and child-care tasks for which he feels unprepared.

Additional testing necessary for assessment of the high-risk condition can require time that interferes with work or family responsibilities.

If the woman is hospitalized, there is a significant increase in stress on her and her family from separation of family members, social isolation of the woman, and an increased financial burden.

 ## RESPONSES

Responses to the uncertainty of a high-risk pregnancy may differ among individuals according to the significance placed on the pregnancy, understanding of the condition itself, past experiences, previous coping mechanisms, and the amount of family or professional support received.

Some responses include fear, anxiety, frustration, anger, and denial. These emotional reactions can influence some women to be noncompliant. There may be a threat to self-esteem and blaming of self and others.

Many responses are part of the process of grieving for the loss of a normal pregnancy, the expected birth experience, or a perfect baby.

 Because of additional stressors that accompany a high-risk situation, the woman also has an increased risk of postpartum depression.

Disruption of maternal and paternal tasks occurs when there is a high-risk pregnancy. Complications in the first trimester can heighten feelings of ambivalence as well as delay validation and acceptance of the pregnancy.

The attachment process can be affected by a delay in establishing a relationship with the fetus because of fear for the survival of the infant. In some circumstances this fear can lead to rejection.

Also, when there is uncertainty about the infant's survival, it is difficult for the couple to develop an identity as parents.

The restrictions of medical management can interfere with parents' being able to prepare the home for the infant or to attend childbirth classes, activities that can enhance development of the parenting role. One of Rubin's maternal tasks, ensuring safe passage, is difficult to achieve when complications threaten the health of the mother or the fetus.

NURSING INTERVENTIONS

Nurses play a vital role in assessing client and family responses to a high-risk pregnancy and assisting in the development of appropriate coping strategies.

Fear and anxiety are the most common emotional responses to a high-risk situation and must be dealt with before the family can be receptive to explanations or other teaching. It is important for the nurse to acknowledge the grief they are experiencing, to discuss the impact on the entire family, and to provide opportunities for the woman and her family to express their feelings. One of Rubin's maternal tasks of pregnancy is learning to give of oneself on behalf of the child. The nurse can encourage development of Rubin's task by acknowledging the woman's sacrifices and providing positive reinforcement for her efforts to protect the fetus.

In collaboration with primary health care providers, the nurse clarifies information about the high-risk condition, treatment options, test results, and possible outcomes to help the family have a realistic perception of the high-risk situation.

Having adequate knowledge about a high-risk situation will diminish the woman's anxiety, increase her self-esteem, decrease frustration, and encourage compliance.

Nurses play a vital role in assessing client and family responses to a high-risk pregnancy and assisting in the development of appropriate coping strategies.

The nurse can encourage development of Rubin's task by acknowledging the woman's sacrifices and providing positive reinforcement for her efforts to protect the fetus.

In collaboration with primary health care providers, the nurse clarifies information about the high-risk condition, treatment options, test results, and possible outcomes to help the family have a realistic perception of the high-risk situation.

Whenever possible, the nurse encourages the woman to participate in care and decision making by allowing her to choose her own food, administer her own medications if appropriate, and state her preferences for scheduling of activities.

Many women in high-risk situations have activity restrictions and are often on bedrest; feelings of isolation, boredom, and loss of control can result. Diversional activities become important when activity is restricted. Crafts, reading, games, puzzles, movies, journal writing, or other activities provide distraction, keep the mind alert, and contribute to a sense of accomplishment.

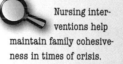

Diversional activities become important when activity is restricted. Crafts, reading, games, puzzles, movies, journal writing, or other activities provide distraction, keep the mind alert, and contribute to a sense of accomplishment.

When possible, the nurse encourages the woman to continue some family roles such as bill-paying, reading to children, or planning meals. Also, some types of employment allow the woman to continue with aspects of her job responsibilities.

The woman and her family continue to prepare to give birth and become parents. The nurse can provide childbirth education and parenting information by methods appropriate to the woman's activity level such as videos or private sessions.

Nursing interventions help maintain family cohesiveness in times of crisis. The entire family can be included in the care of the hospitalized woman by encouraging them to visit and telephone frequently, providing flexible visiting times, suggesting that they bring favorite foods from home and eat together, and any other ways to incorporate the woman into daily family life. Appropriate referrals to social worker, pastoral care provider, nutritionist, or a support group are made when indicated.

Nursing interventions help maintain family cohesiveness in times of crisis.

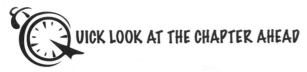
If the woman experiencing miscarriage, stillbirth, or neonatal death does not work through her grief successfully, her ability to invest in another pregnancy and attach to a future infant are jeopardized.

Pregnancy losses within the first 20 weeks may produce a variety of feelings, ranging from relief to intense sadness and grief.

Death of the fetus at the second stage of the pregnancy or the death of a newborn infant can elicit a strong grief reaction.

Grief is also part of the emotional dynamics when adoption or elective abortion is decided, and this grief can be complicated by feelings of guilt.

Anticipatory grief is the preparation for a possible loss while still hoping for the infant's survival. Acute grief develops when a loss occurs. The family experiencing complicated grief is unable to progress through the grief process, and usually requires professional help.

Women tend to express grief through talking and crying. Men usually express their grief through physical activity or work. However, they may be angry, and need permission to grieve. Sibling children react according to their age, and move through the grief process more quickly than adults.

There are differences in response to loss among various cultures.

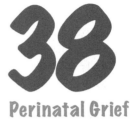

38

Perinatal Grief

While providing physical care when there are complications of pregnancy or birth, the nurse also offers psychological support for grieving by:

- expressing empathy

- acknowledging grief

- being flexible about family visitation policies

- giving permission to grieve

- giving explanations and providing guidance for expression of grief

- allowing family participation in decision making about care

- encouraging sharing of feelings

- providing momentos or keepsakes

- providing opportunities for the family to have contact with the infant

- ensuring continuity of care

- arranging referrals to support services.

To support the woman and her family during this time of grief, the nurse must be familiar with the grief process, typical responses, and cultural variation in grief expression.

TERMS
- ☐ **grief process**
- ☐ **anticipatory grief**
- ☐ **acute grief**
- ☐ **complicated grief**

Although pregnancy is usually a time of joy and happiness, there can be situations that result in loss and grief. About 30% of pregnancies end in miscarriage, stillbirth, or neonatal death. The **grief process** also can be seen with the loss of the "normal experience" or the loss of the "perfect child" that accompanies a high-risk pregnancy or the birth of an infant who has a congenital anomaly or who is ill or preterm.

If the woman does not work through her grief successfully, her ability to invest in another pregnancy and attach to a future infant will be jeopardized.

TYPES OF PERINATAL LOSS

The impact of the loss on the woman and her family depends on the significance placed on the pregnancy, how emotionally invested they were in the pregnancy, and how emotionally attached they were to the fetus or newborn. Pregnancy losses within the first 20 weeks may produce a variety of feelings ranging from relief to intense sadness and grief. Although acceptance of the fetus as a separate individual may not have occurred yet, attachment to the fetus often has begun.

> Pregnancy losses within the first 20 weeks may produce a variety of feelings ranging from relief to intense sadness and grief.

In the second half of the pregnancy, the woman and her family have seen changes in her body, have felt fetal movement, and the fetus is real to them; they have begun to anticipate and prepare for the newborn. Death of the fetus at this stage of the pregnancy or the death of a newborn infant can elicit a strong grief reaction.

Grief is also part of the emotional dynamics of choosing to give up the baby for adoption or terminate a pregnancy through elective abortion. Such grief experienced by the woman, her partner, and family may also be complicated by feelings of guilt.

> Grief is also part of the emotional dynamics of choosing to give up the baby for adoption or terminate a pregnancy through elective abortion. Such grief experienced by the woman, her partner, and family may also be complicated by feelings of guilt.

TYPES OF GRIEF

Grief tends to follow a series of typical phases. (See Table 38-1.) **Anticipatory grief** is preparation for a possible loss while still hoping for the infant's survival. The family may experience the early phases of grief and may begin to work through the grief before the loss occurs. In so doing, they may continue to have ambivalence about the pregnancy and may not be able to attach to the fetus or newborn. **Acute grief** develops when a loss occurs.

When **complicated grief** occurs, the family is unable to progress through the grief process and usually requires professional intervention. Some signs of complicated grief are persistent thoughts of self-destruction; excessive weight gain or loss; continued social isolation; use of alcohol, nicotine, or illegal drugs; and inability to maintain the activities of daily life.

Table 38-1   Phases of the Grief Process

Phase	Definition	Psychological Manifestations	Physical Manifestations
Shock and numbness	Initial reaction that allows the person to adjust and to manage the grief, usually peaks in about 2 weeks.	Feelings of disbelief, unreality, looking at oneself from outside.	Tight throat, heavy chest, sighing, "heavy heart," "empty arms," crying, trembling, loss of appetite, sleep disturbance.
Searching and yearning	Desire to talk about the events, need to find answers to what happened, reality of loss beginning to impact daily life.	Dreaming of the infant, nightmares. Feelings of anger, frustration, oversensitivity, conflict, guilt, and shame.	Crying, acting out in anger, sleeplessness, change in eating habits, enormous energy.
Disorganization	Confronting the reality of the loss. Depression is the most common reaction during this time. Most grief work happens in this phase; if unable to process the grief—would be unable to move from this phase.	Feelings of loneliness, isolation, powerlessness, or despair. Choosing to move forward, stay in grieving, or not survive. Family at risk for divorce, alcohol/drug abuse, or suicide.	Continued sleep disturbances, with fatigue, lack of energy, more susceptible to infection from weakened immune system, inability to concentrate, over- or undereating.
Reorganization	Healing of heart and mind begins with a decision to go on with life. May take up to one year to reach this phase.	Forgives oneself and others. Searches for meaning to the event. May reach out to help others. Has hope for the future. Has a sense of control.	Normal energy, sleep, and eating patterns and immune system restored.

Adapted from Gilbert, E.S., & Harmon, J.S. (2003). *Manual of high risk pregnancy and delivery.* (3rd ed.). St. Louis: Mosby.

FAMILY RESPONSES TO GRIEF

Since mothers and fathers may not be at the same level of attachment to the infant and usually express their grief in different ways, they may be at different phases of the grief process.

Because partner differences in experiencing grief can have a negative impact on their relationship, they are addressed by the nurse in anticipatory guidance.

During perinatal loss, women often experience a sense of failure. Women tend to express grief through talking and crying and are usually more receptive to attending a grief support group. Men usually express their grief through physical activity or immersing in work. However, they may demonstrate anger, and may need permission to grieve.

Siblings respond to the loss depending on their age. Children less than 3 cannot comprehend death; from 3 to 5 years of age, they may believe they caused the event; from 6 to 10 years, they attempt to find a reason for the death; and by 10 to 12 years, they have an adult concept of death.

Children less than 3 cannot comprehend death; from 3 to 5 years of age, they may believe they caused the event; from 6 to 10 years, they attempt to find a reason for the death; and by 10 to 12 years, they have an adult concept of death.

Very young children react more to the sadness of the parents and to the disruption in family environment. Older children, who have developed an attachment to the expected baby, experience their own grief as well as react to the change in family dynamics.

Children progress through the grief process more quickly than adults. Grandparents experience their own grief, for the loss of the expected grandchild, as well as responding to their child's grief.

CULTURAL VARIATIONS

Grief is a universal experience; however, there are differences in response to pregnancy loss among various cultures. The nurse assesses each family to determine their cultural preferences and to provide culturally sensitive care during perinatal loss.

The nurse assesses each family to determine their cultural preferences and to provide culturally sensitive care during perinatal loss.

- At what point in the pregnancy is the fetus thought to be a person?
- What is the significance of pregnancy and having children to the woman and to the man?
- How do members of the culture express grief? Is it different for men and women?
- What kinds of care would provide comfort? Foods? Touch? Visitors? Keepsakes or momentos?
- What death rituals are appropriate for a perinatal loss?

IMMEDIATE STRATEGIES FOR NURSING INTERVENTION

While providing physical care when there are complications of pregnancy or birth, the nurse includes psychological support for grieving in the following ways.

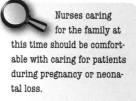

Nurses caring for the family at this time should be comfortable with caring for patients during pregnancy or neonatal loss.

Nurses caring for the family at this time should be comfortable with caring for patients during pregnancy or neonatal loss.

- Expressing empathy through presence, voice, and touch.
- Acknowledging their grief and avoiding insensitive comments.
- Keeping the family together by being flexible about visitation policies.
- Giving permission to grieve and allowing adequate time to grieve.
- Helping the family to understand by giving repeated, simple explanations and providing anticipatory guidance about expression of grief.
- Allowing participation in decision making about care.
- Encouraging sharing of feelings with family, friends, spiritual leaders, or other support people.
- Providing momentos or keepsakes such as ultrasound images, pictures, footprints, or locks of hair.
- Providing opportunities for the family to have contact with the infant.
- Ensuring continuity in care by assigning the same nurse whenever possible and communicating plans from shift to shift.
- Arranging referrals to support services such as grief support groups, pastoral counseling, or grief counseling.

PART VII · QUESTIONS

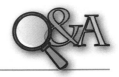

1. A client, who is G2 P1, goes to her physician's office for prenatal care. What history collected during the nursing assessment would indicate that she is at risk for preterm labor?
    a. Age 26 years at the time of conception.
    b. Blood type B, Rh negative.
    c. First pregnancy delivered at 33 weeks gestation.
    d. Married for 6 years.

2. For what obstetrical complication is there more risk for a pregnant woman with diabetes mellitus?
    a. Placenta previa.
    b. Postpartum depression.
    c. Postpartum hemorrhage.
    d. Gestational hypertension.

3. Which of Rubin's maternal tasks of pregnancy is most difficult to achieve when a high-risk condition threatens fetal well-being?

    _____

4. A pregnant woman has just received the diagnosis of a high-risk condition. When the nurse enters the room, the client begins to cry. What first response by the nurse would be most appropriate?
    a. "Did you understand what your doctor told you?"
    b. "I am sure that everything will work out."
    c. "Is there someone you would like me to call?"
    d. "Let me get you a tissue. It is all right to cry."

5. A postpartum client and her family have returned from the special care nursery. The nurse learns that their premature infant has just died. What statement by the nurse would be most therapeutic?
    a. "I am sorry for your loss, what can I do to help you?"
    b. "I know just how you feel. I have taken care of other women who have lost babies."
    c. "The baby would have been very ill and probably would not have developed normally."
    d. "You just have to focus on taking care of your other children."

6. A woman attends a perinatal loss support group for the first time.
   She reports that she had a stillbirth 6 months earlier, still dreams
   frequently of the infant, cries often, doesn't sleep well, and can't
   concentrate at work. She thinks that she is "going crazy." What
   would be the most appropriate action of the nurse leading the
   support group?
   a. Determine that she is experiencing complicated grief.
   b. Explain to the woman that her behaviors are part of the normal
      grief process and will resolve with support.
   c. Make a referral to a psychologist for in-depth grief counseling.
   d. Tell her that although these reactions are normal, she can
      expect to experience them for the rest of her life.

PART VII • ANSWERS AND RATIONALES

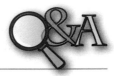

1. **The answer is c.** A history of previous preterm labor or birth increases the risk of experiencing the same complication. Option a is incorrect because maternal age below 16 or above 35 are risk factors for preterm labor. Option b is incorrect because blood type and Rh do not influence the incidence of preterm labor. Option d is incorrect because the socioeconomic factor of unwed status increases risk of preterm labor.

2. **The answer is d.** Having diabetes mellitus places a woman at greater risk for gestational hypertension. A history of diabetes mellitus does not increase the risk for the complications listed in options a, b, and c.

3. **The answer is *ensuring safe passage*.** Although all of Rubin's maternal tasks of pregnancy are affected by a high-risk situation, the task of ensuring safe passage is most difficult to achieve because the outcome is unpredictable and not within the woman's control.

4. **The answer is d.** It is important for the nurse to acknowledge the grief being experienced and to allow the woman to express her feelings. Option a is incorrect because the emotional responses must be addressed before any explanation or teaching is done. Option b gives false reassurance. Option c would be appropriate after initial emotional support by the nurse.

5. **The answer is a.** Option a acknowledges the family's loss, expresses empathy and concern, and therefore is therapeutic. In option b, the nurse does not know how this woman and her family feel; every grief experience is different. In option c, the comment makes a judgment and minimizes the loss. In option d, the comment does not give permission to grieve by denying the loss.

6. **The answer is b.** The behaviors that are described are symptoms of the normal phases of the grief process. The grief process usually takes up to 1 year to reach the reorganization phase. Options a and c are incorrect because she not experiencing complicated grief and does not need in-depth grief counseling at this time. Option d is incorrect because, with support, the manifestations described will *not* persist indefinitely.

VIII

Major Obstetrical Complications of Pregnancy

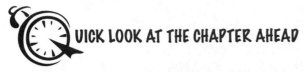

Although most pregnancies result in a healthy infant, approximately 20% of pregnancies end in the first 20 weeks. The usual cause of loss is spontaneous abortion or ectopic pregnancy.

Spontaneous abortion (miscarriage) is the ending of a pregnancy before week 20. In a threatened abortion, the viability of the pregnancy needs to be determined by examining elevations in serial hCG levels and visualizing a gestational sac or fetal heart beat with utltrasound.

In an imminent or incomplete abortion, a dilatation and currettage (D&C) or suction evacuation is suggested. If the abortion is complete, no surgical intervention is necessary.

A missed abortion will usually be expelled spontaneously. In septic abortion, antibiotic therapy is ordered in addition to other interventions. Genetic studies are recommended if recurrent abortions occur.

Ectopic pregnancy occurs when the fertilized ovum implants at a site other than the endometrial lining of the uterus. A woman of childbearing age who complains of abdominal pain needs to be evaluated by a health care provider. Hemorrhage from a ruptured ectopic pregnancy is the leading cause of maternal mortality in the first trimester.

Diagnosis of an ectopic pregnancy is based on a careful history, findings on examination, hCG and progesterone levels to verify the pregnancy, and transvaginal ultrasound. Once the ectopic pregnancy is confirmed, low doses of methotrexate may be used. If methotrexate is not an

39

Early Pregnancy Loss: Spontaneous Abortion and Ectopic Pregnancy

option, surgical intervention is performed. For the woman who is Rh negative and not sensitized, RhoGAM is given.

It is very important to provide adequate explanations of medical management recommendations for the woman and her family to make informed decisions, and offer emotional support as they address their fear, anxiety, and grieving.

After one miscarriage, the risk is no greater than the general population; however, after two or more successive miscarriages, the risk increases. The risk of recurrence of ectopic pregnancy is about 15%. After most early pregnancy losses, couples should wait at least 3 months to plan another pregnancy.

The nurse needs to be able to recognize women who are at risk for these losses, understand the possible causes, assess for signs and symptoms, know current medical management, and be able to provide nursing care to meet the physical and emotional needs of women and their families.

TERMS

- ☐ spontaneous abortion (miscarriage)
- ☐ threatened abortion
- ☐ imminent or incomplete abortion
- ☐ complete abortion
- ☐ missed abortion
- ☐ septic abortion
- ☐ recurrent abortion
- ☐ ectopic pregnancy

SPONTANEOUS ABORTION (MISCARRIAGE)

Definition and Etiology

Spontaneous abortion (miscarriage) is the ending of a pregnancy before week 20. (Pregnancy loss after 20 weeks is considered a stillbirth.) (See Table 39-1.)

Chromosomal abnormalities cause most spontaneous abortions in the first trimester. Other causes in the first trimester include maternal hormonal imbalances, chronic disease, infection, implantation abnormalities, and exposure to teratogenic chemicals in the environment.

Spontaneous abortion between 14 and 20 weeks of gestation is often associated with cervical insufficiency, infection, uterine defects such as bicornate uterus, or fibrous tumors of the uterus.

Signs and Symptoms

Cramping or backache from uterine contractions and vaginal bleeding are the most common signs of spontaneous abortion. The amount of bleeding may range from minimal spotting to heavy bleeding, and

Table 39-1 Types of Spontaneous Abortion (Miscarriage)

Type	Definition
Threatened	Bleeding or cramping present, but cervix is closed. May resolve or progress to miscarriage.
Imminent or inevitable	Bleeding or cramping present; cervix dilates; membranes may rupture.
Incomplete	Some fetal or placental tissue is retained within the uterus.
Complete	All fetal and placental tissue has been expelled.
Missed	Fetus dies but is not expelled.
Septic	A miscarriage with presence of infection.
Recurrent	Three or more consecutive miscarriages.

the color varies from bright red to brown. Symptoms are influenced by gestational age and may include rupture of membranes, with leakage of a small amount of fluid and passage of clots or tissue. Assessments during prenatal visits that indicate pregnancy loss include a uterus that has not continued to enlarge, a woman's report of a lessening of pregnancy symptoms, inability to hear fetal heart tones with a Doppler, and absence of fetal heart motion during ultrasound.

> Assessments during prenatal visits that indicate pregnancy loss include a uterus that has not continued to enlarge, a woman's report of a lessening of pregnancy symptoms, inability to hear fetal heart tones with a Doppler, and absence of fetal heart motion during ultrasound.

Medical Management

In a **threatened abortion**, the viability of the pregnancy needs to be determined by examining elevations in serial hCG levels and visualizing a gestational sac or fetal heart beat with utltrasound. If the embryo or fetus is alive, bedrest and avoidance of sexual stimulation and intercourse are often recommended. Research does not demonstrate that bedrest and avoidance of sex prevents miscarriage. Also, the administration of the hormone progesterone has not been shown to prevent miscarriage.

> Research does not demonstrate that bedrest and avoidance of sex prevents miscarriage. Also, the administration of the hormone progesterone has not been shown to prevent miscarriage.

In an **imminent** or **incomplete abortion**, a dilatation and currettage (D&C) or suction evacuation is suggested. If the abortion is **complete**, no surgical intervention is necessary.

A **missed abortion** will usually expel the dead fetus spontaneously.

> If the dead fetus is not expelled within 1 month, disseminated intravascular coagulation (DIC) may develop in the woman.

To prevent DIC, a surgical procedure to empty the uterus is suggested in the first trimester; induction of labor is performed in the second trimester.

In **septic abortion**, antibiotic therapy is ordered.

Genetic studies are recommended if **recurrent abortions** occur. For the woman who is Rh negative and not sensitized, RhoGAM is given within 72 hours of the miscarriage.

ECTOPIC PREGNANCY

Definition and Etiology

Ectopic pregnancy occurs when the fertilized ovum implants at a site other than the endometrial lining of the uterus. The most common place is the fallopian tube; other sites are ovary, cervix, or abdominal cavity. The incidence is about 2%.

Risk factors include previous tubal infections with pelvic inflammatory disease (PID), previous tubal or pelvic surgery, congenital abnormalities of the tube, hormonal imbalance, advanced maternal age, use of IUD, high estrogen levels from taking the morning-after pill, use of ovulation-stimulating-drugs, and heavy smoking.

A woman of childbearing age who complains of abdominal pain needs to be evaluated by a health care provider to determine if an ectopic pregnancy is present. Hemorrhage from a ruptured ectopic pregnancy is the leading cause of maternal mortality in the first trimester.

Signs and Symptoms

The typical symptoms of early pregnancy may be experienced by the woman before she begins to develop signs of a complication.

- Abdominal tenderness and pain in the affected area, vaginal bleeding or spotting, and a palpable pelvic mass may indicate an unruptured tubal pregnancy.
- When the tube ruptures, the pain becomes more generalized and may be referred to the right shoulder.
- Faintness, dizziness, and signs of shock occur if the bleeding is severe.

Medical Management

Diagnosis of an ectopic pregnancy is based on a careful history, findings on examination, hCG and progesterone levels to verify the pregnancy, and transvaginal ultrasound. Once an ectopic pregnancy is confirmed, low doses of methotrexate may be used in a stable

Diagnosis of an ectopic pregnancy is based on a careful history, findings on examination, hCG and progesterone levels to verify the pregnancy, and transvaginal ultrasound.

client to dissolve an ectopic mass less than 3 cm in diameter in an unruptured tube or other location. The woman is instructed on how to monitor herself for signs of rupture and hemorrhage. Follow-up with hCG titers show a progressive decrease in levels as the ectopic mass resolves. The average length of time for resolution is 7 weeks.

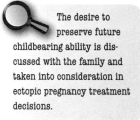

The desire to preserve future childbearing ability is discussed with the family and taken into consideration in ectopic pregnancy treatment decisions.

If methotrexate is not an option, surgical intervention to remove the ectopic mass is performed. The desire to preserve future childbearing ability is discussed with the family and taken into consideration in ectopic pregnancy treatment decisions. For the woman who is Rh negative and not sensitized, RhoGAM is given.

NURSING CARE FOR EARLY PREGNANCY LOSS

Physical and emotional components of nursing care are addressed with women and their families experiencing an early pregnancy loss. Assessment of the number of weeks gestation, the amount of pain and bleeding, status of the embryo or fetus, and the emotional response is done during the initial contact with the health care system. Primary concerns are for excessive bleeding or signs of shock or infection.

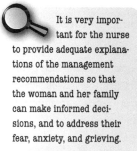

It is very important for the nurse to provide adequate explanations of the management recommendations so that the woman and her family can make informed decisions, and to address their fear, anxiety, and grieving.

Based upon assessment findings, decisions are made about medical management. If decisions are made for a surgical procedure, the nurse gives appropriate preoperative and postoperative care. It is very important for the nurse to provide adequate explanations of the management recommendations so that the woman and her family can make informed decisions, and to address their fear, anxiety, and grieving.

Appropriate teaching after early pregnancy loss is as follows:

- After a miscarriage, the woman is advised to limit activity for at least 24 hours and to avoid douching, tampons, or sexual intercourse until bleeding has stopped to prevent infection.
- A vaginal discharge is normal from 1 to 2 weeks and varies in color from red to brown.

- The woman is instructed to report any heavy bleeding or signs of infection such as fever, chills, foul-smelling vaginal discharge, or abdominal tenderness.

If methotrexate is ordered for ectopic pregnancy, teaching includes

- side effects of the medication
- signs and symptoms of possible rupture and hemorrhage
- avoidance of alcohol, folic acid, and sexual intercourse until ectopic pregnancy is resolved.

If surgery was done for ectopic pregnancy, discharge instructions are similar to any postoperative client.

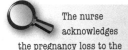

The nurse acknowledges the pregnancy loss to the client and her family, offers anticipatory guidance for the grieving process, and gives information about available resources to help them cope.

The nurse acknowledges the pregnancy loss to the client and her family, offers anticipatory guidance for the grieving process, and gives information about available resources to help them cope. See Chapter 38 on perinatal grief for details on psychological support.

Couples often express concern about the risk of loss for a future pregnancy. After one miscarriage, the risk is no greater than the general population; however, after two or more successive miscarriages, the risk increases. The risk of recurrence of ectopic pregnancy is about 15%.

The couple may ask when they can plan another pregnancy. They should be instructed to wait until physical recovery is complete. Depending upon the procedures used, this time will vary. After most early pregnancy losses, couples should wait at least 3 months. With ectopic pregnancy or recurrent miscarriage, concerns about future fertility are also discussed.

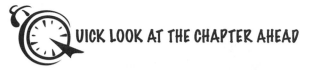

Preterm labor (PTL) is defined as uterine contractions producing cervical change occurring between 20 and 37 completed weeks of pregnancy.

Risk assessment for PTL is done by taking a careful history for risk factors. However, 50% of women who experience preterm labor have no identifiable risk factors. Early detection of preterm labor continues to be the best strategy to improve outcomes.

A biochemical marker used to predict women at high risk for preterm labor is fetal fibronectin.

Women with a shortened cervical length or some funneling may have a condition called cervical insufficiency and have a greater risk of preterm birth.

One attempt to prevent preterm birth is the use of progesterone, either by injection or vaginal suppository.

The medical diagnosis of preterm labor is made when there are four or more contractions in a 20-minute period, with cervical dilation of more than 1 cm or cervical effacement of 80% or more.

Tocolytic drugs are used to stop contractions by relaxing smooth muscles of the uterus. Tocolytics delay birth for the 24 to 48 hours needed to use corticosteroids to promote lung maturation in the fetus and prevent neonatal respiratory distress syndrome. Pregnant women with urinary or genital tract infections should be treated with antibiotics.

When possible, birth of a preterm infant should take place in a hospital with a newborn intensive care unit. Membranes should be left intact when possible.

40

Preterm Labor: Overview

TERMS
- [ ] **preterm labor (PTL)**
- [ ] **fetal fibronectin**
- [ ] **transvaginal ultrasound**
- [ ] **cervical insufficiency**
- [ ] **progesterone**
- [ ] **tocolytic drugs**
- [ ] **corticosteroids**

The preterm birth rate is 12% in the United States. The neonatal intensive care nursery is one of the most expensive services in the health care system. Although technological and pharmacological advances have been made in treatment, the rate of preterm labor continues to increase. Prevention of preterm labor and birth has become a national health care priority, and is the most important component in the management of pregnancies with more than one fetus.

DEFINITION AND ETIOLOGY

Preterm labor (PTL) is defined as uterine contractions producing cervical change occurring between 20 and 37 completed weeks of pregnancy. Several risk factors are related to the incidence of PTL. (See Table 40-1.) A history of prior preterm birth can triple the risk of preterm labor. The rate of preterm birth is 40% in a twin pregnancy and 80% in triplets or higher order multiples. African-Americans, Native Americans, and Hispanics have a higher rate of PTL than Caucasians. The rate of PTL is higher among lower socioeconomic groups.

SIGNS AND SYMPTOMS

Sometimes it is difficult for the pregnant woman to recognize signs and symptoms of preterm labor because they are similar to the usual sensations of pregnancy. Regular uterine contractions detected by palpation or with uterine monitoring are the most significant symptom, and may occur with or without pain.

Other signs and symptoms of preterm labor include menstrual-like cramps, back or abdominal discomfort, pelvic pressure, and increased vaginal discharge. Urinary frequency or diarrhea may also occur with preterm labor.

RISK ASSESSMENT AND PREVENTION

Although risk assessment for PTL is done by taking a careful history for risk factors, current risk assessment tools are not adequate in identifying, predicting, or preventing preterm births: Fifty percent of women who experience preterm labor have no identifiable risk factors.

Table 40-1   Risk Factors for Preterm Labor

Obstetric History	Current Obstetrical Status
Prior preterm labor and birth	Multiple gestation
Prior induced abortions	Premature rupture of the membranes
Cervical biopsy or surgery	Cervical effacement or dilation < 32 weeks
Cervical insufficiency or incompetent cervix	First trimester bleeding
Diethylstilbestrol (DES) exposure	Placenta previa or abruption
Infertility	Vaginal or cervical infections
Pregnancy spacing of less than 1 year	Chorioamnionitis
	Hydramnios
	Fetal malformations
	In-vitro fertilization
	Abdominal surgery or trauma
	Poor weight gain

Medical History	Social-Personal Characteristics
Urinary tract infection	Late or no prenatal care
Diabetes	Nonwhite ethnicity
Hypertension	Low socioeconomic status
Heart disease	Age < 18 or > 35 years
Anemia	Unmarried
Febrile illness	Low pre-pregnancy weight
	Smoking > 10 cigarettes/day
	Use of alcohol or illicit drugs
	High physical or emotional stress
	Domestic violence
	Physically demanding lifestyle

Early detection of preterm labor continues to be the best strategy to improve outcomes. Biochemical markers and transvaginal ultrasound may be performed if there is a history of prior preterm birth, or if current symptoms of preterm labor are present.

One biochemical marker used to predict women at high risk for preterm labor is **fetal fibronectin**. This is a protein normally found in cervicovaginal fluid in the first half of pregnancy. It should be no longer detectable after 22 weeks of pregnancy and is present again within 2 weeks prior to the onset of labor.

The test may be done for a woman who is between these points, and who has significant risk factors or signs and symptoms of preterm labor.

A swab of vaginal and cervical secretions is analyzed every 2 weeks. A positive finding suggests that cervical changes indicating onset of labor are likely to occur within the next 1 to 2 weeks; a negative finding predicts that preterm birth in the next 1 to 2 weeks is not likely.

Transvaginal ultrasound of the cervix is performed to determine cervical length and the presence of funneling or dilation of the internal cervical os. Cervical length varies, with a median length of 35 mm. Women with a shortened cervical length or some funneling may have a condition called **cervical insufficiency** and have a greater risk of preterm birth. Specific criteria for length of the cervix and the amount of funneling that are predictive of preterm delivery have not yet been determined by research.

> ✓ A positive finding suggests that cervical changes indicating onset of labor are likely to occur within the next 1 to 2 weeks; a negative finding predicts that preterm birth in the next 1 to 2 weeks is not likely.

> ✓ Women with a shortened cervical length or some funneling may have a condition called **cervical insufficiency** and have a greater risk of preterm birth. Specific criteria for length of the cervix and the amount of funneling that are predictive of preterm delivery have not yet been determined by research.

PREVENTION

A strategy to prevent preterm birth is the use of **progesterone,** either by injection or vaginal suppository. The American College of Obstetricians and Gynecologists now recommends that pregnant women with a documented history of prior spontaneous preterm birth be given this hormone.

MEDICAL MANAGEMENT

The medical diagnosis of preterm labor is made when there are four or more contractions in a 20-minute period, with cervical dilation of more than 1 cm or cervical effacement of 80% or more. Among the usual treatment options for preterm labor are bedrest and hydration, but research has not demonstrated benefits from either of these interventions.

> ✓ Among the usual treatment options for preterm labor are bedrest and hydration, but research has not demonstrated benefits from either of these interventions.

Tocolytic drugs are used to stop contractions by relaxing smooth muscles of the uterus. These drugs are used if membranes are intact, cervical dilation is less than 4 cm, and there is no evidence of complications such as hemorrhage, intrauterine infection, fetal distress, severe fetal abnormalities, severe intrauterine growth restriction, or severe maternal medical or obstetrical problems. Commonly used tocolytics are magnesium sulfate, terbutaline, ritodrine, nifedipine, and indomethacin, but there are side effects with each of these drugs.

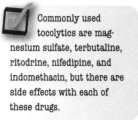

Commonly used tocolytics are magnesium sulfate, terbutaline, ritodrine, nifedipine, and indomethacin, but there are side effects with each of these drugs.

Studies have shown that tocolytics may stop contractions temporarily, but do not prevent preterm birth or improve perinatal outcomes. However, tocolytics do delay birth for at least the 24 to 48 hours needed for corticosteroids to be administered for the promotion of lung maturation in the fetus. **Corticosteroids**, such as betamethasone and dexamethasone, given to the mother between 24 and 34 weeks of gestation have been shown to be successful in preventing neonatal respiratory distress syndrome.

Because urinary or genital tract infections have been associated with the increased likelihood of preterm birth, pregnant women with these infections should be treated with antibiotics.

When possible, birth of a preterm infant should take place in a hospital with a newborn intensive care unit. Because many preterm fetuses are in breech position, cesarean delivery is often indicated. Preterm infants in vertex presentation may be delivered vaginally. Because preterm infants are more vulnerable to head trauma during labor and birth than term infants, membranes should be left intact when possible.

When possible, birth of a preterm infant should take place in a hospital with a newborn intensive care unit. Because many preterm fetuses are in breech position, cesarean delivery is often indicated. Preterm infants in vertex presentation may be delivered vaginally. Because preterm infants are more vulnerable to head trauma during labor and birth than term infants, membranes should be left intact when possible.

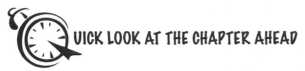

Strategies for preventing preterm birth include education for signs and symptoms of preterm labor; awareness of increased risk for PTL with multifetal pregnancy; not smoking, drinking alcohol, or using drugs; the dangers of domestic violence; and encouraging adequate prenatal care of fetus and self.

Patients are admitted to the hospital for diagnosis of PTL, initiation of tocolytic agents, and evaluation of mother and fetus. If PTL is successfully stopped, the woman may be discharged with oral tocolytic therapy at home.

Corticosteroids stimulate the production of surfactant in the fetal lungs. Contraindications to this therapy are inability to delay birth, L/S ratio at least 2:1, or need to deliver the fetus.

Uterine contractions and fetal heart rate are assessed continuously until contractions have stopped. Women are observed for fever, uterine tenderness, changes in vaginal discharge, and increase in white blood cell count. The emotional state of the woman and her family as well as their understanding of the therapy are evaluated. Nonstress tests and biophysical profiles are done periodically to determine fetal well-being and decision making about continuance of tocolytic therapy.

Though unproven and with many negative side effects, bedrest is a common recommendation. PTL nursing care addresses the side effects.

Recovery after birth may be different because the mother will be recuperating from the labor and birth as well as the effects of extended bedrest.

Home management tasks, child care issues, and finances are affected when the woman cannot maintain her usual role. Emotional support from family and friends is vital. Health care providers need to assess the level of support available to the family and make appropriate referrals.

41

Preterm Labor: Nursing Care

TERMS
- [ ] **magnesium sulfate**
- [ ] **beta-mimetics**
- [ ] **Betamethasone**
- [ ] **Dexamethasone**
- [ ] **side effects of bedrest**

PREVENTION

Many strategies for preventing preterm birth often fall within the scope of nursing practice:

- Educating all pregnant women about the signs and symptoms of preterm labor, including how to detect uterine contractions and what to do if signs of premature labor occur. (See Table 41-1.)
- Educating women with multifetal pregnancy about increased risk for PTL.
- Identifying women who smoke, drink alcohol, or use drugs, and providing interventions for cessation.
- Assessing pregnant women for domestic violence and providing appropriate referrals.
- Encouraging adequate prenatal care, appropriate weight gain, well-balanced diet, stress management, and adequate rest.

 TOCOLYSIS

Patients are admitted into the hospital for diagnosis of PTL, initiation of tocolytic agents, and evaluation of mother and fetus. See Table 41-2 for the nursing implications of the administration of tocolytic drugs. Intravenous

Table 41-1 Teaching for Detection of PTL

Topic	Content
Warning signs of PTL	Contractions every 10 minutes or more often may be painless. Menstrual-like cramps, back or abdominal discomfort, pelvic pressure, and increased vaginal discharge. Leakage of fluid from the vagina.
How to detect uterine contractions	Place both hands on the sides of the abdomen over the uterus to feel if the uterus tightens. If you suspect you are having contractions, feel your abdomen for at least 15 minutes. If you are being treated for PTL, you may be instructed to monitor yourself 2 to 3 times a day for 30–60 minutes at a time.
What to do if symptoms occur	Call your health care provider. You may be asked to empty the bladder, lie down on the left side for 1 hour, drink 3 glasses of water or juice, and report symptoms in 1 hour.

magnesium sulfate is often the tocolytic of choice because it has fewer side effects than the **beta-mimetics**.

If beta-mimetics are used, intravenous fluids are administered cautiously, and the woman is assessed for signs of pulmonary edema such as tachypnea, dypnea, cyanosis, or crackles heard when assessing breath sounds.

If PTL is successfully stopped, in some circumstances the woman may be discharged with oral tocolytic therapy at home. The woman is taught how to count her pulse prior to taking medication.

CORTICOSTEROID THERAPY

Corticosteroids, such as **Betamethasone** or **Dexamethasone**, stimulate the production of surfactant in the fetal lungs. Intramuscular injections in the gluteal muscle are given to the mother for 2 days; for best results birth should be delayed for at least 24 hours after completing the 2 days of therapy. A current review of medical literature does not support repeating this course of therapy weekly. Containdications to this therapy include inability to delay birth, L/S ratio at least 2:1, or a medical or obstetrical condition that makes it necessary to deliver the fetus.

 If the woman is also receiving beta-mimetics, she is assessed carefully for pulmonary edema and hyperglycemia.

MATERNAL AND FETAL ASSESSMENT

- Uterine contractions and fetal heart rate are assessed continuously until contractions have stopped.
- Medication administration protocols established by hospitals determine the frequency of taking vital signs, uterine and fetal monitoring, and other assessments.
- Because premature labor can be associated with infection, women are observed for fever, uterine tenderness, changes in vaginal discharge, and increase in white blood cell count.
- Evaluation of the emotional state of the woman and her family as well as their understanding of the therapy is ongoing.
- Nonstress tests and biophysical profiles are done periodically to

Table 41-2 Tocolytic Therapy

Drug and Action	Maternal Side Effects	Nursing Implications
Beta-mimetics: Terbutaline and Ritodrine Stimulates beta receptors, causing relaxation of smooth muscle in the uterus, bronchial tract, and blood vessels, and stimulation of the cardiac muscle.	Hypotension Widening of pulse pressure Light-headedness Tremors Anxiety Restlessness Tachycardia Heart palpitations Hyperglycemia Decreased serum potassium	Explain possible side effects and reassure patient that they will resolve when medication is stopped. Assess maternal blood pressure and pulse and fetal heart rate before giving. Do not administer with fetal heart rate above 180 beats per minute, maternal heart rate greater than 120 beats per minute, blood pressure below 90/60, cardiac dysrhythmias, or reports of chest pain. Assess breath sounds for signs of pulmonary edema. Assess blood sugar and potassium as ordered. Monitor intake and output.
Magnesium Sulfate Central nervous system depressant. Relaxes smooth muscle by preventing the release of acetylcholine, thereby blocking nerve transmission to the muscle.	With initial therapy, patient may have hot flashes, nausea, vomiting, drowsiness, headaches, blurred vision, and muscle weakness. These usually subside when dose is lowered. Signs of magnesium toxicity include respiration rate < 12 per minute, absence of deep tendon reflexes, severe hypotension, and extreme muscle relaxation.	Explain possible side effects and reassure patient that they will resolve when the dose is lowered. Assess vital signs, especially blood pressure and respiration rate. Assess that urinary output is at least 30 cc per hour to ensure that magnesium is being excreted. Assess deep tendon reflexes at least every 4 hours. Monitor magnesium lab values. Assess fetal heart rate.
Calcium channel blocker: Nifedipine Reduces smooth muscle contractility by blocking calcium movement into the intracellular space.	Common side effects are related to arterial vasodilation: hypotension, tachycardia, headache, facial flushing, dizziness, fatigue, and peripheral edema.	Explain possible side effects and reassure patient that they will resolve when medication is stopped. Assess blood pressure and pulse before giving. Do not administer if heart rate is greater than 120 beats per minute and blood pressure is below 90/60. Assess for peripheral edema. Assess fetal heart rate.
Prostaglandin inhibitor: Indomethacin Inhibits prostaglandin synthesis, thereby decreaseing uterine contractility.	Common side effects include nausea, heartburn, vomiting, depression, and dizzy spells.	Use is limited to 24–48 hours because of the association with diminished production of amniotic fluid and premature closure of the fetal ductus arteriosus. Administer with meals to decrease GI side effects.

determine fetal well-being. Results of these tests contribute to decision making about continuance of tocolytic therapy.

BEDREST

Although research has not demonstrated benefits of bedrest in the treatment of preterm labor, it continues to be a common recommendation.

Some of the side effects of prolonged bedrest are increased risk of deep vein thrombosis, muscle weakness and atrophy, bone loss, diuresis from a shift in body fluids, orthostatic hypotension, decreased peristalsis leading to constipation, changes in circadian rhythms resulting in abnormal sleep patterns, increased stress, and a sense of isolation contributing to depression and boredom.

Nursing care given to women with preterm labor addresses the **side effects of bedrest**.

- For skeletal muscle effects, the health care provider may order limited ambulation when possible, isometric exercises, and massage.
- The nurse encourages proper body alignment in bed using pillows or supports.
- Because of possible orthostatic hypotension, the nurse should be aware of safety when the woman is allowed to ambulate.
- To decrease the likelihood of constipation, dietary fiber and adequate fluids are encouraged and stool softeners may be ordered.
- Sleep-pattern disturbances and feelings of isolation or depression can be lessened by maintaining a routine; keeping occupied with diversional activities such as reading, keeping a journal, or crafts; home management activities; and using support groups in the hospital or online.

The nurse encourages behaviors to help the woman develop a sense of control and keep focused on the goal of maintaining bedrest to prevent preterm delivery. Recovery after birth may be different because she will be recuperating from the labor and birth as well as the effects of extended bedrest.

Because of muscle weakness or a feeling of dizziness, the woman is cautioned about risk for falling when caring for herself and the baby. The woman may also feel fatigue and be unable to resume activities of daily living as soon as other women.

Bedrest has many effects on family functioning. Anxiety about maternal/fetal outcomes and difficulty assuming responsibilities usually undertaken by the woman strain human and financial resources. Home management tasks, child-care issues, and finances are affected when the woman cannot maintain her usual role. Emotional support from family and friends is vital in helping the family cope. Health care providers need to assess the level of support available to the family and make appropriate referrals.

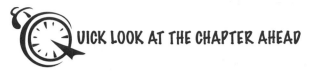

The two most common reasons for maternal hemorrhage are placenta previa and placental abruption. Placenta previa occurs when the placenta attaches to the lower portion of the uterus at or near the cervix. Medical management includes hospitalization, bedrest, close observation for bleeding and labor, and determining the status and gestational age of the fetus. The goal is to delay birth until the fetus is mature.

A cesarean birth is scheduled if the placenta previa is complete or partial; a vaginal birth is possible with a marginal placenta previa. Heavy bleeding or fetal distress, however, requires an emergency cesarean birth.

Nursing care of placenta previa involves monitoring of mother and fetus to minimize complications. There should be no vaginal exams. Clear explanations with emotional support are necessary.

Placental abruption is the premature separation of a normally implanted placenta. Classification of placental abruption is determined by the amount of bleeding: mild, moderate, or severe. Medical management depends on severity of bleeding and the status and maturity of the fetus. Replacement of blood volume is of utmost importance.

Nursing care of women with placental abruption includes frequent monitoring of mother and fetus to detect complications from hemorrhage.

The symptoms displayed by the patient may not correlate with the amount of visible bleeding if there is a central, concealed abruption.

42

Placenta Previa and Placental Abruption

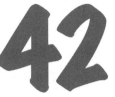

TERMS
- [ ] placenta previa
- [ ] placental abruption
- [ ] marginal separation
- [ ] mild abruption
- [ ] moderate abruption
- [ ] severe abruption
- [ ] disseminated intravascular coagulation (DIC)

The blood loss following placental abruption can trigger the development of disseminated intravascular coagulation (DIC). To detect development, repeated DIC panels are ordered. If DIC develops, clotting factors and blood volume are replaced.

Often a placental abruption occurs suddenly, and the lives of the mother and fetus are threatened. In a severe placental abruption, fetal death is common. Explanations and emotional support need to be provided throughout.

 The perinatal nurse needs an understanding of the differences in detection and management of these complications. (See Table 42-1.)

Table 42-1 Comparison of Placenta Previa and Placental Abruption

Characteristic	Placenta Previa	Placental Abruption
Type of bleeding	Always visible, initially slight, then more profuse in recurrent episodes	Sudden, may be concealed or visible
Pain	Painless	Constant pain, uterine tenderness on palpation
Uterus	Usually not in labor	Continuous tetanic contractions with minimal or no relaxation between contractions, rigid and board-like abdomen
Fetal distress	When there is heavy blood loss	Usually present
Fetal presentation and station	May be breech or transverse lie, engagement is absent	No relationship with the fetal presentation or station
Related factors	Greater than 4 previous pregnancies, closely spaced pregnancies, previous abortion, previous cesarean delivery, multiple gestations, advanced maternal age, anemia, abnormal fetal presentation, congenital malformations, tumors of the uterus, endometritis, male fetus, cigarette smoking	Maternal hypertension and vascular disease, previous abruption, high parity, poor nutrition, especially folic acid deficiency, cigarette smoking, cocaine use, trauma, sudden loss of a large amount of amniotic fluid

PLACENTA PREVIA

Placenta previa occurs when the placenta attaches to the lower portion of the uterus at or near the cervix. Placenta previa is categorized by how much of the internal os of the cervix is covered by placental tissue: marginal when the placenta extends to the edge of internal os, partial or incomplete when the cervix is partially covered, and total or complete when the cervix is completely covered by the placenta. Bleeding occurs in the third trimester when the cervix begins to efface and dilate. The medial diagnosis is usually made by ultrasound to determine placental location.

Medical management of placenta previa includes hospitalization, bedrest, close observation for bleeding and labor, and determining the status and gestational age of the fetus. Medical management is determined by severity of bleeding and maturity of the fetus. The goal is to delay birth until the fetus is mature. A cesarean delivery is scheduled if the placenta previa is complete or partial; a vaginal birth is possible with a marginal placenta previa. Heavy bleeding or fetal distress, however, requires an emergency cesarean delivery.

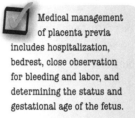

Medical management of placenta previa includes hospitalization, bedrest, close observation for bleeding and labor, and determining the status and gestational age of the fetus.

Nursing care of placenta previa involves monitoring of mother and fetus to minimize complications. The nurse assesses bleeding by recording amount of blood and number of perineal pads used per day. Hemoglobin and hematocrit values are reviewed for presence of anemia. Frequency for taking vital signs depends on the amount of bleeding.

There should be **no vaginal exams** of a patient with placenta previa.

Monitoring for contractions and fetal heart patterns is done frequently. Bleeding episodes can produce fear and anxiety in the woman and her family. Clear explanations with emotional support are necessary. Also, supportive techniques for enduring extended bedrest are the same as with preterm labor. See Chapter 41 for details of bedrest support.

PLACENTAL ABRUPTION

Placental abruption is the premature separation of a normally implanted placenta. A separation at the edge of the placenta is called a **marginal separation**, and vaginal bleeding is evident. If the separation is in the central portion of the placenta, the blood is trapped and concealed behind the edges of the placenta.

If blood is forced into the uterine musculature during abruption, the muscle is damaged and cannot contract properly. This contributes to a greater risk for postpartum uterine atony, leading to postpartum hemorrhage.

Classification of placental abruption is determined by the amount of bleeding: mild, moderate, or severe. In a **mild abruption**, the woman has a small amount of bleeding with minor uterine tenderness and no signs of maternal or fetal distress.

In a **moderate abruption**, the woman experiences uterine tenderness and prolonged contractions with or without vaginal bleeding. There may be some changes in maternal vital signs and there is usually evidence of fetal distress.

In **severe abruption**, moderate to heavy bleeding occurs and uterine contractions are continuous and very painful. Maternal vital signs are unstable and there is severe fetal distress. Increasing pain and increasing uterine tone indicate increased severity of the placental abruption.

The medical diagnosis of placental abruption is made on the basis of presenting signs and symptoms. An ultrasound may be done to determine placental location and to detect the presence of a clot behind the placenta. The diagnosis is confirmed after birth when the placenta is examined.

Medical management is dependent on the severity of the bleeding and the status and maturity of the fetus. If the bleeding is mild, there is no fetal distress, and the fetus is less than 36 weeks of gestation, the pregnancy is maintained and the woman is monitored closely for complications. If the bleeding is heavy or there are signs of fetal distress, a cesarean delivery is performed regardless of gestational age. Replacement of blood volume is of utmost importance in the management of women experiencing placental abruption.

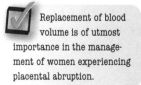

Replacement of blood volume is of utmost importance in the management of women experiencing placental abruption.

Nursing care of women with placental abruption includes frequent monitoring of mother and fetus to detect complications from hemorrhage such as shock, renal failure, fetal distress, and disseminated intravascular coagulation (DIC). The amount of blood loss is evaluated by changes in maternal vital signs, fetal heart pattern, and hemoglobin and hematocrit values. Perineal pad count and evaluation of increased uterine tenderness, firmness, and size are additional assessments.

Nursing care of women with placental abruption includes frequent monitoring of mother and fetus to detect complications from hemorrhage such as shock, renal failure, fetal distress, and disseminated intravascular coagulation (DIC). The amount of blood loss is evaluated by changes in maternal vital signs, fetal heart pattern, and hemoglobin and hematocrit values. Perineal pad count and evaluation of increased uterine tenderness, firmness, and size are additional assessments.

The signs of hypovolemic shock are increased pulse, decreased blood pressure, cold and clammy skin, anxiety, and a drop in hemoglobin and hematocrit levels.

The symptoms displayed by the patient may not correlate with the amount of visible bleeding if there is a central, concealed abruption.

If perfusion to the kidneys is inadequate, renal failure may result and urine output decreases to less than 30 cc/hour.

The severity of fetal distress depends on the amount of placental separation and is demonstrated by late decelerations from uteroplacental insufficiency.

The blood loss following placental abruption can trigger the development of **disseminated intravascular coagulation (DIC).** Because of the changes in the blood-clotting mechanism with DIC, the woman may have bruising, petechiae, bleeding gums, bleeding from IV sites, and heavy vaginal bleeding. DIC can develop before, during, or after birth.

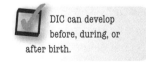

DIC can develop before, during, or after birth.

To detect the development of DIC, repeated DIC panels are ordered. This blood work consists of a complete blood count with platelets and fibrinogen, prothrombin time, partial thromboplastin time, and fibrinogen degradation products.

If DIC develops, replacement of clotting factors and blood volume is part of the usual treatment.

Often a placental abruption occurs suddenly and the lives of the mother and fetus are threatened. In a severe placental abruption, fetal death is common. Because of the emergency situation, the woman and her family can be very anxious and fearful. Explanations are given as quickly and simply as possible; further details would be offered after the birth. Emotional support needs to be provided throughout this time.

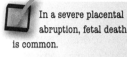

Often a placental abruption occurs suddenly and the lives of the mother and fetus are threatened.

In a severe placental abruption, fetal death is common.

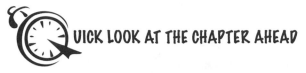
Hypertension is the most common medical complication of pregnancy and the second leading cause of maternal death.

Hypertensive disorders of pregnancy are classified as chronic hypertension or gestational (pregnancy-induced) hypertension. Women with chronic hypertension can develop preeclampsia/eclampsia, placental abruption, preterm labor, intrauterine growth restriction, or fetal death. Care includes more frequent prenatal visits with close monitoring.

Gestational hypertension is the development of hypertension after week 20 of pregnancy. Preeclampsia is hypertension with proteinuria and/or pathologic edema occurring after week 20 of pregnancy. Eclampsia is the occurrence of seizures in a preeclamptic woman.

The development of preeclampsia/eclampsia in a woman with chronic hypertension is defined as chronic hypertension with superimposed preeclampsia.

Mild or severe preeclampsia is diagnosed when specific clinical signs are present.

Pathologic edema is edema of the face and hands, or in feet and ankles nonresponsive to 12 hours of bedrest, and suggests the development of mild preeclampsia.

At this time, there is no reliable method of predicting preeclampsia. Therefore, early identification of the condition is vitally important.

43

Hypertensive Disorders of Pregnancy: Overview

Currently there is no proven intervention to prevent a woman from developing these disorders.

A diagnosis of preeclampsia increases the likelihood of placental abruption, preterm birth, uteroplacental insufficiency, uterine growth restriction, and fetal distress.

A major complication of preeclampsia is progression to eclampsia with seizures. The focus of treatment is controlling the blood pressure and detecting signs that indicate the possibility of seizures.

The key components of the complication HELLP syndrome are hemolysis, elevated liver enzymes, and low platelet count.

Signs of HELLP syndrome include epigastric pain or right upper quadrant tenderness, nausea or vomiting, headache, flu-like symptoms, jaundice, and hematuria.

 At every prenatal visit, the pregnant woman is evaluated for the classic signs of hypertensive disorders: elevated blood pressure, protein in the urine, and pathologic edema.

 Hypertensive disorders of pregnancy occur in 7 to 10% of all pregnancies and can result in life-threatening complications for mother and infant. (See Figure 43-1.)

TERMS

- ☐ chronic hypertension
- ☐ gestational hypertension
- ☐ pregnancy-induced hypertension (PIH)
- ☐ preeclampsia
- ☐ eclampsia
- ☐ chronic hypertension with superimposed preeclampsia
- ☐ mild preeclampsia
- ☐ severe preeclampsia
- ☐ HELLP syndrome

Figure 43-1 Pathophysiology of hypertensive disorders of pregnancy.

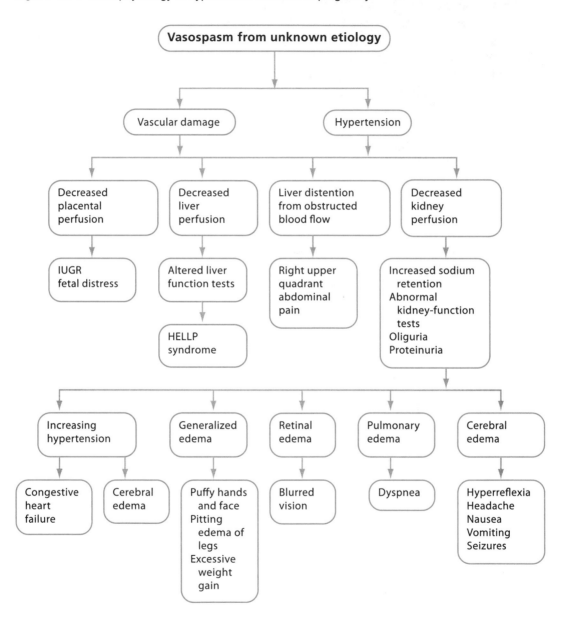

Source: Adapted from Olds, S.B., London, M.R., Ladewig, P.W., and Davidson, M.R. (2004). *Maternal Newborn Nursing & Women's Health Care* (7th Ed.). Upper Saddle River, NJ: Pearson Prentice Hall.

DEFINITIONS AND CLASSIFICATIONS

Hypertension occurring prior to pregnancy or before week 20 of pregnancy is defined as **chronic hypertension.** Women with chronic hypertension are at increased risk for developing further hypertensive complications such as preeclampsia/eclampsia, placental abruption, preterm labor, intrauterine growth restriction, or fetal death. Nursing care for chronic hypertension includes more frequent prenatal visits, with close monitoring for complications.

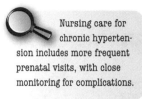

Nursing care for chronic hypertension includes more frequent prenatal visits, with close monitoring for complications.

   Gestational hypertension is triggered by pregnancy and appears after week 20. It replaces the term **pregnancy-induced hypertension (PIH)**. **Preeclampsia** is the development of hypertension with proteinuria and/or pathologic edema after week 20 of pregnancy. **Eclampsia** is the occurrence of seizures in a preeclamptic woman. The development of preeclampsia/eclampsia in a woman with chronic hypertension is defined as **chronic hypertension with superimposed preeclampsia**. The terms gestational hypertension, PIH, and preeclampsia are often used interchangeably.

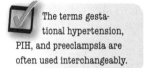

The terms gestational hypertension, PIH, and preeclampsia are often used interchangeably.

   The symptoms of gestational hypertension may be evident for the first time during labor or in the early postpartum period.

   Mild preeclampsia is diagnosed when there is an increase in blood pressure equal to or above 140/90 mm Hg on two occasions 6 hours apart, and proteinuria on dipstick between +2 and +3 on a midstream clean-catch or catheterized urine specimen. In a 24-hour urine collection, protein of 200 mg or more per liter indicates mild preeclampsia. Pathologic edema of the face and hands or in feet and ankles nonresponsive to 12 hours of bedrest suggests the development of mild preeclampsia.

   Severe preeclampsia is diagnosed when blood pressure is equal to or above 160/110 mm Hg or there is a 30 mm Hg rise in systolic or a 15 mm Hg rise in diastolic pressures on two occasions 6 hours apart when the woman is at bedrest on her left side. In addition, any of the following clinical signs may be present: proteinuria on dipstick between +3 and +4 or 5 grams or more in a 24-hour urine specimen, urinary output of less than 500 ml in 24 hours, cerebral or visual disturbances, epigastric pain, pulmonary edema, impaired liver functioning, thrombocytopenia, oligo-hydramnios, or fetal growth restriction.

RISK FACTORS AND PREVENTION

Current research on the presence of two molecules in the blood prior to the development of preeclampsia raises the possibility of predicting preeclampsia during pregnancy. At this time, there is no reliable method of predicting preeclampsia. Therefore, early identification of the condition is vitally important. Women who are considered to be at risk are carefully monitored.

> Current research on the presence of two molecules in the blood prior to the development of preeclampsia raises the possibility of predicting preeclampsia during pregnancy.

Risk factors for preeclampsia include first pregnancy, age younger than 19 or older than 40 years, multiple gestation, African-American or Hispanic ethnicity, personal or family history of PIH, and obesity. Preexisting diseases such as chronic hypertension, diabetes mellitus, or renal disease are additional risk factors.

Currently there is no proven intervention to prevent a woman from developing these disorders. Research does not support sodium restriction or the administration of diuretics, calcium supplements, low dose aspirin, or prophylactic antihypertensives.

COMPLICATIONS

A diagnosis of preeclampsia increases the likelihood of placental abruption, preterm birth, uteroplacental insufficiency, uterine growth restriction, and fetal distress. A major complication of preeclampsia is progression to eclampsia with seizures. The focus of treatment is controlling blood pressure, and detecting signs that indicate the possibility

> A diagnosis of preeclampsia increases the likelihood of placental abruption, preterm birth, uteroplacental insufficiency, uterine growth restriction, and fetal distress.

of seizures: severe frontal headache, epigastric pain, hyperreflexia with clonus, and visual disturbances.

The key components of the **HELLP syndrome** are **h**emolysis, **e**levated **l**iver enzymes, and **l**ow **p**latelet count. In the HELLP syndrome, red blood cells are damaged as they pass through constricted blood vessels, causing hemolysis. Obstructed blood flow causes damage to the liver, resulting in elevated liver enzymes. As vascular damage occurs with vasospasm, platelets aggregate at the damaged areas, leading to the low platelet count. Signs of HELLP syndrome include epigastric pain or right upper quadrant tenderness, nausea or vomiting, headache, flu-like symptoms, jaundice, and hematuria.

Laboratory values consistent with HELLP syndrome show a decrease in hematocrit, increase in aspertate transaminase (AST) and alanine transaminase (ALT), and decrease in platelet count.

> The key components of the **HELLP syndrome** are **h**emolysis, **e**levated **l**iver enzymes, and **l**ow **p**latelet count.

> Signs of HELLP syndrome include epigastric pain or right upper quadrant tenderness, nausea or vomiting, headache, flu-like symptoms, jaundice, and hematuria.

On rare occasions, HELLP syndrome progresses to include disseminated intravascular coagulation (DIC). See Chapter 42 for a discussion of DIC.

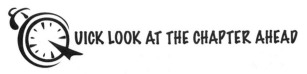

QUICK LOOK AT THE CHAPTER AHEAD

Delivery of the infant is the only cure for pre-eclampsia. In management of a pregnancy less than 37 weeks of gestation, the mother receives treatment to control the preeclampsia, prevent complications, and allow the fetus to mature.

With gestational hypertension or mild preeclampsia, nursing care includes supporting the woman through activity restriction; encouraging her to rest in the left lateral position several times a day; and education about reporting symptoms such as severe headaches, visual changes, and right upper quadrant or epigastric pain.

Explanations and opportunities for the woman and her family to express fears, anxieties, and other reactions are provided by the nurse.

Much of the nursing care focuses on the assessments necessary with the administration of magnesium sulfate. In the event of a seizure, nursing interventions prevent maternal injury and the nurse observes the seizure activity. The physician is notified immediately. Following the seizure, maternal and fetal oxygenation is a priority. Once the mother and fetus have been stabilized, delivery is done.

During the intrapartum period, the woman continues to receive magnesium sulfate, with ongoing assessments and nursing care. Induction of labor with oxytocin is often necessary. Higher doses of pitocin may be needed. Pain management during labor is important. General anesthesia is avoided. Intravenous fluids are given but carefully monitored to prevent fluid overload. Fetal heart monitoring during labor may show loss of variability.

44

Hypertensive Disorders of Pregnancy: Management

For up to five days postpartum, the woman with hypertensive disorders of pregnancy continues to be at risk for HELLP syndrome, liver rupture, or seizures. Magnesium sulfate and close monitoring is continued for at least 24 hours postpartum. Psychological needs for mother and family must be addressed. The newborn may exhibit hypotonia and depressed respirations as side effects of magnesium sulfate.

TERMS
- ☐ home management
- ☐ inpatient management
- ☐ magnesium sulfate
- ☐ corticosteroids
- ☐ activity restriction
- ☐ seizure

MEDICAL MANAGEMENT

Because there are no diagnostic laboratory tests, the medical diagnosis of hypertensive disorders of pregnancy can be made only if symptoms are present, especially increased blood pressure. Delivery of the infant is the only cure for preeclampsia. The decision about when to deliver is based upon fetal gestational age, status of the fetus, and severity of the mother's condition. If the hypertensive disorder develops after 37 weeks of pregnancy, the recommended management is delivery of the infant by induction of labor or cesarean delivery.

In management of a pregnancy less than 37 weeks of gestation, the mother receives treatment to control the preeclampsia, prevent complications, and allow the fetus to mature.

A woman with mild preeclampsia whose blood pressure improves with bedrest may have **home management**. Education of the patient and family for home management includes blood pressure monitoring every 4 hours, with daily assessment of weight, urine dipstick for protein, and fetal movement counts. Nonstress tests are done twice a week and the primary care physician would be seen weekly. If the woman's blood pressure does not improve with bedrest or there are signs of severe preeclampsia, she is treated in the hospital.

> Education of the patient and family for home management includes blood pressure monitoring every 4 hours, with daily assessment of weight, urine dipstick for protein, and fetal movement counts. Nonstress tests are done twice a week and the primary care physician would be seen weekly.

Inpatient management includes blood pressure monitoring every 4 hours both day and night, daily evaluation of patellar reflexes, weight, urine dipstick for protein, and fetal movement. Nonstress tests are done twice weekly and biophysical profile with amniotic fluid index weekly. Complete blood count, creatinine, and liver enzyme tests are done twice weekly to determine the progression of the disease.

The medication of choice to control blood pressure and prevent seizures is **magnesium sulfate**. Antihypertensive and diuretic drugs may be used in the control of severe hypertension. **Corticosteroids** are ordered to promote lung maturity in the fetus of less than 34 weeks of gestation. Plans for delivery are made if the preeclampsia worsens, diagnostic tests indicate kidney or liver dysfunction or HELLP syndrome, seizures occur, or fetal distress develops.

NURSING MANAGEMENT

With gestational hypertension or mild pre-eclampsia, nursing care includes supporting the woman through **activity restriction**; encouraging her to rest in the left lateral position several times a day; and providing education about reporting symptoms such as severe headaches, visual changes, and right upper quadrant or epigastric pain.

Explanations about fetal movement counts, nonstress tests, biophysical profiles, frequent blood pressure readings, laboratory blood and urine tests, and frequent questioning about the presence of any symptoms all increase patient compliance with the management program.

> With gestational hypertension or mild preeclampsia, nursing care includes supporting the woman through **activity restriction**; encouraging her to rest in the left lateral position several times a day; and providing education about reporting symptoms such as severe headaches, visual changes, and right upper quadrant or epigastric pain.

Opportunities for the woman and her family to express fears, anxieties, and other reactions are provided by the nurse.

Much of the nursing care for hypertension focuses on the assessments necessary for the administration of magnesium sulfate. (See Table 44-1.)

- Calcium gluconate needs to be readily available as an antidote for magnesium toxicity.
- Seizure precautions are initiated, which include having oxygen, suction equipment, and pads for the siderails available.
- Frequent assessments for signs of impending seizure such as epigastric pain, visual disturbance, or hyperreflexia with clonus are done.
- A quiet environment with limited lighting is maintained.

In the event of a **seizure**, nursing interventions are done to prevent maternal injury and to observe the seizure activity for accurate documentation. The physician is notified immediately. Following the seizure, maternal and fetal oxygenation is a priority. Once the mother and fetus have been stabilized, delivery is initiated.

During the intrapartum period, the woman continues to receive magnesium sulfate, along with ongoing assessments and nursing care. Induction of labor with oxytocin is often necessary. Because magnesium

Table 44-1   Nursing Assessments with Magnesium Sulfate Administration

Assessment	Range		Implications
Serum magnesium levels	4–7 mEq/L (5–8 mg/dL)		Therapeutic range
	8–10 mEq/L (9–12 mg/dL)		Loss of deep tendon reflexes
	10–12 mEq/L (12–15 mg/dL)		Respiratory depression
	12–15 mEq/L (15–18 mg/dL)		Respiratory arrest
	15–20 mEq/L (18–25 mg/dL)		Bradycardia, arrhythmia, heart block
	20–25 mEq/L (25–30 mg/dL)		Cardiac arrest
Deep tendon reflexes (DTR)	Reflexes absent	0	Reflexes should be checked hourly. DTR are a good indicator of magnesium toxicity. The goal of magnesium therapy is for DTR to be decreased but not absent. A sudden change in DTR or absence of reflexes warrants discontinuation of the medication.
	Less than normal or		
	diminished	+1	
	Low normal	+2	
	High normal, brisk	+3	
	Brisk with clonus	+4	
Respirations	12–20 breaths per minute		If respiratory rate is below 12 breaths per minute, medication is discontinued and the physician notified.
Pulse	60–100 beats per minute with no arrhythmia		A significant drop in pulse is reported to the physician and medication is discontinued if pulse is less than 60 beats per minute.
Blood pressure	100–140 mm Hg systolic		Blood pressure needs to be maintained at a systolic level of 100 mm Hg for placental perfusion. A significant drop in blood pressure is reported to the physician. The accuracy of the measurement is essential; the arm should be at the heart level and an appropriately sized cuff used.
	60–90 mm Hg diastolic		
Fetal heart rate	120–160 beats per minute, regular		Decreased variability occurs. Signs of fetal distress are reported to the physician. No evidence of adverse effects if maternal magnesium levels are within therapeutic range.
Urine output	At least 30 cc per hour		A Foley catheter is inserted for accurate measurement of output. Magnesium is excreted through the kidneys. Women with hypertensive disorders of pregnancy may have decreased kidney functioning that contributes to an increased risk of magnesium toxicity. If urinary output decreases, the patient is assessed for hyporeflexia more frequently.
Side effects	Facial flushing, hot flashes, nausea, vomiting, headaches, muscle weakness, drowsiness		These symptoms are more pronounced with the rapid infusion of loading doses. Explanations to patient and family are essential. Marked lethargy or decreased level of consciousness is reported to physician.

sulfate relaxes smooth muscle, uterine contractility may be diminished and higher doses of pitocin needed.

Pain can increase blood pressure; therefore, pain management during labor is important. See Chapter 22 for discussion of intrapartal pain management.

General anesthesia is avoided if possible because hypertension can rise with the administration of this type of anesthesia. If epidural or spinal anesthesia is used, intravenous fluids are given to control possible hypotensive side effects.

Intravenous fluid intake during induction of labor and anesthesia needs to be carefully monitored to prevent fluid overload that could lead to pulmonary edema. Also, fetal heart monitoring during labor may show loss of variability.

For up to five days postpartum, the woman with hypertensive disorders of pregnancy continues to be at risk for HELLP syndrome, liver rupture, or seizures.

Magnesium sulfate and close monitoring are continued for at least 24 hours postpartum. Psychological needs for mother and family must be addressed, especially if the mother was not alert during the birth experience or the newborn is in the special-care nursery.

> Psychological needs for mother and family must be addressed, especially if the mother was not alert during the birth experience or the newborn is in the special-care nursery.

The newborn may exhibit hypotonia and depressed respiration as side effects of the use of magnesium sulfate.

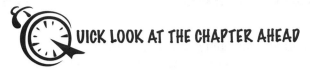

NE LOOK AT THE CHAPTER AHEAD

QUICK LOOK AT THE CHAPTER AHEAD

Premature rupture of membranes (PROM) occurs
if the amniotic sac ruptures before the onset of
labor. Rupture of the membranes before week
37 of gestation is preterm premature rupture of
membranes (pPROM). Prolonged rupture of the
membranes (prolonged ROM) occurs when the
membranes rupture more than 24 hours before
birth.

Factors thought to contribute to PROM include
vaginal or uterine infections, hydramnios, incompetent cervix, cervical cerclage, placenta previa
or abruption, multiple gestation, amniocentesis,
genital tract abnormalities, fetal anomalies, a history of PROM in a previous pregnancy, a history
of cervical conization, smoking, substance abuse,
and lower socioeconomic status.

Premature rupture of membranes is usually
reported by the client as a persistent leaking of
fluid from the vagina in a gush or trickle. A sterile speculum exam, use of nitrazine paper, and a
microscopic exam are diagnostic tests for PROM.
A direct digital exam of the cervix is not done.

Spontaneous labor usually occurs within hours or
days after PROM. If the pregnancy is close to or at
term, induction of labor is the usual intervention.
If the pregnancy is less than 36 weeks of gestation and there are no signs of infection, the pregnancy will be preserved until spontaneous labor
to allow for fetal lung maturity.

When labor begins either spontaneously or with
induction, fetal status is monitored very carefully
for cord compression.

45

Premature Rupture
of Membranes

Women with PROM are monitored for signs of infection. Good handwashing and perineal hygiene are stressed. Women are instructed to change the perineal pad frequently and avoid use of tampons.

Monitoring the fetus is an integral part of assessment of the woman with PROM.

The woman may be on modified bedrest with bathroom privileges and may shower.

Nursing care to meet the psychological needs of the woman and her family includes clear explanations of the treatment plan, help in expressing fears and concerns, and appropriate referrals to a social worker or spiritual counselor.

TERMS
- [ ] **premature rupture of membranes (PROM)**
- [ ] **preterm premature rupture of membranes (pPROM)**
- [ ] **prolonged rupture of membranes (prolonged ROM)**
- [ ] **expectant management**
- [ ] **intrauterine infection**

In 10% of pregnancies, membranes rupture before labor begins. If rupture occurs before week 37 of pregnancy, it is a contributing factor to preterm labor and birth. When membranes rupture and the barrier to infection is broken, the risk for intrauterine infection or fetal infection increases.

 # DEFINITIONS AND ETIOLOGY

Premature rupture of membranes (PROM) occurs if the amniotic sac ruptures before the onset of labor. Rupture of the membranes before week 37 of gestation is defined as **preterm premature rupture of membranes (pPROM). Prolonged rupture of the membranes (prolonged ROM)** occurs when the membranes rupture more than 24 hours before birth.

Although the cause is unknown, factors thought to contribute to PROM include

- vaginal or uterine infections
- hydramnios
- incompetent cervix
- cervical cerclage
- placenta previa or abruption
- multiple gestation
- amniocentesis
- genital tract abnormalities
- fetal anomalies
- a history of PROM in a previous pregnancy
- a history of cervical conization.

Smoking, substance abuse, and lower socioeconomic status have also been associated with premature rupture of membranes.

 # ASSOCIATED RISKS

Maternal risks associated with premature rupture of the membranes are intra-amniotic infection as a result of ascending vaginal organisms and more frequent occurrence of placental abruption.

 Ascending vaginal organisms are microorganisms moving up the vagina, through the cervix, and into the amniotic sac.

Fetal and neonatal risks include complications of prematurity and increased risk for infection. Diminished amounts of amniotic fluid can lead to fetal distress from cord compression or prolapse. Limb and facial deformities, amniotic band syndrome, and pulmonary hypoplasia can also occur with severe oligohydramnios.

MEDICAL MANAGEMENT

Premature rupture of membranes is usually reported by the client as a persistent leaking of fluid from the vagina in a gush or trickle. A sterile speculum exam confirms the diagnosis of ruptured membranes if there is pooling visible behind the cervix.

Nitrazine paper moistened with vaginal fluid indicates PROM if it turns from yellow to dark blue. This occurs because amniotic fluid has an alkaline pH.

A ferning pattern seen on microscopic exam of vaginal fluid is another diagnostic test for PROM.

> Direct digital exam of the cervix is **not** done after PROM because it increases the risk for infection and could stimulate labor in the woman who is preterm.

Spontaneous labor usually occurs within hours or days after PROM. Decision making regarding medical management weighs the risks of infection and the consequences of prematurity. If the pregnancy is close to or at term and labor does not begin within 12 to 24 hours, induction is the usual intervention. If the pregnancy is less than 36 weeks of gestation, expectant management is the usual option.

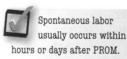
Spontaneous labor usually occurs within hours or days after PROM.

The woman remains hospitalized until birth and is observed for signs of labor and infection. As long as there are no signs of infection, the pregnancy will continue until spontaneous labor to allow for fetal lung maturity.

Expectant management usually includes the administration of antibiotics to prevent infection and corticosteroids to promote fetal lung development. Although rupture of membranes is usually a contraindication to the use of tocolytic drugs, these medications may be given to prolong the pregnancy for 48 hours to enhance the benefit of cortico-steroid therapy.

When labor begins either spontaneously or by induction, fetal status is monitored very carefully for changes in the fetal heart rate pattern, indicating cord compression. An amnioinfusion with normal saline solution may be administered to increase amniotic fluid volume and relieve pressure on the umbilical cord.

NURSING CARE

The primary nursing concern for the mother and fetus is risk for infection if membranes rupture more than 24 hours before birth. Women with PROM are monitored for signs of **intrauterine infection**. (See Table 45-1.) The temperature and pulse are taken at least every 2 hours.

Maternal tachycardia is an early sign of intra-amniotic infection. Fever is the most reliable indicator of infection, but occurs late.

Blood is drawn for complete blood count and c-reactive protein every 12 to 24 hours. The woman is evaluated for abdominal tenderness and foul-smelling vaginal discharge.

Good handwashing and perineal hygiene are stressed in patient teaching. Women are instructed to change the perineal pad frequently and avoid use of tampons.

> The primary nursing concern for the mother and fetus is risk for infection if membranes rupture more than 24 hours before birth.

> Maternal tachycardia is an early sign of intra-amniotic infection. Fever is the most reliable indicator of infection, but occurs late.

> Good handwashing and perineal hygiene are stressed in patient teaching. Women are instructed to change the perineal pad frequently and avoid use of tampons.

Table 45-1 Signs of Intrauterine Infection

Fever
Maternal tachycardia
Fetal tachycardia
Uterine tenderness
Foul odor of vaginal discharge
Increase in white blood cell (WBC) count
Presence of serum c-reactive protein (CRP)

Monitoring the fetus is an integral part of assessment of the woman with PROM. Fetal heart rate is evaluated for tachycardia and signs of cord compression or fetal distress. Fetal tachycardia is an early sign of infection. Continuous fetal monitoring is recommended for at least the first 24 hours; then intermittent monitoring if there are no signs of labor or fetal distress. A nonstress test to rule out cord compression and fetal sepsis may be ordered daily. Biophysical profiles, ultrasounds, and an amniocentesis may be done to determine the most appropriate time for delivery.

Monitoring the fetus is an integral part of assessment of the woman with PROM.

Fetal tachycardia is an early sign of infection.

The woman with PROM may be on modified bedrest with bathroom privileges and may shower. See Chapter 41 for a discussion of bedrest during pregnancy. Nursing care to meet the psychological needs of the woman and her family includes use of clear explanations of the treatment plan, interventions to facilitate the expression of fears and concerns, and appropriate referrals to a social worker or spiritual counselor.

PART VIII • QUESTIONS

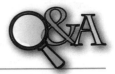

1. The nurse interviews a woman at her first prenatal visit. Which element of her past places this client at risk for an ectopic pregnancy?
   a. Appendectomy at age 17.
   b. History of high blood pressure.
   c. Pelvic inflammatory disease treated at age 27.
   d. Report of oral contraceptive failure.

2. A client is being admitted to the outpatient surgical area for a dilatation and currettage for an incomplete spontaneous abortion. What nursing assessment has highest priority?
   a. Amount of bleeding.
   b. Level of discomfort.
   c. Stage of the grief process.
   d. Understanding of the procedure.

3. Identify the medical condition associated with the characteristics listed in Table Q-1 by checking the appropriate box.

Table Q-1

Characteristic	Placenta previa	Placental abruption
Pain present		
Bleeding always visible		
Associated with breech presentation		
Associated with cocaine use		
Tetanic contractions		

4. A woman who is 34 weeks of gestation comes to the emergency room with vaginal bleeding. Which usual admission procedure would be omitted by the nurse?

a. Assessing uterine contraction pattern.

b. Counting fetal heart rate.

c. Determining cervical dilation.

d. Obtaining maternal vital signs.

5. List four signs of preterm labor that the nurse would teach to all pregnant women.

a._____

b._____

c._____

d._____

6. The nurse is reviewing prenatal records for risk assessment for preterm labor. Which prenatal client is at greater risk for developing preterm labor?

a. Age at conception is 29 years.

b. Diagnosis by ultrasound of twin pregnancy.

c. Pregnancy spacing more than 2 years.

d. Weight gain at 40 weeks of gestation is 27 pounds.

7. The nurse assesses a client receiving terbutaline for tocolysis of preterm labor. The following data are collected: BP 118/72, P 128, R 16. Based on these findings, what should the nurse do?

a. Administer the ordered dose of terbutaline.

b. Delay administration of the dose for 1 hour.

c. Notify the physician of the collected data.

d. Withhold the ordered dose of terbutaline.

8. The nurse is caring for a woman who gave birth 36 hours ago. She was on bedrest for 7 weeks during pregnancy. For what potential problem is the woman most at risk?

a. Constipation.

b. Fainting.

c. Heavy bleeding.

d. Postpartum depression.

9. Which nursing assessment data would support a diagnosis of intrauterine infection?

a. Fetal heart rate of 188 beats per minute.

b. Ruptured membranes.

c. Straw-colored discharge on underwear.

d. Temperature of 99.1°F (37.3°C).

10. When the nurse reviews a prenatal record, what information places the pregnant woman most at risk for premature rupture of membranes?
    a. Chlamydia infection.
    b. First pregnancy.
    c. Pregnancy-induced hypertension.
    d. Single-fetus pregnancy.

11. What question would the nurse ask a client with gestational hypertension to assess for cerebral edema?
    a. Are you experiencing any difficulty breathing?
    b. Do you have a headache?
    c. Do you have swelling of your hands?
    d. How much weight have you gained this week?

12. Identify the key components of the HELLP syndrome.

    _____

    _____

    _____

13. A woman with gestational hypertension is receiving magnesium sulfate therapy. Nursing assessments include deep tendon reflexes absent, respirations 14, pulse 60, blood pressure 100/62, and urinary output 20 cc/hour. What is the priority nursing action?
    a. Continue magnesium therapy.
    b. Decrease the dosage.
    c. Discontinue the magnesium therapy.
    d. Notify physician of findings.

14. A woman hospitalized with preeclampsia complains of pain in her upper abdomen and blurred vision. What is the first nursing action?
    a. Administer corticosteroids.
    b. Check seizure precaution equipment.
    c. Prepare for cesarean delivery.
    d. Review lab reports of liver function tests.

PART VIII · ANSWERS AND RATIONALES

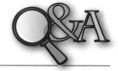

1. **The answer is c.** A history of pelvic inflammatory disease increases the risk of ectopic pregnancy because of potential scarring of the fallopian tubes. The other options do not reflect risk factors for ectopic pregnancy.

2. **The answer is a.** Vaginal bleeding during a spontaneous abortion may range in amount from spotting to heavy. Because hemorrhage is a concern, assessment for bleeding takes highest priority. The other options address important assessments that would be done later by the nurse.

3. **The answers are in Table Q-2.**

Table Q-2

Characteristic	Placenta previa	Placental abruption
Pain present		X
Bleeding always visible	X	
Associated with breech presentation	X	
Associated with cocaine use		X
Tetanic contractions		X

4. **The answer is c.** In the presence of vaginal bleeding, no vaginal exams would be done. A vaginal exam could stimulate excessive bleeding.

5. The responses could be any four of the following signs of preterm labor:
    * contractions every 10 minutes or more often
    * painless contractions
    * menstrual-like cramps
    * back or abdominal discomfort
    * pelvic pressure
    * increased vaginal discharge
    * leakage of fluid from the vagina.

6. **The answer is b.** Multiple gestation is a major risk factor for

preterm labor. Of twin pregnancies, 40% result in preterm birth. The other options do not increase the risk of preterm labor and birth.

7. **The answer is d.** Betamimetics such as terbutaline are not administered if the maternal heart rate is greater than 120 beats per minute.

8. **The answer is b.** Orthostatic hypotension leading to dizziness and faintness is a major side effect of prolonged bedrest. Although constipation can occur with prolonged bedrest, it is not the most significant problem. Prolonged bedrest does not increase the risk for postpartum hemorrhage or postpartum depression.

9. **The answer is a.** Fetal tachycardia is an early sign of intrauterine infection. Although ruptured membranes are a risk factor for infection, this does not indicate that an infection has occurred. The straw-colored discharge on underwear is most likely urine. The temperature given is within the normal range.

10. **The answer is a.** Vaginal infections such as chlamydia increase the risk for premature rupture of membranes. The other options are not risk factors for PROM.

11. **The answer is b.** Headache is a clinical manifestation of cerebral edema. Generalized edema can cause swollen hands, face, legs, and excessive weight gain. Dyspnea or difficulty breathing is a sign of pulmonary edema.

12. **Hemolysis, elevated liver enzymes, and low platelet count.**

13. **The answer is c.** Deep tendon reflexes are a good indicator of magnesium toxicity. Reflexes are absent when magnesium levels are above the therapeutic range. The medication should be discontinued first; then the physician notified. Respiration, pulse, and blood-pressure measurements are within the normal range. Urinary output is below the normal 30 cc per hour and would contribute to high magnesium levels.

14. **The answer is b.** Upper abdominal or epigastric pain and visual disturbances such as blurred vision are signs of impending seizure. Oxygen, suction equipment, and padding for the siderails are part of seizure precautions. This equipment should be readily available. Corticosteroids are not indicated in this situation. Delivery of the infant would not occur until the mother's condition is stable. Upper right quadrant abdominal pain may occur if the HELLP syndrome is present; however, the possibility of seizure is more immediate.

IX

Significant Medical Complications of Pregnancy

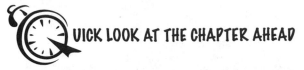

Diabetes mellitus, which complicates 3–5% of all pregnancies, is a metabolic disorder of carbohydrate metabolism caused by insufficient production or use of insulin.

Type 1 is an autoimmune destruction of the pancreatic cells that produce insulin. Type 2 occurs when receptor sites at the tissue level are not responsive, thus causing resistance to the insulin that is produced.

Diabetes mellitus existing prior to pregnancy is *pregestational* diabetes. Diabetes arising during pregnancy is *gestational* diabetes. White's system is most commonly used to classify the pathology associated with gestational diabetes.

Women with gestational diabetes are at increased risk for a number of complications.

Many of the problems experienced by the fetus and neonate are directly related to high maternal blood glucose levels.

All pregnant women should be screened for gestational diabetes between weeks 24 and 28.

Women with a history of high-risk factors for diabetes should be scheduled for screening at the first prenatal visit.

 Good control of the blood sugars through diet, exercise, and insulin if necessary significantly reduces the risks to mother and fetus. The nurse needs to provide appropriate education and referrals to increase patient and family compliance with medical management.

46

Diabetes Mellitus: Overview

TERMS
- [ ] **diabetogenic effect of pregnancy**
- [ ] **diabetes mellitus—type 1 and type 2**
- [ ] **pregestational diabetes**
- [ ] **gestational diabetes**

Diabetes mellitus complicates 3 to 5% of all pregnancies and contributes to serious problems in both mother and fetus. About 90% of pregnant women with diabetes develop the disease during pregnancy.

DEFINITION AND ETIOLOGY

Diabetes mellitus is a metabolic disorder of carbohydrate metabolism resulting from insufficient production or use of insulin. **Type 1** is an autoimmune destruction of the pancreatic cells that produce insulin. **Type 2** occurs when receptor sites at the tissue level are not responsive, thus causing resistance to the insulin produced.

During pregnancy, the needs of the growing fetus increase glucose production by the maternal liver. The placental hormones stimulate the pancreas to produce increased insulin. The placental hormones also increase insulin resistance, requiring additional insulin production. In the nondiabetic woman, the pancreas can adjust insulin production to meet the increased demands for insulin. This delicate balance in carbohydrate metabolism during pregnancy puts a stress on the pancreas known as the **diabetogenic effect of pregnancy**.

Diabetes mellitus occurring prior to pregnancy is defined as **pregestational diabetes**. Diabetes identified during pregnancy is called **gestational diabetes**. Because of the diabetogenic effect of pregnancy, the pancreas cannot produce enough insulin and hyperglycemia develops. Insulin needs change throughout the perinatal period. (See Table 46-1.)

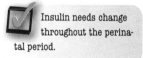
Insulin needs change throughout the perinatal period.

White's classification system is most commonly used to classify the pathology associated with diabetes during pregnancy. It is based upon age of onset, duration of the disease, and the presence of vascular disease.

MATERNAL RISKS

Women with diabetes during pregnancy are at increased risk for miscarriage, pregnancy-induced hypertension, preterm labor, hydramnios, infection, hypoglycemia, ketoacidosis, retinopathy, and intrapartal complications such as difficult labor, induction of labor,

Table 46-1 Perinatal Insulin Needs

Time	Insulin Requirements	Implications
First trimester	Decreased due to inhibition of anterior pituitary hormones, growth of the embryo, and decreased maternal intake.	Insulin dosage and diet must be adjusted for the pregestational diabetic. Blood sugar can be unstable. Nocturnal hypoglycemia can occur. Morning sickness can influence oral intake. Unstable glucose levels increase the risk of miscarriage.
Second trimester	Gradually increases (10–20% for Type 1 and 30–90% for Type 2) due to insulin-resistant properties of placental hormones.	Insulin dosage may need to be adjusted every 5 to 10 days. Monitor blood sugar frequently, at least fasting, before and after lunch, before dinner, and at bedtime. If fasting blood sugar is high, test blood sugar between 2 and 3 a.m. Adequate glucose level is needed for fetal growth.
Third Trimester	Continues to increase until week 36, reaches a plateau, and then may decrease slightly as placental functioning diminishes.	Same as the second trimester.
Labor and delivery	Decreases during active labor due to increased metabolism.	Monitor blood glucose level and urine for ketones every 1 to 2 hours. Adjust IV fluids according to blood sugar. IV fluids with glucose are needed if blood glucose falls below 70 mg/dL. Some women may require insulin infusion adjusted according to blood sugar and ketones.
Postpartum	Markedly and rapidly decreases because of loss of placental hormones.	Pregestational diabetics should continue to monitor their blood glucose and urine ketones. Insulin needs will return to about two-thirds of the prepregnancy dosage by postpartum day 4. Gestational diabetics should monitor blood sugar and ketones for at least 24 hours and usually do not require insulin postpartum.
Breastfeeding	Considerably decreased because of carbohydrate use in milk production.	Breastfeeding should be encouraged. 500 to 800 additional calories needed. Close blood glucose monitoring needed. Expect fluctuations during weaning. Increased risk of nipple infection and mastitis.

and cesarean delivery. Miscarriage is related to inadequate glucose control during the first 7 weeks of pregnancy.

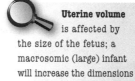

Miscarriage is related to inadequate glucose control during the first 7 weeks of pregnancy.

Pregnant women with diabetes have twice the risk of developing pregnancy-induced hypertension, especially when diabetes-related vascular changes already exist.

The pregnant woman with diabetes has an increased risk for developing preterm labor when there is increased uterine volume from a macrosomic infant, hypertensive disorder, kidney or urinary tract infections, or vascular compromise. Although the mechanism for hydramnios is not fully understood, it may result from excessive fetal urination because of fetal hyperglycemia.

Uterine volume is affected by the size of the fetus; a macrosomic (large) infant will increase the dimensions of the uterus.

Hyperglycemia and glycosuria increase the risk of vaginal and urinary tract infections. Also, insulin-dependent diabetic women are five times more likely to develop postpartum endometriosis or a wound infection.

Hypoglycemia is most likely to occur in the first trimester, during early postpartum, and when breastfeeding. Ketoacidosis may develop if hypoglycemia or hyperglycemia triggers an increase in ketone bodies in the blood when fatty acids are metabolized. Retinopathy may worsen in women with diabetes during pregnancy, especially if hypoglycemia develops.

Intrapartal complications such as a difficult labor, induction of labor, fetal distress, or cesarean delivery are more likely, and are associated with a macrosomic infant and uteroplacental insufficiency.

FETAL AND NEONATAL RISKS

Many of the problems experienced by the fetus and neonate are directly related to high maternal blood glucose levels.

 With severe ketoacidosis, there is a 50% chance of fetal death.

Some stillbirths are unexplained and others are associated with vascular complications or placental abruptions. Congenital anomalies occur in infants of diabetic mothers four times more frequently and are the

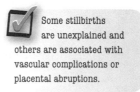

Some stillbirths are unexplained and others are associated with vascular complications or placental abruptions.

major cause of infant death. The most common anomalies are cardiac defects, central nervous system abnormalities, and skeletal malformations.

Typically, infants of diabetic mothers are large for gestational age (LGA) due to high levels of fetal insulin production triggered by high glucose levels crossing the placenta from the mother. This increases growth and fat deposition.

In women with class D or higher diabetes who have existing vascular disease before pregnancy, placental insufficiency may lead to intrauterine growth restriction (IUGR).

Delayed lung maturity may occur because of interference with production of surfactants from high blood sugar levels.

The infant of a diabetic mother may develop hypoglycemia within 2 to 4 hours after birth. The fetal pancreas has been producing large quantities of insulin. The abrupt decrease in blood glucose, previously supplied by the mother through the placenta, triggers hypoglycemia.

Additional neonatal complications include birth trauma, hyperbilirubinemia, hypocalcemia, polycythemia, and transient respiratory distress. See Chapter 63 for a discussion of the infant of the diabetic mother.

SCREENING

All pregnant women should be screened for gestational diabetes between 24 and 28 weeks of gestation. Screening is done with a 1-hour glucose challenge test. A blood glucose level less than 140 mg/dL is considered normal. When results are above normal, a 3-hour glucose tolerance test is done.

Diagnosis of gestational diabetes is defined by the National Diabetes Data Group as two or more values exceeding the normal limits in mg/dL: fasting—105, 1 hour—190, 2 hour—165, and 3 hour—145.

Women with a history of high risk factors for diabetes are scheduled for screening at the first prenatal visit. Risk factors include

- a family history of diabetes
- a history of gestational diabetes in a previous pregnancy
- unexplained stillbirth, fetal anomaly, or recurrent miscarriage
- delivery of infant weighing 9 pounds or more
- obesity of the mother
- hypertensive disorder

- recurrent monilial vaginitis
- hydramnios in current pregnancy
- glycosuria in two consecutive prenatal visits
- Native American, Hispanic American, Asian American, African American, or Pacific Islander ethnicity
- age over 40.

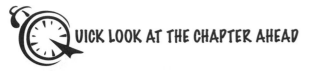

For a woman who is already diabetic, planning before conception and control of blood sugar are essential for a positive pregnancy outcome.

Management of diabetes during the second and third trimesters is similar for the pregestational and the gestational diabetic.

Careful attention to caloric distribution throughout the day and regular exercise are important to maintain desired blood glucose levels and to control weight.

The oral hypoglycemic agent glyburide is safe to use during pregnancy because it does not cross the placenta. If insulin is necessary, combinations of short, intermediate, and long-acting insulins are used.

An increased need for insulin does not mean the disease is getting worse. It means the placenta is healthy and producing insulin-resistant hormones.

It is important for blood glucose levels to be stable to prevent ketoacidosis, which can lead to coma or death of mother and fetus.

Women with gestational diabetes need to be monitored more frequently for preeclampsia, preterm labor, and polyhydramnios.

Fetal surveillance with nonstress testing, ultrasound, kick counts, and biophysical profile is essential.

47

Diabetes Mellitus: Medical and Nursing Management

If the pregnant woman with diabetes mellitus develops preterm labor, insulin dosages need to be adjusted.

Magnesium sulfate or indomethacin is preferred for tocolysis; they do not affect blood sugar.

Women with good control of their diabetes and no signs of complication are allowed to continue until term. Induction or cesarean delivery is scheduled if problems occur.

It is important to continue postpartum medical management of the woman with pregestational diabetes.

Breastfeeding is encouraged because it influences weight loss postpartum and lowers insulin requirements.

Maintaining a normal weight, appropriate nutritional intake, and regular exercise reduce the risk of future diabetes.

A woman with diabetes must take it into account in selecting a method of birth control.

Appropriate teaching of the woman with diabetes and her family is an integral part of medical management. Compliance is essential for a successful outcome.

TERMS
- [ ] **glyburide**
- [ ] **insulin**
- [ ] **ketoacidosis**
- [ ] **hypoglycemia**
- [ ] **hyperglycemia**

PRECONCEPTION AND EARLY PREGNANCY

For a woman who is a pregestational diabetic, preconception planning and blood sugar control during pregnancy are essential for a positive pregnancy outcome. There are implications for preconception and early pregnancy control. In order to prevent fetal abnormalities, maintaining the blood sugar in the normal range for 1 to 2 months before conception is recommended. Any negative health behaviors such as smoking, alcohol use, inappropriate diet, or inadequate exercise should be addressed prior to attempting a pregnancy.

The normal signs and symptoms of early pregnancy such as fatigue, morning sickness, and sensitivity to odor and taste can affect the diet/exercise regimen and the insulin requirements of the woman with pregestational diabetes. Fluctuations in blood

 Fluctuations in blood glucose levels increase the risk of miscarriage and fetal anomalies in the first trimester.

glucose levels increase the risk of miscarriage and fetal anomalies in the first trimester. More frequent self-monitoring of blood glucose levels with additional testing after meals and during the night is required. Diabetic management during the first trimester may require hospitalization to adjust insulin dosages.

LATER PREGNANCY

Management of diabetes during the second and third trimesters is similar for the pregestational and the gestational diabetic. The essential components of diabetic management include diet, exercise, self-monitoring of blood sugar levels, and insulin or oral hypoglycemic agents if necessary.

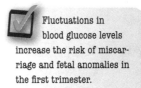 Management of diabetes during the second and third trimesters is similar for the pregestational and the gestational diabetic.

Total caloric intake and the distribution of the calories among carbohydrates, proteins, and fats should be considered when planning daily intake. Careful attention to caloric distribution throughout the day, including a bedtime snack, is important.

A regular exercise program is encouraged to maintain desired blood sugar levels and weight control.

Self-monitoring of blood glucose levels determines the effectiveness of blood glucose management. Elevated blood sugar levels indicate a need for increased insulin.

If the gestational diabetic is following the recommended diet but more than half of her daily blood sugar levels are elevated, insulin or oral hypoglycemic therapy is indicated.

The pregestational diabetic may be on insulin therapy or oral hypoglycemic agents before the pregnancy begins and require adjustment of the dosage.

Recent research has indicated that the oral hypoglycemic agent glyburide is safe to use during pregnancy because it does not cross the placenta. **Glyburide** is comparable to insulin in controlling blood glucose, and has a lower rate of causing maternal hypoglycemia. If **insulin** is necessary, combinations of short, intermediate, and long-acting insulins are used to control blood sugar levels. The insulin pump may be used during pregnancy. It is important for the pregnant diabetic woman to understand that an increased need for insulin does not mean the disease is getting worse. It means the placenta is healthy and producing the insulin-resistant hormones.

Recent research has indicated that the oral hypoglycemic agent glyburide is safe to use during pregnancy because it does not cross the placenta.

It is important for the pregnant diabetic woman to understand that an increased need for insulin does not mean the disease is getting worse. It means the placenta is healthy and producing the insulin-resistant hormones.

It is important for blood glucose levels to be stable to prevent ketoacidosis. **Ketoacidosis** occurs when ketone bodies are released in fatty acid metabolism. If **hypoglycemia** occurs, there are insufficient carbohydrates for energy sources, and fatty acids are metabolized. In **hyperglycemia**, insufficent amounts of insulin to transport carbohydrates into the cells require fats to be used instead of carbohydrates.

Ketoacidosis is very dangerous to mother and fetus and can lead to coma or death.

Eliminating nocturnal hypoglycemia by having a bedtime snack, close monitoring and control of blood sugars while awake, and attention to insulin dosage related to food intake and exercise are part of the educational plan to prevent ketoacidosis.

Women with diabetes during pregnancy need to be monitored more frequently for the obstetrical complications of preeclampsia, preterm labor, and polyhydramnios. Fetal surveillance techniques of nonstress test, ultrasound, kick counts, and biophysical profile are an essential part of prenatal care. The most common complications to be detected are macrosomia and decreased uteroplacental perfusion. See Chapter 13 for details of fetal surveillance.

> Eliminating nocturnal hypoglycemia by having a bedtime snack, close monitoring and control of blood sugars while awake, and attention to insulin dosage related to food intake and exercise are part of the educational plan to prevent ketoacidosis.

If the pregnant woman with diabetes mellitus develops preterm labor, traditional management of PTL can influence blood sugar control. Beta-sympathomimetics and corticosteroids affect carbohydrate metabolism and increase blood sugar levels. Therefore, insulin dosages need to be adjusted when these drugs are used. Magnesium sulfate or indomethacin is preferred for tocolysis because neither affects the blood sugar.

TIMING OF BIRTH

Decisions about the timing of birth are based upon results of assessments of maternal and fetal well-being. Women with good control of their diabetes and no signs of complications are allowed to continue the pregnancy until term. Induction or cesarean delivery is scheduled if problems occur. Because fetal lung maturity is delayed with diabetes mellitus, assessment of surfactant production is recommended to help determine delivery time.

POSTPARTUM CONSIDERATIONS

The woman with pregestational diabetes who is not breastfeeding typically returns to her prepregnancy management regimen within 6 weeks of the birth. If she is breastfeeding, insulin and nutritional requirements will be affected as long as she is producing breastmilk. The increase in metabolism required to produce breastmilk usually offsets the increased nutritional needs and lowers insulin requirements. It is important to continue with medical management of her diabetic condition.

The woman with gestational diabetes will require ongoing long-term follow-up because of the high risk of developing type 2 diabetes within the next 20 years. Maintaining a normal weight, appropriate nutritional intake, and regular exercise reduce the risk of future diabetes. Breastfeeding is encouraged for the woman with gestational diabetes because it influences weight loss postpartum and lowers insulin requirements. (See Table 46-1.)

 Breastfeeding is encouraged for the woman with gestational diabetes because it influences weight loss postpartum and lowers insulin requirements.

Women with diabetes resuming sexual intercourse can use low-dose combined oral contraceptives if there is no evidence of vascular compromise. Barrier methods are safe, effective, and inexpensive options.

 Because of the increased risk of infection in women with diabetes, the intrauterine device is not recommended.

Many couples who do not desire more children choose permanent sterilization.

TEACHING AND SUPPORT

Appropriate teaching of the woman with diabetes and her family is an integral part of management. (See Table 47-1.) Compliance with the management plan is essential for the diabetic woman to have a successful pregnancy outcome.

Appropriate teaching of the woman with diabetes and her family is an integral part of management.

Health care providers need to incorporate cultural and family preferences when planning diet and activity.

The woman with pregestational diabetes is already familiar with the disease; has received education about diet, exercise, and insulin regimen; and has learned techniques for self-monitoring blood glucose levels and insulin administration. Reviewing this information, discussing the effect of pregnancy on the diabetic condition, providing emotional support,

Reviewing this information, discussing the effect of pregnancy on the diabetic condition, providing emotional support, and encouraging compliance with changes in routines by the nurse assists the pregestational diabetic to cope with a revised management plan.

and encouraging compliance with changes in routines by the nurse assists the pregestational diabetic to cope with a revised management plan.

For the gestational diabetic and her family, the diagnosis of diabetes often comes as a shock. The information about the disease, and the need for self-monitoring of blood sugars, diet, exercise, and the administration of insulin can be overwhelming. The gestational diabetic and her family have to cope with major lifestyle changes. Emotional support from the nurse is essential to allow time for the gestational diabetic to assimilate the implications of the disease and the large amount of information.

> Emotional support from the nurse is essential to allow time for the gestational diabetic to assimilate the implications of the disease and the large amount of information.

Table 47-1 Teaching About Diabetes and Pregnancy

Topic	Content
Understanding diabetes	Explain definition; pathophysiology; signs and symptoms; effects on mother, fetus, and neonate; and medical management. Describe need for compliance and that it may be difficult to maintain stable blood sugars because needs of growing fetus cannot be accurately predicted.
Understanding the high-risk nature of this pregnancy	Explain effects of diabetes on pregnancy and the increased risk of certain obstetrical complications. Discuss need for more frequent prenatal visits and increased tests for maternal and fetal well-being. Teach signs and symptoms of pregnancy-induced hypertension and preterm labor.
Self-monitoring of blood glucose	Describe the technique of blood glucose monitoring and have the woman demonstrate proper technique. Explain frequency for testing and importance of an accurate record of blood sugars that is brought to each prenatal visit. The desired ranges of blood glucose levels in mg/dL are: fasting 60–90; before meals 60–105; 2 hours after meals 90–120; bedtime 90–120; nocturnal 60–120.
Diet	Encourage weight gain of 25 to 35 pounds during the pregnancy if she is within a normal weight range. Based upon her current weight, caloric intake is calculated. The distribution of calories is 45% carbohydrate, 20% protein, and 35% fat. 25% of calories are consumed at breakfast, 30% at lunch, 30% at dinner, and 15% at bedtime. Discuss ways of managing intake such as exchange system or carbohydrate counting.
Exercise	Recommend exercise 3 to 4 times weekly for 20 to 30 minutes. An ideal exercise is brisk walking.

Table 47-1 Teaching About Diabetes and Pregnancy (continued)

Topic	Content
Insulin administration	Explain types of insulin, classifications, dosages, times and methods of administration, rotation of injection sites, and adjustments to dosages based upon blood sugar readings. Demonstrate insulin administration and have the woman and her family demonstrate proper techniques.
Recognizing and treating hypoglycemia	Teach signs of hypoglycemia: shakiness, irritability, sweating, hunger, headache, blurred vision, pallor, and clammy skin. Explain that symptoms may develop more rapidly during pregnancy. Stress the importance of early recognition because seizures, coma, and death can occur if left untreated. If symptomatic, the woman should test her blood sugar. If it is less than 65 mg/dL, she should ingest 20 grams of carbohydrates and wait 20 minutes and retest her glucose level. If blood sugar has not returned to a normal range, she should repeat the carbohydrate snack. Stress the importance of having a snack and glucagon available at all times. Family members should be taught how to administer glucagon if the woman is unconscious. Report frequent hypoglycemic episodes to health care provider.
Recognizing and treating hyperglycemia	Teach the signs of hyperglycemia: slow onset, thirst, frequent urination, dry mouth, fatigue, nausea, abdominal cramps, headache, drowsiness, flushed skin, rapid deep breathing, and "fruity" odor to the breath. Hyperglycemia is detected through the monitoring of blood sugars and is usually treated with adjustments to diet, exercise, and insulin dosage. If there are frequent elevated blood sugar levels, the health care provider should be notified.

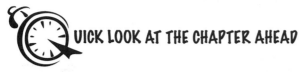

Any condition that interferes with maternal oxygenation can lead to decreased fetal oxygenation.

During pregnancy, the respiratory system adapts to the increased oxygenation needs of mother and fetus.

If the pregnant woman has chronic or acute respiratory disease, she can develop respiratory acidosis.

Asthma is the most common form of lung disease in pregnant women, occurring in 1–4% of pregnancies.

There is no significant increase in adverse perinatal outcomes for women with mild, well-controlled asthma.

Medications used for management of asthma are considered safe during pregnancy and lactation.

Cystic fibrosis (CF), a genetic defect resulting in abnormal production of mucus, primarily affects the respiratory, gastrointestinal, and genitourinary systems.

Women with CF may have problems with infertility, but conception does not worsen the disease and does not affect long-term survival rates.

The incidence of tuberculosis (TB) is increasing in women of childbearing years. Pregnant women in high-risk groups should be screened.

An inactive TB infection is not reactivated by pregnancy and has no detrimental effect on the mother or fetus.

48

Respiratory Complications in Pregnancy

After birth, a mother with inactive TB may breastfeed and care for her infant. If the disease is active, the mother does not care for her newborn until she is noninfectious.

Bronchitis and the common cold are the most common respiratory infections during pregnancy. Management of symptoms is the usual treatment.

Treatment of pneumonia during pregnancy includes the administration of a broad-spectrum antibiotic, followed by specific antibiotics.

If a woman develops severe acute respiratory syndrome (SARS) during pregnancy, the goal is treatment of the disease with careful monitoring of the fetus.

Mild hypoxemia in the fetus increases the risk for intra-uterine growth restriction; severe hypoxemia may result in fetal death.

The nurse must understand the normal adaptations of the pulmonary system during pregnancy, recognize signs of pulmonary complications, and provide education and support to the woman and her family as they participate in the therapeutic regimen for management of acute or chronic respiratory diseases. Preconceptual health care and stabilization of the respiratory condition are essential for a successful pregnancy outcome.

TERMS

- ☐ **respiratory acidosis**
- ☐ **asthma**
- ☐ **cystic fibrosis (CF)**
- ☐ **tuberculosis (TB)**
- ☐ **bronchitis**
- ☐ **common cold**
- ☐ **pneumonia**
- ☐ **severe acute respiratory syndrome (SARS)**

NORMAL PHYSIOLOGIC CHANGES

During pregnancy, the respiratory system adapts to the increased oxygenation needs of mother and fetus. See Chapter 10 for a discussion of these changes. The greatest stress to the respiratory system occurs after 24 weeks of gestation because of the increasing size of the fetus and placenta.

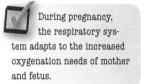

During pregnancy, the respiratory system adapts to the increased oxygenation needs of mother and fetus.

Because the woman must exhale carbon dioxide produced by the fetus, she will have mild hyperventilation and may feel slight shortness of breath. This increased ventilation produces a slight respiratory alkalosis. There is an increase in the binding capacity of maternal hemoglobin and a rise in maternal blood oxygen levels.

PATHOPHYSIOLOGY

If the pregnant woman has chronic or acute respiratory disease, she can develop **respiratory acidosis**. Conditions such as asthma, cystic fibrosis, tuberculosis, pneumonia, or bronchitis can cause obstruction from increased secretions or constriction of smooth muscles of the respiratory tract, and decrease the ability to exhale sufficient amounts of carbon dioxide. Therefore, carbon dioxide accumulates in the blood, blood pH decreases, and respiratory acidosis occurs.

ASTHMA

Asthma is the most common form of lung disease in pregnant women, occurring in 1 to 4% of pregnancies. Asthma is an allergic-type inflammatory response of the respiratory tract to various stimuli causing constriction of the airways. It is characterized by cough, chest tightness, dyspnea, and wheezing. The severity of the condition improves in one-third of pregnant women, remains unchanged in one-third, and worsens in one-third.

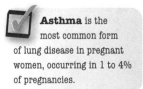

Asthma is the most common form of lung disease in pregnant women, occurring in 1 to 4% of pregnancies.

Almost half of pregnant women with asthma require adjustments in their therapy during pregnancy. Although asthma during pregnancy has been associated with an increase in perinatal mortality, premature birth, low birth weight, and hypoxia at birth, current research suggests there is no significant difference in preterm birth rate or other adverse perinatal outcomes in women with mild, well-controlled asthma.

If the woman needs steroid therapy to control asthma, she has an increased risk for developing gestational diabetes that may require insulin for control.

If asthma is severe or not properly treated, increases in cesarean deliveries and in intrauterine growth restriction have been demonstrated.

Medications used for management of asthma are considered safe during pregnancy and lactation, and women are encouraged to continue using the medications prescribed.

CYSTIC FIBROSIS

Cystic fibrosis (CF), a genetic defect resulting in abnormal production of mucus, primarily affects the respiratory, gastrointestinal, and genitourinary systems. CF is a severe chronic lung disease, controlled by vigorous pulmonary hygiene and administration of antibiotics. The goals of respiratory care are to decrease the amount of mucus in the lung fields to promote adequate oxygenation and to prevent pulmonary infections. With cystic fibrosis, the enzymes necessary to digest fats and proteins are not secreted by the pancreas, and essential nutrients are not absorbed. Therefore, pancreatic enzyme supplements are administered with all meals and snacks.

Because of improved medical treatment, more women with CF reach childbearing age. Women with CF may have problems of conception because of increased amounts of thick cervical mucus, but pregnancy does not worsen the disease and does not affect long-term

> The goals of respiratory care are to decrease the amount of mucus in the lung fields to promote adequate oxygenation and to prevent pulmonary infections.

> With cystic fibrosis, the enzymes necessary to digest fats and proteins are not secreted by the pancreas, and essential nutrients are not absorbed. Therefore, pancreatic enzyme supplements are administered with all meals and snacks.

survival rates. However, management techniques such as position for postural drainage need to be modified to accommodate the enlarging uterus, and nutritional intake, maternal weight gain, and fetal growth must be closely monitored.

RESPIRATORY INFECTIONS

The incidence of **tuberculosis (TB)** is increasing in women of childbearing years. Pregnant women in high-risk groups should be screened, which includes recent immigrants from countries in Central and South America, Africa, and Asia with a high prevalence of TB; members of low-income groups or ethnic/racial minorities; women with HIV; alcohol abusers; IV drug users; and women who have close contact with an infected person. An inactive TB infection is not reactivated by pregnancy and has no detrimental effect on the mother or fetus.

> An inactive TB infection is not reactivated by pregnancy and has no detrimental effect on the mother or fetus.

A pregnant woman with a positive skin test discovered during pregnancy has a shielded chest X ray to determine if active disease is present.

Medications used for treatment of TB include isoniazid, rifampin, ethambutol, and pyrazinamide. All of these drugs except pyrazinamide are considered safe for use during pregnancy.

> Pyrazinamide should be used only when necessary.

Supplemental vitamin B_6 is recommended with the administration of isoniazid.

After birth, the mother may breastfeed and care for her infant if the TB is inactive. If the disease is active, the mother should not care for her newborn until she is noninfectious.

Bronchitis and the **common cold** are the most common respiratory infections during pregnancy. Management of symptoms is the usual treatment: increased fluids, rest, use of air humidifier, and medications for cough and nasal congestion, as ordered by primary health care provider. Antibiotics should never be given for viral infections. Antihistamines are safe to use at any time during the pregnancy; oral decongestants should not be given during the first trimester.

Treatment of **pneumonia** during pregnancy includes the administration of a broad-spectrum antibiotic, followed by specific antibiotics after the sensitivity of the organism is known. Measures to relieve symptoms include cough suppressants, increased fluid intake, and antipyretics for fever.

 With globalization and rapid transportation, the threat of an international outbreak of an infectious disease such as **severe acute respiratory syndrome (SARS)** is greater than ever before. Therefore, health care providers must be vigilant in history taking and review of symptoms for the possibility of an exotic infection.

If a woman develops SARS during pregnancy, the goal is treatment of the disease with careful monitoring of the fetus. During the symptomatic part of the disease, contact and airborne precautions are necessary. While the woman is recuperating and asymptomatic, blood, breastmilk, and stool can contain the SARS corona virus.

It is important to implement universal precautions when caring for SARS patients.

Once she has recovered from the disease, routine prenatal care continues. Follow up of five infants born to women who had SARS during pregnancy did not reveal any evidence of SARS in the neonates.

The nurse must recognize the signs and symptoms of respiratory emergencies that can occur in the pregnant woman and take appropriate action. (See Table 48-1.)

Follow up of five infants born to women who had SARS during pregnancy did not reveal any evidence of SARS in the neonates.

Table 48-1 Respiratory Emergencies

Condition	Description
Adult Respiratory Distress Syndrome (ARDS)	Rare occurrence with possible etiology linked to DIC or inhalation of gastric contents during anesthesia. Progressive respiratory distress with dyspnea and tachypnea, progressive hypoxemia despite oxygen therapy, bilateral consolidation of lungs on X ray.
Amniotic fluid embolism	Very rare, but second leading cause of maternal death. During the birth process, a bolus of amniotic fluid enters the maternal circulation and moves to the lungs. Acute onset of respiratory distress with dyspnea, chest pain, cyanosis, loss of consciousness, pulmonary edema, circulatory collapse, coagulopathy, and death.

Table 48-1 Respiratory Emergencies (continued)

Condition	Description
Pulmonary embolism (PE)	Uncommon. Associated with thromboembolitic disease. Symptoms depend on the size and location of the obstruction and include chest pain, dyspnea, and tachypnea. A massive embolus causes sudden collapse, crushing substernal chest pain, shock, cyanosis, diaphoresis, loss of consciousness, and death.
Status asthmaticus	Rare. Acute, severe, prolonged asthma symptoms that do not respond to vigorous therapeutic measures. Worsening of cough, dyspnea, cyanosis, and hypoxemia. May lead to cardiac dysrhythmias, asphyxia, respiratory failure, and death.

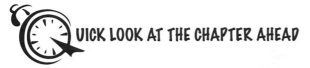

QUICK LOOK AT THE CHAPTER AHEAD

Cardiac disease is the leading nonobstetrical cause of maternal death.

The fetus of a woman with congenital heart disease has an increased risk of congenital cardiac abnormality.

The pregnant woman is most vulnerable for cardiac complication from gestation weeks 28 to 32 and in the first 48 hours postpartum.

For a woman with cardiac disease, counseling is important so that she can make an informed decision about maintaining the pregnancy.

Medical and nursing management focuses on preventing cardiac complications.

Vaginal birth is preferred because there are fewer hemodynamic changes than with cesarean delivery. After 36 weeks of gestation, labor may be induced if fetal lungs are mature.

The postpartum woman with cardiac disease should be monitored frequently.

Women with cardiac disease can breastfeed if they are careful.

Anemia during pregnancy decreases the oxygen-carrying capacity of the blood. Iron deficiency anemia is the most common type. It is treated with dietary counseling and iron supplements.

Folic acid deficiency anemia is similar to iron deficiency anemia, may occur with iron deficiency anemia, and is treated with folic acid supplements.

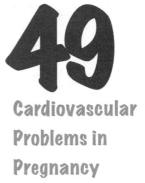

49

Cardiovascular Problems in Pregnancy

Sickle-cell anemia is an inherited autosomal recessive defect in hemoglobin formation. Treatment includes a good diet with iron and folic acid supplements.

Thalassesemia is another autosomal recessive defect in hemoglobin formation. Pregnant women with mild thalassesemia are treated with folic acid supplements.

The risk for thrombophlebitis with deep vein thrombosis (DVT) increases during pregnancy, but the highest incidence occurs postpartum. Anticoagulation therapy with heparin is safe, along with bedrest and elevation of the affected extremity.

 Nurses need to understand the normal hemodynamic changes and common cardiovascular complications that can occur during the perinatal period. Normal hemodynamic changes and adaptations in the perinatal period that increase the work required of the heart are discussed in Chapter 10.

TERMS

- ☐ cardiac disease
- ☐ maternal hypoxemia
- ☐ cardiac decompensation
- ☐ cardiac valvular disease
- ☐ anemia: iron-deficiency, folic acid deficiency, sickle-cell
- ☐ sickle-cell crisis
- ☐ thalassesemia
- ☐ thrombophlebitis
- ☐ deep vein thrombosis (DVT)
- ☐ pulmonary embolism (PE)

CARDIAC DISEASE

Cardiac disease occurs in up to 2% of pregnant women. Classification of heart disease is usually based upon the functional capacity of the heart. (See Table 49-1 for descriptions and pregnancy implications.)

 Cardiac disease is the leading nonobstetrical cause of maternal death.

Mortality risk associated with cardiac defects and pregnancy depends upon the specific type of cardiac lesion, functional capacity of the heart, and the development of pregnancy-related complications.

Maternal hypoxemia in women with cardiac complications increases the incidence of miscarriage, IUGR, fetal hypoxemia, preterm labor and birth, and stillbirth. The fetus of a woman with congenital heart disease has an increased risk of congenital cardiac abnormality.

In a woman with cardiac disease, the increased workload of pregnancy can stress the heart, resulting in symptoms of **cardiac decompensation**: fatigue, dyspnea, palpitations, and edema. The pregnant woman is most vulnerable for this complication from 28 to 32 weeks of gestation and in the first 48 hours postpartum.

Table 49-1 Functional Classification of Cardiac Disease

Class	Description	Pregnancy Implications
I	Cardiac disease present and asymptomatic with any activity.	Usually experiences normal pregnancy, labor, and birth. No activity restrictions.
II	Ordinary activity causes symptoms of fatigue, dyspnea, palpitations, or anginal pain.	Pregnancy, labor, or birth may worsen symptoms. Needs careful monitoring for decreased functional capacity of the heart. Slight activity restriction may be advised and excessive weight gain should be avoided.
III	Symptomatic with less than ordinary activity, comfortable at rest.	Marked restriction of physical activity is advised. Can have severe cardiac complications during pregnancy, labor, delivery, or early postpartum.
IV	Symptomatic at rest. Unable to perform any physical activity because of cardiac insufficiency.	Pregnancy would not be recommended because of increased maternal and fetal morbidity and mortality.

For a woman with cardiac disease, counseling is important so that she can make informed decisions about maintaining the pregnancy in relation to health risks.

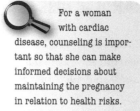

For a woman with cardiac disease, counseling is important so that she can make informed decisions about maintaining the pregnancy in relation to health risks.

Medical and nursing management focuses on prevention of cardiac complications. Antepartum care includes control of weight gain, activity restriction or bedrest to control cardiac symptoms, detection and treatment of anemia or hypertension, fetal surveillance for signs of hypoxia, and treatment of preterm labor with magnesium sulfate if necessary.

Tocolysis with terbutaline is contraindicated with maternal cardiac disease because it increases the pulse rate and the cardiac workload.

Drugs used in the treatment of cardiac disease include heparin, furosemide, and digitalis; these drugs are safe to use during pregnancy.

Intrapartal management includes conservation of energy through adequate pain control, careful positioning during labor, prevention of hypotension, and use of forceps or vacuum extractor during birth to prevent maternal fatigue.

Women with **cardiac valvular disease** are usually given prophylactic antibiotics during labor to prevent bacterial endocarditis.

Vaginal birth is preferred because there are fewer hemodynamic changes than with cesarean delivery. Induction of labor after 36 weeks of gestation may be indicated if fetal lungs are mature.

In the first 48 hours postpartum, blood flow to the heart and cardiac output increase, putting great stress on the heart. See Chapter 23 for cardiovascular changes in postpartum. The postpartum woman with cardiac disease needs to be monitored frequently and assessed for signs of cardiac decompensation. A gradual return to usual activities with periods of rest is recommended. Follow-up care and family planning are important.

Women with cardiac disease can breastfeed if they are careful to prevent fatigue and if the medications they are taking are not harmful to the infant.

ANEMIA DURING PREGNANCY

Anemia during pregnancy decreases the oxygen-carrying capacity of the blood. Symptoms include pallor, fatigue, and activity intolerance. Anemia complicates up to 25% of pregnancies and can be caused by maternal adaptation to the pregnant state, inadequate nutrition, or genetic defects in red blood cell production. The increase in blood volume that occurs during pregnancy can lead to physiologic anemia. The medical diagnosis of anemia is determined by a hemoglobin less than 11 g/dL and hematocrit less than 35%. See Chapter 10 for a description of physiologic anemia of pregnancy.

> Anemia during pregnancy decreases the oxygen-carrying capacity of the blood. Symptoms include pallor, fatigue, and activity intolerance.

Iron deficiency anemia is the most common type of anemia during pregnancy. It increases the risk for infection, delays healing time, and decreases the energy level postpartum. The fetus will receive necessary iron for growth and development, while maternal iron stores become depleted, leading to symptoms of anemia. Treatment includes dietary counseling and iron supplementation.

Folic acid deficiency anemia is similar to iron deficiency anemia, may occur with iron deficiency anemia, and is treated with folic acid supplements.

Sickle-cell anemia is an inherited autosomal recessive defect in hemoglobin formation, resulting in red blood cells that are elongated and crescent-shaped. It is more common in people of African American or Mediterranean descent.

Painful **sickle-cell crises** occur because the crescent-shaped red blood cells cause stasis and clumping that leads to blockage of the blood vessel. The woman with sickle-cell anemia during pregnancy has increased risk for infection, gestational hypertension, preterm birth, placental insufficiency, and IUGR. Sickle-cell crises occur more frequently during the second half of pregnancy and may be very severe. Strategies to prevent sickle-cell crises include screening for and treating infections, preventing dehydration, and reducing stress. If a crisis occurs, it is managed with pain control, hydration, oxygen therapy, and

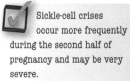

> Sickle-cell crises occur more frequently during the second half of pregnancy and may be very severe.

blood transfusion if necessary. Treatment includes a good diet with iron and folic acid supplements.

Thalassesemia, an autosomal recessive disorder, is another defect in hemoglobin formation causing a shortened life span of the red blood cells. It is seen most often in people of Mediterranean or Southeast Asian descent. Women with a severe form of this disease are usually infertile. Pregnant women with a mild form of thalassesemia are treated with folic acid supplements; iron supplements are not given.

 Strategies to prevent sickle-cell crises include screening for and treating infections, preventing dehydration, and reducing stress. If a crisis occurs, it is managed with pain control, hydration, oxygen therapy, and blood transfusion if necessary. Treatment includes a good diet with iron and folic acid supplements.

THROMBOEMBOLYTIC DISEASE

Pregnancy predisposes women to the development of thromboses because of increased levels of clotting factors and increased stasis in the lower extremities. Although the risk for **thrombophlebitis** with **deep vein thrombosis (DVT)** increases during pregnancy, the highest incidence of this complication occurs during the postpartum period. Pregnant women at greatest risk are those with a history of thromboembolytic disease, obesity, advanced maternal age, increased parity, cesarean delivery, or prolonged bedrest. See Chapter 25 for signs and symptoms of thrombophlebitis.

During diagnostic radiologic procedures, exposure of the fetus to radiation is minimized by shielding the pelvis when possible.

When a DVT is diagnosed, anticoagulation therapy with heparin is safe for use during pregnancy and breastfeeding. Additional management includes bedrest with elevation of the affected extremity. A severe complication, **pulmonary embolism (PE)**, may occur. See Chapter 48 for a description of this respiratory emergency.

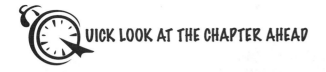

Perinatal infections affect both mother and fetus. Here are the ones that present the greatest risk.

Bacterial vaginosis (BV) is usually treated with oral metronidazole (Flagyl).

All pregnant women should be screened for chlamydia and gonorrhea because most cases are asymptomatic. Chlamydia is treated during pregnancy with erythromycin. Gonorrhea should be treated in both sexual partners with a cephalosporin antibiotic.

All infants are treated with erythromycin ophthalmic ointment to prevent conjunctivitis and ophthalmia neonatorum.

Group B streptococcus (GBS) is the most common cause of life-threatening neonatal infection. If a woman is identified as a GBS carrier, prophylactic antibiotics are given at the onset of labor or with rupture of membranes.

Pregnant women are given counseling and offered screening for human immunodeficiency virus (HIV) as part of routine prenatal care. With antiretroviral therapy, transmission to the fetus is about 8%. Breastfeeding is contraindicated for HIV-infected women.

Human papillomavirus (HPV) does not have an adverse effect on the growth or development of the fetus and does not increase the risk of obstetrical complications.

50

Infections During Pregnancy

All pregnant women should be screened for syphilis as part of their prenatal care and treated with penicillin if positive.

A TORCH screen may be done to detect the presence of five teratogenic perinatal infections: toxoplasmosis, hepatitis B, rubella, cytomegalovirus, and herpes simplex.

Pregnant women are at higher risk for the development of urinary tract infection (UTI), and are screened at the initial prenatal visit, at 32 to 34 weeks of gestation, and if there are complaints of any signs or symptoms. UTIs are treated with appropriate antibiotics.

TERMS

- ☐ bacterial vaginosis (BV)
- ☐ chlamydia
- ☐ gonorrhea
- ☐ group B streptococcus (GBS)
- ☐ human immunodeficiency virus (HIV)
- ☐ syphilis
- ☐ TORCH
- ☐ urinary tract infection (UTI)

Exposure in the first trimester to perinatal infections increases the risk for miscarriage or congenital fetal defects. Infections later in pregnancy increase the risk of intrauterine growth restriction, central nervous system abnormalities, stillbirth, and neonatal death.

About 15% of all pregnancies are complicated by active maternal infection. There is an increased incidence of genitourinary tract infections. Moreover, the organisms are becoming more drug resistant. Although a pregnant woman may have any type of infection, only the ones that present the greatest risk to the fetus or newborn are discussed in this chapter.

BACTERIAL VAGINOSIS (BV)

Bacterial vaginosis occurs in up to 20% of all pregnancies because of the disturbances in the natural flora due to changes in the pH of vaginal secretions. It increases the risk of miscarriage, premature rupture of membranes, preterm labor, postpartum endometritis, and neonatal septicemia. Treatment is usually with oral metronidazole (Flagyl). If treated during breastfeeding, the woman is instructed to pump and discard the breastmilk for 24 hours after receiving the medication.

CHLAMYDIA

Chlamydia is the most common sexually transmitted disease in the United States. Thirty percent of pregnant women are infected with the organism. All pregnant women should be screened for it because 75% of cases are asymptomatic.

Untreated chlamydia infections can lead to pelvic inflammatory disease (PID).

Treatment for chlamydia during pregnancy is administration of erythromycin; tetracycline, doxycycline, and ofloxacin are contraindicated during pregnancy because of harmful effects on the development of fetal teeth and cartilage.

Infants born to women with chlamydial infection have an increased risk of developing pneumonia or conjunctivitis leading to blindness.

Erythromycin ophthalmic ointment is administered to all newborns to prevent conjunctivitis.

GONORRHEA

Pregnant women should also be screened for **gonorrhea**, an often asymptomatic sexually transmitted disease. Untreated gonorrhea increases the risk for miscarriage, PID, preterm labor, premature rupture of the membranes, intrauterine infection, and urinary tract infections. The treatment of choice is a cephalosporin antibiotic. It is important to treat both sexual partners to prevent reinfection. All infants are treated with erythromycin ophthalmic ointment to prevent ophthalmia neonatorum that can cause blindness.

GROUP B STREPTOCOCCUS

Group B streptococcus (GBS) is the most common cause of life-threatening neonatal infection. GBS is found in the maternal genital and lower intestinal tract and may be transmitted to the infant at the time of birth.

> **Group B streptococcus (GBS)** is the most common cause of life-threatening neonatal infection.

The Centers for Disease Control recommends that all pregnant women be screened for GBS in vaginal and rectal cultures between 35 and 37 weeks of gestation. If a woman is identified as a GBS carrier, prophylactic antibiotics are given at the onset of labor or with rupture of membranes.

If the GBS status in unknown at the onset of labor, intrapartum antibiotics are given to women at less than 37 weeks of gestation, with membranes ruptured 18 or more hours, or with a temperature elevation equal to or greater than 100.4°F (38.0°C).

HUMAN IMMUNODEFICIENCY VIRUS (HIV)

Pregnant women should be given counseling and offered **HIV** screening as part of routine prenatal care. If the woman is found to be HIV positive, appropriate treatment of the disease is initiated to decrease the viral load to an undetectable level. The effect of pregnancy on the progression of

HIV/AIDS is unclear. Women are counseled that most medications used in the treatment of HIV are safe for use during pregnancy.

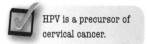

The effect of pregnancy on the progression of HIV/AIDS is unclear.

Transmission of HIV to the fetus is approximately 30% without treatment. With antiretroviral therapy, transmission rate is reduced to about 8%. Cesarean delivery before rupture of membranes reduces the risk of transmission to the newborn and is recommended to women with a viral load greater than 1000.

After birth, infants usually test positive for the HIV antibody for up to 18 months, reflecting the passive transfer of maternal antibodies. If the infant has not been infected, this positive response will convert to negative.

Breastfeeding is contraindicated for HIV-infected women because the virus can be transmitted via breastmilk.

HUMAN PAPILLOMAVIRUS (HPV)

HPV is the most common viral sexually transmitted disease in all women. It does not have an adverse effect on the growth or development of the fetus and does not increase the risk of obstetrical complications. However, genital warts may grow rapidly, can obstruct the vaginal canal, and may bleed heavily during pregnancy or birth due to increased vascularity. Cesarean delivery may be indicated if the warts are very large or the risk of hemorrhage is great. HPV is a precursor of cervical cancer.

HPV is a precursor of cervical cancer.

SYPHILIS

All pregnant women should be screened for **syphilis** as part of their prenatal care and treated with penicillin if positive. Congenital syphilis may lead to spontaneous abortion, preterm labor, stillbirth, or congenital defects. Treatment before 16 weeks of gestation usually prevents congenital syphilis; after this time treatment will eliminate the infection in the mother, but the fetus may already be damaged.

TORCH

A **TORCH** screen may be done to detect the presence of five teratogenic perinatal infections: toxoplasmosis, hepatitis B, rubella, cytomegalovirus, and herpes simplex. (See Table 50-1.)

URINARY TRACT INFECTION (UTI)

Pregnant women are at higher risk for the development of **urinary tract infections** because of structural changes in the urinary tract. See Chapter 10 for changes to the urinary system brought about by pregnancy. No symptoms of a UTI occur in 5 to 10% of women. UTIs are associated with low birth weight, preterm labor and birth, hypertension, preeclampsia, maternal anemia, IUGR, and intrauterine infection. Pregnant women are screened for UTI at the initial prenatal visit, at 32 to 34 weeks of gestation, and if there are complaints of any signs or symptoms. UTIs are treated with appropriate antibiotics.

Table 50-1 TORCH Infections

Infection	Maternal/Neonatal Effects	Implications
Toxoplasmosis	Increased risk of miscarriage and premature labor or birth, IUGR, microcephaly, hydrocephaly, neurological, opthalmological, cognitive effects.	Recommend not eating undercooked or raw meat. Avoid exposure to cat feces since this is a mode of transmission.
Other/ Hepatitis B	Increased risk of premature labor and birth if active disease occurs in the third trimester. Infant may be infected at birth if mother has acute infection or is a carrier and has a 90% chance of becoming a carrier if not treated.	If the mother is positive for hepatitis B, newborn should receive hepatitis B immunoglobulin (HBIG) within 12 hours of birth, in addition to hepatitis B vaccine according to recommended immunization protocol.
Rubella	If mother develops the disease during the first 16 weeks of pregnancy, high incidence of deafness, cataracts, heart or CNS defects, and developmental delays.	Screen all pregnant women with rubella antibody titers. If not immune, recommend rubella vaccination postpartum.
Cytomegalovirus	95% of women are asymptomatic. Newborn exhibits IUGR, microcephaly, CNS abnormalities, deafness, blindness, jaundice, enlarged liver and spleen, or developmental delays.	Recommend good personal hygiene. Transmitted through personal contact with infected saliva, cervical mucus, semen, and urine. No treatment available.
Herpes simplex	Painful lesions on cervix, vagina, or external genitals. If fetus is exposed to active primary lesions during vaginal birth, there is a 50% chance of infection. Recurrent maternal infections have a 3–5% risk of transmission. Infant mortality up to 60% if neonate develops the infection.	If active lesions are present at onset of labor, cesarean delivery is indicated. Antiviral therapy may be given to the mother near term to prevent a recurrence. In 70% of neonatal infections, there is no history of genital herpes or evidence of lesions, so a thorough history and physical examination are important. Infected infants are treated with antiviral medications.

PART IX • QUESTIONS

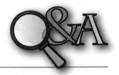

1. When planning dietary management for a pregnant woman with diabetes, the nurse considers perinatal insulin requirements. Which statement about perinatal insulin needs is most accurate?
   a. Insulin requirements in the first trimester are increased due to the influence of anterior pituitary hormones.
   b. In the second and third trimesters, insulin needs increase as placental hormone production increases.
   c. During labor, additional insulin is needed to provide energy for delivery.
   d. Loss of placental hormones after delivery rapidly increases insulin needs.

2. List three obstetrical complications for which there is increased risk in the pregnant diabetic, and give one assessment technique for the detection of each complication.

Table Q-3

Complication	Assessment parameter

3. A pregestational diabetic woman is hospitalized at 10 weeks of gestation for adjustments in insulin dosage. She reports to the nurse that she has a headache and feels shaky and cold. What would be the first action by the nurse?
   a. Check blood sugar level.
   b. Give a carbohydrate snack.
   c. Provide a warm blanket.
   d. Take her blood pressure.

4. When providing postpartum discharge instructions for the gestational diabetic, what information should the nurse include?

a. Breastfeeding will increase insulin requirements for the mother but is recommended for the health of the infant.

b. If she was taking insulin during the pregnancy, she will need to take insulin for the rest of her life.

c. Low-dose combined oral contraceptives are not recommended for family planning.

d. Maintaining a normal weight will decrease the risk of developing type 2 diabetes later in life.

5. A prenatal client at 11 weeks of gestation with a history of steroid-controlled asthma asks the nurse if she should continue to take her medication. What would be the best response by the nurse?

a. "Asthma treatment medications can cause birth defects, so you should wait until after the first trimester to take them."

b. "Because pregnancy often makes asthma worse, you will need your medications more than ever."

c. "There is a higher risk of gestational diabetes because you take steroids for your asthma."

d. "You should continue to take your medications when you need them because you need to maintain control of the asthma."

6. Based on prenatal history information, for which client would the nurse expect a medical order for tuberculosis skin testing?

a. 17-year-old Hispanic G1 P0 who immigrated from Central America 6 months ago.

b. 21-year-old African American G2 P1 who works in a day-care center.

c. 29-year-old Caucasian G5 P3 who works in a clothing store.

d. 32-year-old Asian American G2 P0 who has a history of asthma.

7. When caring for a woman in second-stage labor with Class I cardiac disease, what action by the nurse would be most appropriate?

a. Encourage her to push with contractions.

b. Maintain side-lying position.

c. Monitor maternal oxygen saturation.

d. Prepare for forceps delivery.

8. Which complaint by a postpartum patient with thrombophlebitis is most significant?
   a. "A red area has appeared behind my knee."
   b. "I have noticed pain in back of my calf when I walk."
   c. "My chest hurts when I take a deep breath."
   d. "There is more swelling in my left foot today."

9. Prophylactic antibiotic eye ointment is administered to the newborn shortly after birth to prevent infection from what two organisms?
   a. _____
   b. _____

10. The record of a woman in labor indicates she is positive for group B streptococcus (GBS). What nursing care would be most appropriate?
    a. Administer vaccination postpartum.
    b. Explain contraindications of breastfeeding.
    c. Give prophylactic antibiotics.
    d. Prepare for cesarean delivery.

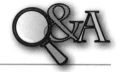

PART IX · ANSWERS AND RATIONALES

1. **The answer is b.** The insulin-resistant properties of placental hormones increase insulin requirements during the second and third trimesters. Option a is incorrect because insulin needs decrease during the first trimester due to the inhibition of anterior pituitary hormones. Option c is incorrect because the increased metabolism during labor decreases insulin need. Option d is incorrect because after delivery of the placenta there is no longer insulin resistance from placental hormones and insulin needs decrease.

2. **Any three of these complications and any one of the assessment techniques for each complication would be an appropriate answer.**

    Table Q-4

Complication	Assessment paramenters
Preeclampsia or pregnancy-induced hypertension (PIH)	Elevated blood pressure, protein in the urine, sudden weight gain, and pathologic edema
Preterm labor	Report of signs and symptoms, vaginal exam or ultrasound to detect cervical changes
Polyhydramnios	Fundal height, biophysical profile (BPP) to measure amniotic fluid volume
Macrosomia	Fundal height, ultrasound for fetal measurements
Uteroplacental insufficiency	Nonstress tests, biophysical profiles (BPP)

3. **The answer is a.** A woman is reporting signs of hypoglycemia. The first nursing action would be to check her blood sugar level. Further interventions would be determined in response to the

blood sugar level. Option b is incorrect because a carbohydrate snack should not be given until a blood sugar is known. Option c is not the most appropriate first choice because it is not related to recognizing that the woman is exhibiting symptoms indicative of hypoglycemia. Option d is incorrect because the blood sugar level is the most significant information to obtain.

4. **The answer is d.** Gestational diabetes increases the risk of developing type 2 diabetes within the following 20 years. Maintaining a normal weight through appropriate diet and exercise reduces this risk. Option a is incorrect; breastfeeding decreases insulin needs because of carbohydrate use in milk production. Option b is incorrect because the woman required insulin due to the insulin-resistant properties of placental hormones, not because the pancreas was unable to produce insulin. Once the placenta is delivered, hormone levels decrease and the resistance to insulin diminishes. Option c is incorrect because low-dose combined oral contraceptives are safe for women if there is no evidence of vascular compromise.

5. **The answer is d.** Pregnant women with asthma are encouraged to continue using the medications prescribed because any condition that interferes with maternal oxygenation can lead to decreased fetal oxygenation. Option a is incorrect because medications used for management of asthma are considered safe during pregnancy. There is no evidence that they cause birth defects. Option b is incorrect because in two-thirds of pregnant women with asthma, pregnancy improves the condition or it remains the same. Only one-third of women with asthma have a worsening of the condition. Option c is not the best choice because although the information is correct, it does not answer the client's question about continuing to take prescribed medications.

6. **The answer is a.** Pregnant women in high-risk groups should be screened for tuberculosis. The client in option a is in a high-risk category because she is a recent immigrant from an area of the world with a high incidence of tuberculosis. The information about the clients in the other options does not indicate that they are members of high-risk groups.

7. **The answer is a.** The woman with Class I cardiac disease can experience normal pregnancy, labor, and birth. She would be encouraged

to push during the second stage of labor. The other options indicate intrapartal labor management for women who have Class II or higher cardiac disease.

8. **The correct answer is c.** Chest pain is indicative of pulmonary embolism, a severe complication of thrombophlebitis. The other options describe worsening of the symptoms of thrombophlebitis (swelling, redness, and pain) but they are not as significant as chest pain.

9. **The correct answers are chlamydia and gonorrhea.**

10. **The correct answer is c.** Prophylactic antibiotics are given at the onset of labor or with rupture of membranes to women positive for group B streptococcus (GBS). Option a is incorrect because there is no vaccination for GBS. Option b is incorrect because breastfeeding would not be contraindicated with GBS. Option d is not the best choice because GBS is not an indication for cesarean delivery, as is an active herpes infection.

X

Complications of Labor, Delivery, and Postpartum

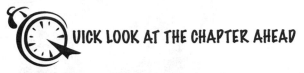

Labor stimulation can be classified as induction or augmentation. Induction initiates uterine contractions before the onset of spontaneous labor. Augmentation stimulates the contraction pattern of a woman in labor.

Risks calling for induction are postterm gestation, maternal diabetes, renal or cardiac disease, hypertensive disorders, premature rupture of membranes, oligohydramnios, intrauterine growth restriction, non-reassuring antenatal testing, isoimmunization, and fetal death.

Contraindications to induction are complete placenta previa, placental abruption, prolapsed cord, acute fetal distress, previous classic uterine incision, cephalopelvic disproportion, and active herpes.

The Bishop scoring system predicts cervical readiness for induction: dilation in centimeters, percentage of effacement, station of presenting part, consistency of cervix, and cervical position, each scored from 0 to 3.

Cervical ripening can be accomplished by using prostaglandin E2 gels, cervical dilators, or a Foley catheter bulb in the cervical canal.

Procedures for stimulation of contractions include stripping the membranes, amniotomy, and administration of oxytocin.

A decision for labor induction may result in a cascade of other interventions that affect the birth process.

51

Stimulation of Labor

Dysfunctional labor may call for augmentation of labor by medical means only after ensuring the bladder is empty, encouraging ambulation if appropriate, and assessing for adequate hydration. The usual medical procedures are amniotomy and oxytocin administration.

 Because stimulation of labor is associated with interventions that increase risks for mother and fetus, the nurse must understand issues related to labor-stimulation techniques when caring for women in labor.

 The incidence of interventions to stimulate labor is increasing in the United States.

TERMS

☐ induction
☐ Bishop scoring system
☐ cervical ripening
☐ amniotomy
☐ oxytocin
☐ uterine dystocia
☐ augmentation

INDUCTION

The American College of Obstetricians and Gynecologists recommends **induction** of labor when the benefits of birth are greater than the risks of continuing the pregnancy.

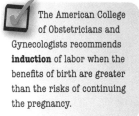

The American College of Obstetricians and Gynecologists recommends **induction** of labor when the benefits of birth are greater than the risks of continuing the pregnancy.

Common indications for induction include postterm gestation, maternal diabetes, renal or cardiac disease, hypertensive disorders, premature rupture of membranes, oligohydramnios, intrauterine growth restriction, non-reassuring antenatal testing, isoimmunization, and fetal death.

Contraindications for induction include complete placenta previa, placental abruption, prolapsed cord, acute fetal distress, previous classic uterine incision, cephalopelvic disproportion, and active herpes.

Cervical Readiness

The success of the induction depends on the ability of the cervix to efface and dilate. A cervix that is soft, anterior, and beginning to efface and dilate is considered ripe for induction.

The **Bishop scoring system** is used to predict the readiness of a woman's cervix for induction of labor. The five parameters of dilation in centimeters, percentage of effacement, station of presenting part, consistency of cervix, and cervical position are each given a score from 0 to 3. The higher the score, the more responsive the cervix would be to induction.

Cervical ripening can be accomplished by using prostaglandin E2 gels, cervical dilators, or a Foley catheter bulb in the cervical canal. Prostaglandins soften and ripen the cervix by increasing water absorption of the tissues, increasing the frequency of prelabor contractions, and increasing the number of oxytocin receptors in the uterine muscle. Cervical dilators made of seaweed or synthetic materials and Foley catheter bulbs provide physical pressure on the internal cervical os, promoting ripeness by softening and dilation.

Stimulation of Contractions

Procedures for stimulation of contractions include stripping the membranes, amniotomy, and administration of oxytocin. When stripping the membranes a physician or certified nurse midwife inserts a finger into the internal cervical os and turns the finger full circle twice. This action loosens the amniotic membranes from the lower uterine segment and may release prostaglandins that stimulate uterine contractions.

Amniotomy is the artificial rupture of the amniotic membranes and may be performed to induce the beginning of labor. The primary health care provider inserts an instrument into the cervix; a small tear is made in the amniotic membrane and fluid is released. Two serious complications of amniotomy are prolapsed cord if the presenting part is not engaged and increased risk of infection if birth does not occur within 24 hours.

Use of Oxytocin

Oxytocin is a hormone secreted by the posterior pituitary that stimulates smooth muscle contractions of the uterus. Oxytocin receptors within the uterus become more sensitive as estrogen levels increase throughout pregnancy. Intravenous administration of oxytocin produces regular contractions and initiates labor.

> Because there are risks to mother and fetus involved in the administration of oxytocin, this drug is used with caution. (See Table 51-1.)

Other Interventions

A decision for labor induction may result in a cascade of other interventions that affect the birth process.

- Restrictions on ambulation because of the intravenous line and continuous electronic fetal monitoring may influence the rate of effacement and dilation, thereby slowing labor.
- Greater pain from contractions stimulated with oxytocin increases the need for epidural anesthesia. See Chapter 22 for side effects of epidural anesthesia.
- Obstetrical procedures such as amniotomy and placement of fetal scalp electrode or intrauterine pressure catheter increase the risk of infection and umbilical cord prolapse.
- When induction of labor occurs, the risk for cesarean delivery significantly increases.

Table 51-1 Key Concepts About Oxytocin Administration

Explain the procedure to the woman and her family. The latent phase of labor is usually shorter because of more frequent contractions. Contractions stimulated by oxytocin may be more painful than contractions associated with spontaneous labor. Once active labor is achieved, there is usually little difference in labor progress.

Before initiation of oxytocin, the fetus is assessed by a baseline 20-minute monitor strip.

Continuous electronic monitoring of fetal heart rate and contraction pattern must be done throughout oxytocin administration.

A primary intravenous line is started and oxytocin is administered through a piggybacked secondary line and controlled by an infusion pump.

The initial dose of oxytocin is low and is gradually increased, based on observation of contraction pattern, fetal heart rate, and maternal blood pressure according to physician order.

The goal of oxytocin administration is a uterine contraction pattern sufficient to accomplish a vaginal birth. The frequency of contractions should be 2 to 3 minutes apart, the duration of contractions should be no more than 90 seconds, and cervical dilation should progress at least 1 centimeter per hour.

Ongoing assessments include frequency, duration, and intensity of contractions; uterine resting tone; fetal heart rate pattern; blood pressure; effacement; and dilation.

Risks associated with the use of oxytocin result from hyperstimulation of the uterus and include placental abruption; fetal hypoxia; trauma to cervix, vagina, perineum, or fetus; uterine rupture; and amniotic fluid embolism. Because oxytocin has an antidiuretic effect, prolonged infusion at a high rate can lead to water intoxication. Also, the administration of oxytocin during labor may increase the risk of uterine atony leading to postpartum hemorrhage. Therefore, oxytocin infusion is usually continued in the early postpartum period to keep the uterus contracted.

The oxytocin infusion is discontinued if late or variable decelerations or bradycardia occur, uterine contractions have a frequency of less than 2 minutes or a duration more than 90 seconds, or if the uterus does not return to the baseline resting tone between contractions. The woman is turned to her left side, the flow rate of the primary intravenous line is increased, oxygen is administered, and the physician is notified.

AUGMENTATION

During the course of labor, **uterine dysto-cia** or ineffective uterine contractions may occur. When dysfunctional labor is present, augmentation of labor may be required. **Augmentation** with medical means is carried out only after noninvasive methods such as ensuring the bladder is empty, encouraging ambulation if appropriate, and assessing for adequate hydration are done.

The two usual medical procedures for augmentation are amniotomy and oxytocin administration. After amniotomy, there is more pressure on the cervix from the fetal presenting part. This may stimulate stronger contractions if the woman is more than 4 centimeters dilated. With augmentation of labor, nursing care is the same as in induction of labor.

Greater sensitivity to the oxytocin may be exhibited since the woman is already producing some oxytocin. Therefore, small increases in oxytocin dosage are used.

Augmentation with medical means is carried out only after noninvasive methods such as ensuring the bladder is empty, encouraging ambulation if appropriate, and assessing for adequate hydration are done.

With augmentation of labor, nursing care is the same as in induction of labor.

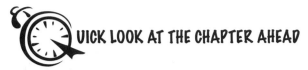
Cesarean is a safe surgical procedure for delivery of the fetus through an incision in the uterus.

A transverse incision in the lower uterine segment is preferred because it allows for a subsequent vaginal birth after cesarean (VBAC). The classic vertical incision is usually done only in an extreme emergency.

Risks to the mother include reactions to anesthesia, infection, hemorrhage, and development of clots or emboli.

The primary risk to the newborn is decreased lung-fluid clearance leading to respiratory distress. Also, the infant may experience prematurity or hypoxia.

Women who had a previous cesarean with a low transverse uterine incision for twins, placenta previa, or breech presentation can be encouraged to attempt labor and vaginal birth after cesarean (VBAC).

VBAC should only be attempted if the facility and staff are prepared, with 24-hour blood banking, electronic fetal monitoring, continuous anesthesia coverage, and adequate perioperative staff.

The most common risk of VBAC is uterine rupture and hemorrhage. Close monitoring during labor is essential.

Prostaglandin agents are not recommended for induction of labor. Oxytocin may be used with extreme caution.

52

Cesarean Delivery: Overview

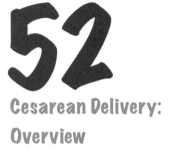

Because maternity nurses may assist at any phase of perioperative care, it is important to understand the techniques and the effects of cesarean delivery on the woman and her newborn.

TERMS
- [ ] transverse incision
- [ ] classic vertical incision
- [ ] vaginal birth after cesarean (VBAC)

Approximately 25% of pregnant women deliver by cesarean procedure in the United States. This rate is influenced by many factors, including the increased use of electronic fetal monitoring, increased rate of elective induction, and fear of malpractice suits.

DEFINITIONS AND INDICATIONS

Cesarean delivery is a surgical procedure for delivery of the fetus through an incision in the uterus. The first cesarean delivery is called a primary cesarean delivery; any additional births by cesarean are called repeat cesareans. In addition, a cesarean may be either scheduled or emergency. In a scheduled cesarean, the woman and her family have time to prepare emotionally for this type of delivery. In an emergency, preparation for and explanations about the procedure take place rapidly.

Incisions in the skin and the uterus can be made either horizontally or vertically. (See Figure 52-1.) The incision in the uterus is significant. A **transverse incision** in the lower uterine segment is preferred because there is less chance of rupture during a subsequent pregnancy and labor, therefore allowing for vaginal birth after cesarean (VBAC). In an extreme emergency, a **classic vertical incision** may be made in the uterus.

Indications for cesarean delivery include fetal distress, fetal abnormality such as myelomeningocele, abnormal fetal presentations such as breech, macrosomia, active genital herpes, cephalopelvic disproportion (CPD), placenta previa, placental abruption, prolapsed umbilical cord, previous

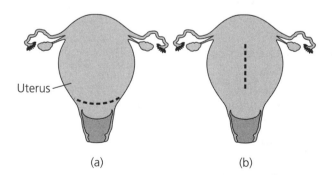

Figure 52-1 Uterine incisions: (a) Low tranverse incision. (b) Classic incision.

cesarean, previous classic uterine incision, or failure to progress in labor. There is controversy about scheduling a cesarean delivery to prevent pelvic-organ prolapse that can lead to pain and urinary incontinence.

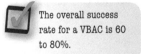 There is controversy about scheduling a cesarean delivery to prevent pelvic-organ prolapse that can lead to pain and urinary incontinence.

 ## MATERNAL AND NEONATAL RISKS

Although a cesarean delivery has higher maternal risks than a vaginal one, it is a safe surgical procedure with few complications. Risks to the mother include reactions to anesthesia, infection, hemorrhage, and development of clots or emboli. Usual blood loss during a cesarean delivery is 400 to 800 ml, twice that of a vaginal one. Greater than 1000 ml blood loss is considered hemorrhage.

The primary risk to the newborn from a cesarean delivery is decreased lung fluid clearance because of lack of chest compression at the time of birth. This may lead to respiratory distress. Also, because a cesarean is often performed when there is a high-risk situation, the infant may experience the problems of prematurity or hypoxia.

 ## VAGINAL BIRTH AFTER CESAREAN (VBAC)

Women who have had a previous cesarean with a low transverse uterine incision for a nonrecurring indication such as twins, placenta previa, or breech presentation may be encouraged to attempt a trial of labor and **vaginal birth after cesarean (VBAC)**. The overall success rate for a VBAC is 60 to 80%.

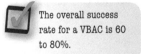 The overall success rate for a VBAC is 60 to 80%.

Contraindications to VBAC include a previous classic uterine incision, previous uterine surgery, more than two previous cesarean deliveries, a contracted pelvis, or a medical or obstetrical complication that would make vaginal birth an inappropriate option.

A VBAC should only be attempted if the facility and staff are prepared for emergency cesarean delivery with 24-hour blood banking, electronic fetal monitoring, continuous anesthesia coverage, and adequate perioperative staff.

The most common risk of VBAC is uterine rupture and hemorrhage. For this reason, close monitoring during labor with assessments of uterine contraction pattern and fetal heart rate is essential.

Signs and symptoms of uterine rupture are a non-reassuring fetal heart rate pattern, acute and continuous abdominal pain, vaginal bleeding, hematuria, irregular contour of the abdominal wall, and hypovolemic shock.

Prostaglandin agents are not recommended for induction of labor. Oxytocin may be used with extreme caution for induction or augmentation of labor during VBAC. Particular attention is given to signs of uterine hyperstimulation, at which time the oxytocin is discontinued immediately.

Although the risk of uterine rupture from a low transverse incision is minimal, it is an emergency when it happens. For this reason, the trend for VBAC has decreased in recent years.

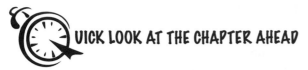

Preparation procedures for a cesarean delivery are: insertion of an intravenous line and an indwelling bladder catheter. Abdomen prepared per agency policy. NPO (nothing by mouth) status maintained. Antacids administered if needed. The fetal heart rate is monitored until the surgery begins.

Epidural or spinal anesthesia is preferred. The woman is tilted to the left side until birth. The abdomen is cleansed and draped.

When possible, a support person is in the birth room to provide emotional support and reassurance. Every effort to promote bonding is made.

Newborn care is the same as after a vaginal birth, with particular attention to assisting infant respiration.

Postpartum care of the woman is similar to a vaginal birth. Interactions with the infant are encouraged and breastfeeding may be initiated during the recovery period.

Ongoing postpartum care after a cesarean delivery includes assessment, pain management, prevention of complications, emotional support, and discharge teaching.

Emotional support can assist the woman and her family to view cesarean delivery as an acceptable alternative to vaginal delivery.

When feeding the infant, the woman is instructed to hold the infant in a position that does not put pressure on the incision: usually support with pillows. In addition, the incision is supported when turning, changing position, ambulating, deep breathing, and coughing.

53

Cesarean Delivery: Nursing Care

When the decision for a cesarean delivery is made, the nurse can provide psychological support to the woman and her family by explaining the reason for the procedure and necessary preoperative preparations; encouraging the presence of support people during and after the birth; and involving the couple in decision making whenever possible. The goals of these interventions are to reduce anxiety and to facilitate a positive birth experience.

PREOPERATIVE NURSING CARE

There are several procedures included in preoperative preparation for a cesarean delivery:

- An intravenous line is inserted for administration of fluids to maintain blood pressure during anesthesia, and to give medications or blood if necessary.
- An indwelling bladder catheter is inserted to keep the bladder empty during the surgery and during the first 12 to 24 hours postpartum. (A full bladder interferes with surgery, prevents the uterus from contracting, and contributes to bleeding postpartum.)
- The abdomen is prepared per agency policy. **NPO** (nothing by mouth) status is maintained to reduce the risk of regurgitation and aspiration.
- Antacids may be administered to neutralize gastric acidity so as to prevent pulmonary irritation if aspiration occurs.
- The fetal heart rate pattern is monitored until the surgery begins.
- The support person is directed to change into surgical clothing, cap, and mask before entering the cesarean delivery room.

INTRAOPERATIVE NURSING CARE

Epidural or spinal anesthesia is preferred over general anesthesia for the operative procedure. General anesthesia can depress the respirations of the newborn.

To maintain uterine blood flow, the woman is tilted to the left side until the birth of the infant. The abdomen is cleansed and draped before the incision is made.

When possible, the support person is in the room to provide emotional support and reassurance. It is important for the parents to see the infant as soon as possible and every effort to promote bonding is made. The support person is encouraged to hold the infant so that the mother can see and touch the infant. Roles of the nurse in the delivery room are scrub nurse, circulating nurse, or infant-care nurse.

Roles of the nurse in the delivery room are scrub nurse, circulating nurse, or infant-care nurse.

The care of the newborn after cesarean delivery is the same as after a vaginal delivery, with particular attention given to establishing and maintainig respiration. There may be need for additional suctioning or chest physiotherapy to remove excess secretions.

IMMEDIATE POSTOPERATIVE NURSING CARE

The postpartum care of the woman who has had a cesarean is similar to the care after a vaginal birth. See Chapters 25 and 26 for details on postpartum physical assessment and nursing care. In the immediate postoperative period, assessments of the uterus,

> ✓ The postpartum care of the woman who has had a cesarean delivery is similar to the care after a vaginal birth.

lochia, and vital signs follow the same frequency for the first 4 hours. The abdominal incision is supported when the uterus is palpated. In addition, assessments for recovery from surgery and anesthesia are made. The dressing is inspected for signs of bleeding.

If general anesthesia was administered, level of consciousness is assessed and the woman is instructed to cough and deep breathe frequently. If regional anesthesia was used, return of sensation and movement is noted.

Intake and output is assessed according to agency protocol, with particular attention to blood in the urine that could indicate surgical trauma to the bladder.

Pain and nausea are assessed and medications administered as ordered.

Interactions with the infant are encouraged and breastfeeding may be initiated during the recovery period, especially while the effects of regional anesthesia are still present.

The woman may remain in the post-anesthesia recovery area for up to 4 hours.

ONGOING POSTPARTUM CARE

Ongoing postpartum nursing care after a cesarean delivery includes assessment, pain management, prevention of complications, emotional support, and discharge teaching. Assessments of vital signs, uterus, lochia, breasts, incision, and legs are done at least every 8 hours. A variety

> Ongoing postpartum nursing care after a cesarean delivery includes assessment, pain management, prevention of complications, emotional support, and discharge teaching.

of analgesic medications are available for pain control to allow the woman to care for herself and her infant postpartum.

> A variety of analgesic medications are available for pain control to allow the woman to care for herself and her infant postpartum.

Ambulation helps prevent respiratory and cardiovascular complications such as pneumonia or emboli formation. It also enhances peristalsis and reduces gas formation that contributes to pain. Other interventions to reduce gas formation are drinking warm fluids, avoiding carbonated beverages, and taking antiflatulant medication.

Deep breathing and coughing are encouraged to clear the lungs of secretions that could lead to pneumonia. When the Foley catheter is first removed, assessment for bladder distention that can interfere with uterine contractility is made until the woman is voiding adequately.

Disappointment, depression, anger, guilt, or grief may follow a cesarean delivery. Emotional support from the nurse can assist the woman and her family to develop positive perceptions of the birth experience. It is important for the couple to have opportunities to discuss their experience and their feelings and to be helped to view cesarean delivery as an acceptable alternative to vaginal delivery. Negative feelings about the birth experience, an increased amount of pain, and fatigue can delay the woman's progression through the postpartum psychological phases of taking-in to taking-hold. Teaching about self- and infant care is postponed until the woman is comfortable, rested, and receptive to learning.

> Disappointment, depression, anger, guilt, or grief may follow a cesarean delivery.

> Emotional support from the nurse can assist the woman and her family to develop positive perceptions of the birth experience. It is important for the couple to have opportunities to discuss their experience and their feelings and to be helped to view cesarean delivery as an acceptable alternative to vaginal delivery.

Recuperation after a cesarean also places some restrictions on the woman's ability to care for herself and her infant in the hospital and at home. When feeding the infant, the woman should hold the infant in a position that does not put pressure on the incision. This usually requires support with pillows. In addition, the incision should be supported when turning, changing position, ambulating, deep breathing, and coughing. Discharge teaching is similar to that for vaginal birth mothers, except for additional assessment of the abdominal incision and activity restrictions. (See Table 53-1.) See Chapter 27 for additional maternal topics and Chapter 35 for infant topics.

Discharge teaching is similar to that for vaginal birth mothers, except for additional assessment of the abdominal incision and activity restrictions. (See Table 53-1.)

Table 53-1 Discharge Teaching After Cesarean Delivery

Topic	Content
Pain management	Prescribed medications may be necessary for pain management in the first week. Support of the incision during movement, correct positioning, and prevention of fatigue decrease pain.
Signs of infection	Incision site should be inspected each day for signs of infection: localized redness, swelling, bruising, pus discharge, separation of incision, or pain when touched.
Personal hygiene	Daily shower, including washing of the incision with soap and water, careful drying, and exposure of incision to air should be done.
Activity and rest	Physical recuperation takes longer and physical activity should be resumed at a slower rate. There should be no lifting of objects heavier than 10 lb for the first 2 weeks, help at home for at least 1 week, and no driving for 2 to 4 weeks.
Postpartum exercise	No abdominal exercises should be done until discussed with physician.
Sexuality	Couples should abstain from intercourse until the abdominal incision is healed and comfortable, and lochial discharge has stopped.
Emotional adjustments	Feelings of disappointment, guilt, or grief may continue after discharge. Fatigue can increase negative emotions. If these symptoms are prolonged or severe, the health care provider should be contacted.

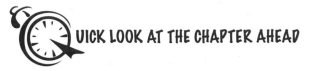
Postpartum hemorrhage causes about one-third of maternal deaths. Early postpartum hemorrhage occurs in the first 24 hours. Late postpartum hemorrhage can occur up to 6 weeks after birth.

Uterine atony, the inablilty of the uterus to remain contracted after delivery, is managed by massaging the uterus until firm, expelling the clots, ensuring that the bladder is empty, and administering oxytocin or methergine as ordered.

Signs and symptoms of lacerations of the uterus, cervix, vagina, or perineum include bright red vaginal bleeding, no clots, and a firm uterus. Management is identification and repair of the laceration.

Hematomas are usually associated with severe perineal pain, feeling of rectal pressure, bruising, swelling, and tenseness of the tissue with a mass bulging at the introitus. Small hematomas not increasing in size can be managed with ice packs and analgesia. Large or expanding hematomas usually require surgical intervention.

When excessive postpartum bleeding persists or signs such as bruising, petechiae, or oozing from a puncture site occur, disseminated intravascular coagulation (DIC) should be suspected.

Prompt recognition and appropriate management of shoulder dystocia can reduce the severity of injuries to mother and infant. After delivery the nurse assesses the infant for signs of trauma. Maternal assessment for trauma includes evaluation for excessive postpartum bleeding and blood in the urine.

54

Intrapartum Emergencies

Umbilical cord prolapse, a medical emergency, occurs following the rupture of membranes. Diagnosis is made by palpation of the umbilical cord on vaginal exam. If a loop of cord is felt, the nurse calls for help while applying upward pressure to lift the presenting part off the cord to relieve compression. This pressure is maintained until the birth of the infant. Additional immediate interventions include placing the woman in the Trendelenburg (knee-chest) postion and administering oxygen.

TERMS

- [ ] postpartum hemorrhage
- [ ] uterine atony
- [ ] lacerations
- [ ] hematoma
- [ ] disseminated intravascular coagulation (DIC)
- [ ] shoulder dystocia
- [ ] umbilical cord prolapse

The intrapartum nurse is always vigilant for possible complications during the four stages of labor. Although complications are rare, they have a significant physical and emotional impact. Assessment for risk factors, recognition of early signs and symptoms, and prompt medical and nursing management influence maternal and fetal outcomes. (See Table 54-1.)

HEMORRHAGE

Bleeding during the intrapartal period is a significant threat to mother and newborn. Postpartum hemorrhage causes about one-third of maternal deaths. Early **postpartum hemorrhage** occurs in the first 24 hours; late postpartum hemorrhage can occur up to 6 weeks after birth.

> Bleeding during the intrapartal period is a significant threat to mother and newborn. Postpartum hemorrhage causes about one-third of maternal deaths.

The major causes of early postpartum hemorrhage are uterine atony; lacerations of the cervix, vagina, or perineum; hematomas; retained placental fragments; injury to the uterus from rupture or inversion; and blood coagulation disorders. Rare causes of postpartum hemorrhage are vasa previa and placenta acreta.

The most frequent causes of late postpartum hemorrhage are retained placental tissue and subinvolution, or failure of healing at the placental insertion site.

Because of the increased blood volume of pregnancy, the woman's vital signs may not change significantly until there is a substantial blood loss of about 2000 ml.

Uterine atony is the inablilty of the uterus to remain contracted after delivery. Overdistention of the uterus from a large fetus, multiple gestation, or hydramnios is the primary risk factor. Other risk factors include grandmultiparity, a full bladder, fast or long labor, use of oxytocin during labor, and retained placental fragments. Signs and symptoms of uterine atony are a boggy, enlarged uterus and bright red bleeding with clots.

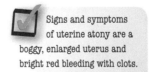

> Signs and symptoms of uterine atony are a boggy, enlarged uterus and bright red bleeding with clots.

Uterine atony is managed by massaging the uterus until firm, expelling the clots, ensuring that the bladder is empty, and administering oxytocin or methergine as ordered. If there are retained placental fragments, the physician will need to remove them surgically.

Table 54-1 Selected Intrapartum Emergencies

Condition	Description
Amniotic fluid embolism	See table of respiratory emergencies in Chapter 48.
Eclamptic seizure	Exact etiology unknown. May be related to cerebral vasospasm, vasoconstriction, edema, and ischemia. See Chapter 44 for discussion of eclamptic seizure.
Hemorrhage	A blood loss of more than 500 ml after vaginal birth or 1000 ml after cesarean delivery. Etiology includes uterine atony, lacerations, hematomas, placental and cord abnormalities, uterine injuries, and coagulation disorders. See text for discussion.
Placental abruption	See Chapter 42 for discussion.
Placenta acreta	Uncommon condition in which a part or all of the chorionic villi of the placenta adhere to the myometrium. The placenta is not able to separate completely after birth and profuse hemorrhage may result.
Shoulder dystocia	Difficulty in delivering the shoulders after delivery of the head. Can result in fetal and maternal injury. See text for discussion.
Umbilical cord prolapse	The umbilical cord comes through the cervix in front of the fetus and is compressed between the fetal presenting part and the maternal pelvis. This leads to fetal distress. See text for discussion.
Uterine inversion	Uterine fundus turns inside out, leading to hemorrhage. Associated factors include excessive traction on the umbilical cord during the third stage of labor, excessive fundal pressure during uterine massage without support of the lower uterine segment, placenta acreta, weakness of the uterine musculature, and decreased uterine tone due to anesthesia or medications.
Uterine rupture	Tear in the uterine wall leading to hemorrhage, fetal distress, and possible expulsion of uterine contents into abdominal cavity. Associated risks include weakened scar in the uterus from previous cesarean delivery or uterine surgery, obstructed labor from fetal malpresentation or cephalopelvic disproportion, grandmultiparity, or use of oxytocin. Signs and symptoms include non-reassuring fetal heart rate pattern, acute and continuous abdominal pain, vaginal bleeding, hematuria, irregular contour of the abdominal wall, and hypovolemic shock.
Vasa previa	The umbilical cord usually attaches directly to the placenta, and then the vessels divide. When the vessels divide before reaching the placenta, there is a greater risk of compression or tearing of the blood vessels. When an umbilical cord blood vessel is in front of the fetus and covers the anterior cervical os, it is called a vasa previa. The most usual sign is sudden bright red bleeding at the time of rupture of membranes, followed by severe fetal distress.

Risk factors for **lacerations** of the uterus, cervix, vagina, or perineum include a very fast labor or birth, and trauma from procedures such as forceps. Signs and symptoms include bright red vaginal bleeding, with no clots, and a firm uterus. Management is identification and repair of the laceration.

A hematoma occurs when a capillary bleeds into the tissues and blood accumulates. **Hematomas** of the vulva or vagina are the most common and may contain as much as 500 ml of blood. Risk factors for hematoma include fast labor and birth, prolonged

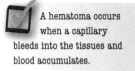
A hematoma occurs when a capillary bleeds into the tissues and blood accumulates.

pushing, macrosomia, forceps or vacuum-assisted delivery, pregnancy-induced hypertension, and birth of a first full-term infant.

Hematomas are usually associated with severe perineal pain, feeling of rectal pressure, bruising, swelling, and tenseness of the tissue, with a mass bulging at the introitus.

Small hematomas that are not increasing in size can be managed with ice packs and analgesia and will resolve over several days. Large or expanding hematomas usually require surgical intervention to drain the hematoma, locate the bleeding vessel, and tie it off.

When excessive postpartum bleeding persists or signs such as bruising, petechiae, or oozing from a puncture site occur, **disseminated intravascular coagulation (DIC)** should be suspected. See Chapter 42 for a discussion of DIC.

SHOULDER DYSTOCIA

Shoulder dystocia has been reported in up to 2% of vaginal births. Failure to progress in labor or a prolonged second stage suggests the possibility of shoulder dystocia. Prompt recognition and appropriate management can reduce the severity of injuries to mother and infant.

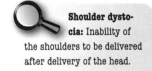
Shoulder dystocia: Inability of the shoulders to be delivered after delivery of the head.

Fetal injuries are fractures of the humerus or clavicle, palsies, injury to the brachial plexus, or asphyxia. Maternal outcomes can be excessive blood loss from uterine atony, lacerations, hematoma, and injury to the bladder.

Antenatal risk factors include macrosomia, abnormal pelvic shape or size, advanced maternal age, diabetes, obesity, excessive weight gain, and history of prior large infants.

Medical Management of Shoulder Dystocia

Medical management begins with timely recognition. When the fetal head retracts or recoils against the maternal perineum after delivery of the head, and external rotation is difficult, this is known as the "turtle sign." It indicates the posterior shoulder did not pass beneath the symphysis pubis.

Gentle pressure is placed on the fetal head to move the posterior shoulder into the hollow of the sacrum and to increase the space for the anterior shoulder to slip under the pubis. If this procedure does not work, shoulder dystocia is diagnosed.

The first intervention is the McRoberts maneuver. Under the direction of the physician or midwife, the nurse assists the woman into a position with the legs sharply flexed against the abdomen to straighten the sacrum and change the maternal pelvic angle. This maneuver is effective more than 90% of the time.

Suprapubic pressure is another noninvasive technique. The nurse may be directed to apply pressure above the symphysis pubis to dislodge and rotate the anterior shoulder. (To prevent bladder trauma, catheterization to empty the bladder is done before using this technique.)

If noninvasive techniques are not successful, the physician may reach through the vagina to rotate the shoulders, deliver the posterior arm, intentionally break the clavicle, or replace the fetal head into the pelvis for cesarean delivery. After delivery the nurse assesses the infant for signs of trauma such as fractured clavicle, Erb's palsy, neurological damage, or neonatal asphyxia. Maternal assessment includes evaluation for excessive postpartum bleeding and blood in the urine from bladder trauma.

 After delivery the nurse assesses the infant for signs of trauma such as fractured clavicle, Erb's palsy, neurological damage, or neonatal asphyxia. Maternal assessment includes evaluation for excessive postpartum bleeding and blood in the urine from bladder trauma.

UMBILICAL CORD PROLAPSE

Umbilical cord prolapse following the rupture of membranes is a medical emergency.

The nurse assesses the fetal heart rate pattern when the membranes rupture to increase the chance of recognizing a prolapsed cord. There may be immediate fetal bradycardia and/or severe variable decelerations from compression of the umbilical cord vessels.

If the heart rate pattern is suggestive of umbilical cord prolapse, a vaginal exam is done. Diagnosis is made by palpation of the umbilical cord.

> The nurse assesses the fetal heart rate pattern when the membranes rupture to increase the chance of recognizing a prolapsed cord. There may be immediate fetal bradycardia and/or severe variable decelerations from compression of the umbilical cord vessels.

If a loop of cord is felt, the nurse calls for help while applying upward pressure to lift the presenting part off the cord to relieve compression. This pressure is maintained until the birth of the infant. Additional immediate interventions include placing the woman in the knee-chest or Trendelenburg position and administering oxygen.

Risk factors include low-birth-weight infants, multiple gestations, hydramnios, high station of fetal presenting part, and malpresentations, especially footing breech and transverse lie. Prolapse may occur after obstetrical interventions such as amniotomy, application of fetal scalp electrode, insertion of intrauterine pressure catheter, or external cephalic version.

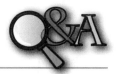

PART X · QUESTIONS

1. Which assessment is most important for the nurse to do before the administration of oxytocin?
    a. Fetal heart rate pattern.
    b. Maternal blood pressure.
    c. Maternal pulse.
    d. Status of the membranes.

2. A woman in labor is receiving oxytocin. Nursing assessment data include contraction frequency every 2 to 3 minutes, contraction duration 75 to 80 seconds, uterine resting tone between contractions not returning to baseline, fetal heart rate 150 to 156 beats per minute, maternal blood pressure 116/72, and maternal pulse 88 beats per minute. What would be the most appropriate nursing action?
    a. Continue the present rate of oxytocin.
    b. Decrease the rate of oxytocin.
    c. Discontinue the oxytocin administration.
    d. Increase the rate of oxytocin.

3. After what type of uterine incision might a woman be able to have a subsequent labor and vaginal birth?

    _____

4. Which statement by a postpartum woman after cesarean delivery indicates that further discharge teaching is needed?
    a. "Being tired may increase the pain I feel."
    b. "I need to hold my incision when I cough."
    c. "My mother will come to help me when I get home."
    d. "The incision needs to be covered with a bandage."

5. What nursing intervention would be most helpful in providing emotional support to a woman and her family after a cesarean delivery?
    a. Encouraging the father to observe the infant's first bath.
    b. Positioning the infant with pillows during feeding.
    c. Providing opportunities to discuss reaction to the birth experience.
    d. Recommending frequent rest periods for the new mother.

6. When assessing a newborn delivered by cesarean delivery, which nursing assessment is of highest priority?
   a. Nutrition.
   b. Respiratory status.
   c. Sleep pattern.
   d. Thermoregulation.

7. The nurse assesses a client after delivery. What data would suggest that this patient is at increased risk for hemorrhage?
   a. Gravida 7 Para 5.
   b. History of gestational diabetes.
   c. Infant birth weight of 7 lbs 11 oz (3487 g).
   d. Length of labor 8 hours.

8. During a vaginal exam, the nurse palpates a loop of umbilical cord at the cervix. What is the immediate intervention?

   _____

   _____

PART X · ANSWERS AND RATIONALES

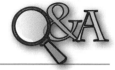

1.   **The answer is a.** Before initiation of oxytocin, the fetal heart rate pattern should be assessed. Oxytocin would not be administered if there are signs of fetal distress. Options b and c are not the best choices because alterations in maternal blood pressure and pulse are not contra-indications to oxytocin use. Option d is incorrect because oxytocin can be administered with either intact or ruptured membranes.

2.   **The answer is c.** The nursing assessment data described indicates hyperstimulation of the uterus because the resting tone does not return to the baseline between contractions. Therefore, the oxytocin should be discontinued. The other options are incorrect.

3.   **The answer is a transverse incision in the lower uterine segment.** There is less chance of rupture of the uterus during labor with a transverse incision. There is a greater possibility of rupture with a classic vertical incision.

4.   **The answer is d.** To prevent infection, the incision should be exposed to air. The other options indicate understanding of discharge teaching.

5.   **The answer is c.** Encouraging discussion of reactions to the birth experience allows expression of negative feelings and helps in the acceptance of the cesarean deliveries. The other options do not directly address the emotional needs of the woman.

6.   **The answer is b.** The primary risk to the newborn from cesarean Birth is decreased lung fluid clearance because of lack of chest compression at the time of birth. This may lead to respiratory distress. Therefore, assessment of respiratory status is of highest priority. The other options are important nursing assessments and would be carried out after respiratory assessment.

7.   **The answer is a.** Grandmultiparity is a risk factor for uterine atony, leading to postpartum hemorrhage. Option b is incorrect because gestational diabetes is not a risk factor for postpartum hemorrhage. Options c and d indicate normal parameters for birth weight and length of labor.

8.   **The answer should indicate applying upward pressure on the presenting part to relieve compression of the umbilical cord while calling for assistance.**

XI

Complex Psychosocial Situations

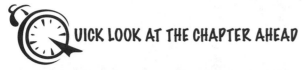
After childbirth, feelings of fatigue, irritability, and loneliness are common. These symptoms are called "baby blues" and diminish in the first 2 weeks. Postpartum depression (PPD), a more serious matter, occurs in 15% of cases.

Because young new mothers often do not have family support, PPD is more prevalent in the United States than in less developed countries. The entire family is affected when a new mother experiences PPD.

Postpartum psychosis can be a progression from or independent of PPD.

Significant risk factors have been identified for PPD, most significantly a history of previous PPD, and possibly a rapid decrease in estrogen and progesterone after birth.

Screening tools to identify risk factors for PPD are the Beck Postpartum Depression Prediction Inventory, the Beck Depression Inventory, the Edinburgh Postnatal Depression Scale, and the Beck Postpartum Depression Checklist.

During pregnancy, the woman should be evaluated each trimester for signs and symptoms of depression, and allowed to express feelings about her labor and delivery.

Ongoing assessment for signs and symptoms of depression should be done at every health care visit throughout the first year postpartum.

To increase self-confidence in the new mother, the nurse teaches child-care skills, provides

55

Postpartum Depression

opportunities to practice skills under guidance, and offers positive reinforcement. Early bonding is facilitated through frequent mother-infant interactions. The new father and other family members are included in the teaching.

The new mother is encouraged to have adequate rest and to use support systems available from her family and the community.

Antidepressant medication may be considered for the woman who develops postpartum depression.

It is important for the nurse to engage women in conversation about their emotional well-being, to screen for symptoms of postpartum depression, and to offer anticipatory guidance, reassurance, counseling, and appropriate referrals.

TERMS
☐ "baby blues"
☐ postpartum depression
☐ postpartum psychosis

After childbirth, emotions may vary from joy to anxiety. Feelings of fatigue, irritability, and loneliness are common. A new mother may be overwhelmed, have difficulty sleeping, may have mood swings, and may feel that she does not have time for herself or her partner. These symptoms are commonly called **"baby blues"** and will diminish within the first 2 weeks. However, about 15% of women will experience **postpartum depression (PPD)**, a more serious mood disorder.

DESCRIPTION OF PPD

In American culture, there are expectations that the new family will be independent and that the fast-paced life of the family will continue after the birth of a baby. The parenting role will be added to other roles already assumed by the mother and father. Because extended family may not be available, and young women may not have support from older, more experienced women, postpartum depression is more prevalent in the United States than in less developed countries.

The entire family is affected when a new mother experiences PPD. The relationship between partners may become strained and marital breakdown can occur. The mother-infant interaction is compromised, and the physical, emotional, and cognitive development of the infant may be adversely affected. Other children in the family may be neglected or may be forced to assume roles beyond their capabilities.

Postpartum psychosis can be a progression from or independent of PPD. It involves extremely disorganized thought with hallucinations or delusions, and can include preoccupation with death of self or infant. Postpartum psychosis is rare but considered an emergency because of the risk of infanticide or suicide.

IDENTIFICATION OF RISK FACTORS

Although it is difficult to predict with certainty women who will develop PPD, significant risk factors have been identified. (See Table 55-1.) The most significant predictor of PPD is a history of previous postpartum

Although it is difficult to predict with certainty women who will develop PPD, significant risk factors have been identified. (See Table 55-1.)

depression. Other significant risk factors include

- a history of depression or bipolar illness
- stressful life events
- child-care stress
- perceived lack of social support
- increased prenatal anxiety
- marital dissatisfaction
- birth of an infant with a difficult temperament
- low self-esteem.

Less significant risk factors include

- lower socioeconomic status
- presence of "baby blues"
- unplanned or unwanted pregnancy
- single marital status
- fatigue continuing for 4 weeks postpartum.

Table 55-1 Profile of the Woman Most at Risk for Postpartum Depression

Single or dissatisfied with marital relationship
Primipara over age 35
Low socioeconomic status
History of depression
Has experienced financial problems, marital problems, death or serious illness in the family, job loss or change, or relocation
Having problems providing infant care or having an infant with health problems
Unplanned or unwanted pregnancy
Had "baby blues" the first week postpartum
Describes her baby as difficult, irritable, or fussy
Does not feel support from partner, family, and friends
Does not feel good about herself as a person
Feels exhausted

The rapid decrease in estrogen and progesterone after birth is thought to be a major contributing factor for a woman at risk for PPD.

Screening tools have been developed to identify risk factors for PPD. The one most commonly used is the Beck Postpartum Depression Prediction Inventory. Tools used to identify the presence of postpartum depression include the Beck Depression Inventory, the Edinburgh Postnatal Depression Scale, and the Beck Postpartum Depression Checklist.

NURSING AND MEDICAL MANAGEMENT OF PPD

During pregnancy, the woman should be evaluated each trimester for signs and symptoms of depression. In the early postpartum period, the primary intervention of the nurse is to allow the new mother to express feelings about her labor and delivery. (See Table 55-2.) Letting her talk while expressing negative and ambivalent feelings helps her integrate the childbirth experience into her life.

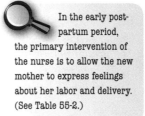

In the early postpartum period, the primary intervention of the nurse is to allow the new mother to express feelings about her labor and delivery. (See Table 55-2.)

If risk factors for postpartum depression or strong negative feelings of guilt or grief are identified during evaluation, the nurse discusses signs and symptoms of postpartum depression and provides a list of resources for further evaluation and treatment. The primary care provider is notified of high-risk factors or symptoms.

Ongoing assessment for signs and symptoms of depression should be done at every health care visit throughout the first year postpartum.

To increase self-confidence in the new mother, the nurse teaches child-care skills, provides opportunities to practice skills under guidance, and offers positive reinforcement. Early bonding is facilitated through

Table 55-2 Helpful Questions to Evaluate Emotional Well-being

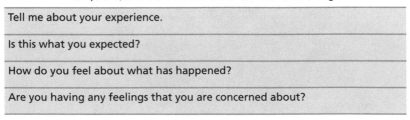

Tell me about your experience.
Is this what you expected?
How do you feel about what has happened?
Are you having any feelings that you are concerned about?

frequent mother-infant interactions. The new father and other family members are included in the teaching.

Because continued fatigue has been identified as a predictor of PPD, the new mother is encouraged to have adequate rest and to use support systems available in her family and the community. See Chapter 7 on community as support. PPD support groups provide opportunities for women to share their experiences, gain insight into their illness, and receive comfort from knowing that they are not alone. The woman's culture also influences her willingness to seek support outside her family.

Antidepressant medication may be considered for the woman who develops postpartum depression. Although the medications are excreted in breastmilk, there is no indication that this is harmful to the infant's development. The medication allows the new mother to interact positively with the infant; the benefits of taking the medication and of breastfeeding the infant outweigh any possible negative effects.

To increase self-confidence in the new mother, the nurse teaches child-care skills, provides opportunities to practice skills under guidance, and offers positive reinforcement. Early bonding is facilitated through frequent mother-infant interactions. The new father and other family members are included in the teaching.

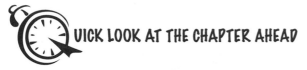

Intimate partner violence (IPV) is a more common experience for pregnant women than most medical complications.

During prenatal visits, the woman may admit to violence if asked and may be open to counseling and referrals.

Women at highest risk for violence during pregnancy are those of low income; less education; and African American, Mexican American, Puerto Rican, or Native American ethnicity.

Other risk factors include history of previous abuse; unmarried status; poor support systems; history of smoking, alcohol or drug abuse; obstetrical history of unexplained preterm birth, spontaneous miscarriage, or bleeding during first or second trimester.

Teenagers are at increased risk for IPV because they are more likely to be unemployed, have low incomes, lack education, and have an unplanned pregnancy.

Screening for intimate partner violence during pregnancy is recommended at the first prenatal visit, at least once each trimester, and at the postpartum checkup. This should be done privately.

When the woman admits to violence from her partner, her degree of threat can be assessed with the Danger Assessment by Campbell.

Battering during pregnancy is likely to continue after the birth. The perpetrator of IPV also has the potential for child abuse.

56

Intimate Partner Violence During Pregnancy

A major nursing responsibility is to assist the woman to develop a safety plan if a quick escape becomes necessary for herself and any children. Nurses should be nonjudgmental if a woman makes the choice to return to the abusive situation.

 Because IPV frequently remains unidentified, nurses need to recognize that pregnancy provides a unique opportunity for women to develop trust with health care providers. During prenatal visits, the woman may admit to violence if asked and may be open to counseling and referrals.

TERMS
- ☐ intimate partner violence (IPV)
- ☐ ABCDES— acknowledgment, belief, confidentiality, documentation, education, safety
- ☐ safety plan

Most studies indicate that 4–8% of pregnant women are abused. Abuse is more common among pregnant women than medical complications such as gestational diabetes or neural tube defects, and it is almost as common as hypertensive disorders of pregnancy.

Intimate partner violence (IPV) may begin or escalate during pregnancy because physical and emotional changes can strain the relationship, and the partner may be threatened by the attention to the fetus.

Women may feel trapped in an abusive relationship because of lack of financial resources, fear for their safety, or the belief that the jealous, controlling behavior of the partner demonstrates love and devotion.

EFFECTS OF ABUSE

Direct effects of the physical trauma from battering during pregnancy include miscarriage, placental abruption, preterm labor or birth, delivery of a low-birth-weight infant, or fetal death. Indirect effects include increased stress, drug and alcohol abuse, suicide attempts, depression, inadequate prenatal care, and increased risk of sexually transmitted diseases including HIV.

RISK FACTORS

Women who are at highest risk for IPV during pregnancy include those of low income; less education; and African American, Mexican American, Puerto Rican, or Native American ethnicity.

Other risk factors include history of previous abuse; unmarried status; poor support systems; history of smoking, alcohol or drug abuse; obstetrical history of unexplained preterm birth, spontaneous miscarriage, or bleeding during first or second trimester.

Teenagers are at increased risk for IPV because they are more likely to be unemployed, have low incomes, lack education, and have an unplanned pregnancy.

SCREENING AND ASSESSMENT

Screening for intimate partner violence during pregnancy is recommended by the American College of Obstetricians and Gynecologists at the first prenatal visit, at least once each trimester, and at the postpartum checkup. Nurses are in a key position to carry out screening for IPV. Women are more likely to report IPV if they are asked. This should be done in an environment with the woman alone. Husband, partner, children, or other family members should not be present. If an interpreter is needed, this interpreter should not be a family member or friend. A tool to identify abuse in the clinical setting has been developed and is available in both English and Spanish. (See Figure 56-1.) Women's health, maternity, and pediatric professional organizations have position statements about violence against women and guidelines for IPV screening.

Screening for intimate partner violence during pregnancy is recommended by the American College of Obstetricians and Gynecologists at the first prenatal visit, at least once each trimester, and at the postpartum checkup.

Nurses are in a key position to carry out screening for IPV.

A tool to identify abuse in the clinical setting has been developed and is available in both English and Spanish. (See Figure 56-1.)

Clinical Manifestations and Behaviors of IPV

Clinical manifestations of IPV include dizziness, hearing loss, detached retina, sexually transmitted infections, depression, anxiety, eating disorders, sleep disturbances, substance abuse, malnutrition, poor pregnancy weight gain, and somatic disorders such as chronic pelvic pain, migraines, or gastrointestinal complaints.

Women's health, maternity, and pediatric professional organizations have position statements about violence against women and guidelines for IPV screening.

Behaviors brought on by IPV include suicide attempts, noncompliance with medical recommendations, missed appointments, vague explanations of injuries, lack of eye-to-eye contact, and a partner who does not want to leave the woman alone, or answers all questions for the woman. Health care providers should suspect IPV against a pregnant woman who has a cluster of these manifestations or behaviors.

During physical assessment, particular attention should be made to target body parts: head, breasts, abdomen, and genitalia. Bruises, cuts, burns, or other injuries are evidence of battering, and should be carefully documented.

1. **WITHIN THE LAST YEAR,** have you been hit, slapped, kicked, or   **YES   NO**
   otherwise physically hurt by someone?

   If YES, by whom?_____

   Total number of times _____

2. **SINCE YOU'VE BEEN PREGNANT,** have you been hit, slapped, kicked, or   **YES   NO**
   otherwise physically hurt by someone?

   If YES, by whom?_____

   Total number of times _____

**MARK THE AREA OF INJURY ON THE BODY MAP AND SCORE EACH
INCIDENT ACCORDING TO THE FOLLOWING SCALE:**   SCORE

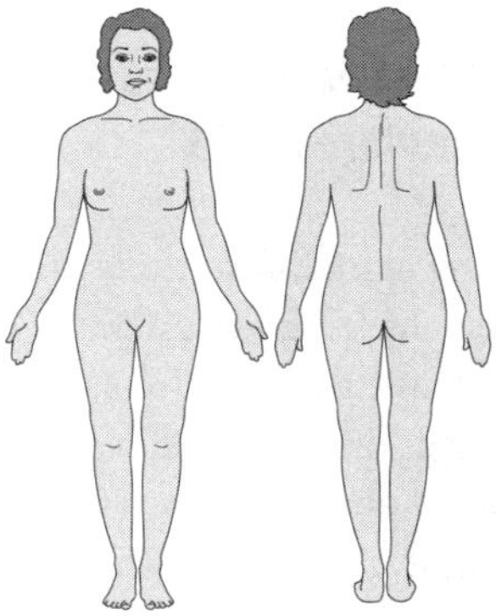

1 = Threats of abuse including use of a weapon   _____

2 = Slapping, pushing; no injuries and/or lasting pain   _____

3 = Punching, kicking, bruises, cuts, and/or continuing pain   _____

4 = Beating up, severe contusions, burns, broken bones   _____

5 = Head injury, internal injury, permanent injury   _____

6 = Use of weapon; wound from weapon   _____

If any of the descriptions for the higher number apply, use the higher number.

3. **WITHIN THE LAST YEAR,** has anyone forced you to have sexual activities?   **YES   NO**

   If YES, by whom?_____

   Total number of times _____

Figure 56-1 Abuse Assessment Screen. Developed by the Nursing Research Consortium on Violence and Abuse. Barbara Parker, Judith McFarlane, Karen Soeken, et al. (1993). "Physical and Emotional Abuse in Pregnancy: A Comparison of Adult and Teenage Women." *Nursing Research, 42*(3), 173–178.

The Campbell Danger Assessment

When a woman admits to violence from her partner, her degree of threat can be assessed with the Danger Assessment by Campbell. This self-administered tool is designed to determine the presence of risk factors associated with homicide.

The woman records the incidence and frequency of abuse for the past year and rates the severity of each incident, then identifies behaviors in the partner associated with homicide.

The higher the score on this tool, the higher the threat of homicide to the woman. Research is being conducted on identifying Campbell scores that accurately predict a woman's degree of homicide risk.

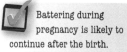 Research is being conducted on identifying Campbell scores that accurately predict a woman's degree of homicide risk.

NURSING INTERVENTIONS

A framework for nursing interventions for women who experience IPV has been described as the **ABCDES**:

- **Acknowledgment** that the woman is not alone.
- **Belief** that it is happening, that violence is not acceptable, and that it is not her fault.
- **Confidentiality** at all times.
- **Documentation,** including the woman's consent, an accurate description of injuries using a body map or photographs, the woman's statements in quotation marks, and any referrals or information given.
- **Education** about the abuse cycle, developing a safety plan, legal issues, and referrals to a battered women's shelter and social services.
- **Safety** as a priority, whether she stays with or leaves the abuser.

Battering during pregnancy is likely to continue after the birth.

The perpetrator of IPV also has the potential for child abuse. A major nursing responsibility is to assist the woman to develop a **safety plan** if a quick escape becomes necessary for herself and any

Battering during pregnancy is likely to continue after the birth.

children. The time of greatest danger is when the woman leaves the abusive situation.

If possible, a bag with copies of important documents such as birth certificates, cash or credit cards, clothing and personal items, and an extra set of house and car keys is packed and hidden in the house or left with a trusted neighbor.

> A major nursing responsibility is to assist the woman to develop a **safety plan** if a quick escape becomes necessary for herself and any children.

In addition, the woman has information about contacting the police for arrest of the abuser and obtaining a restraining order, and telephone numbers for 24-hour hotlines and local battered women's services.

Any literature given to the woman is not identified as IPV information; if found by the abuser, violence could escalate.

Nurses should be nonjudgmental if a woman makes the choice to return to the abusive situation. The woman has been given information and support so that she is better able to assess the amount of danger, and can develop a safety plan when and if she makes the decision to leave.

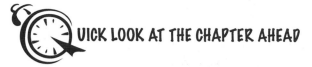

Substance abuse during pregnancy has adverse effects on the health of the mother, fetus, and newborn.

The pregnant woman may be receptive to treatment because of her concern for the well-being of the fetus.

A routine screening for substance abuse of every pregnant woman should be done at the initial prenatal visit.

Tobacco use during pregnancy has many adverse effects on the mother and fetus. Cessation of smoking at any time during the pregnancy has positive health benefits.

Ask all women if they use tobacco. Advise a women who smokes to quit. Assess her willingness to quit. Assist her to modify her smoking behaviors. Arrange for follow-up care.

Pregnant women are advised not to drink any alcohol during pregnancy or while breastfeeding.

Maternal complications of alcohol use during pregnancy are increased risk of miscarriage, stillbirth, placental abruption, and preterm labor.

Birth defects related to prenatal exposure to alcohol can occur early in the first trimester, often before the woman knows she is pregnant.

Binge drinkers or alcoholics are at increased risk of having an infant with fetal alcohol syndrome (FAS), diagnosed when the child manifests problems of growth restriction, facial anomalies, and central nervous system involvement.

57

Substance Abuse During Pregnancy: Part 1

TERMS
- ☐ substance abuse
- ☐ tobacco
- ☐ smoking cessation counseling
- ☐ alcohol
- ☐ teratogen
- ☐ fetal alcohol syndrome (FAS)
- ☐ CAGE—cut, annoyed, guilty, eye opener

391

In the United States, almost 20% of pregnant women smoke cigarettes, more than 13% of pregnant women report drinking alcohol, and approximately 5.5% of pregnant women use illicit drugs. **Substance abuse** during pregnancy has adverse effects on the health of the mother, fetus, and newborn. The pregnant woman may be receptive to reporting substance abuse and receiving treatment because of her concern for the well-being of the fetus.

SCREENING FOR SUBSTANCE ABUSE

Nurses and other health care providers play a unique role in identifying and treating substance abuse during pregnancy. Prenatal care is a time for positive health promotion and provides opportunities for ongoing support of the woman as she makes lifestyle changes. Education about the benefits of reducing or stopping the use of tobacco, alcohol, and illicit drugs is offered.

A routine screening of every pregnant woman is done at the initial prenatal visit. Pregnant women should be asked if they have used drugs or alcohol in the past or during this pregnancy.

Pregnant women should be asked if they have used drugs or alcohol in the past or during this pregnancy.

The issue of substance abuse should be addressed throughout the pregnancy, since the woman might be more willing to disclose information as a trusting relationship is developed. It is important for the nurse to become comfortable asking screening questions. Women are more receptive to questions asked in a nonjudgmental, nonthreatening manner. The nurse can set the tone by introducing the subject with an introductory statement such as, "Because it is important to the health of the mother and her baby, we ask all of our patients these questions."

It is important for the nurse to become comfortable asking screening questions. Women are more receptive to questions asked in a nonjudgmental, nonthreatening manner. The nurse can set the tone by introducing the subject with an introductory statement such as, "Because it is important to the health of the mother and her baby, we ask all of our patients these questions."

If screening results are negative for substance abuse, the health care provider reviews with the woman the benefits of avoiding tobacco, alcohol, and illicit drugs during pregnancy.

If screening results are positive for substance abuse, the health care provider can express concern for mother and baby and the belief that the mother wants her baby to be healthy. Possible strategies to help her stop using tobacco, alcohol, or illicit drugs such as counseling and treatment programs are discussed and appropriate referrals made. Ongoing encouragement and support with praise for accomplishments are provided.

TOBACCO

Tobacco use during pregnancy has many adverse effects on the mother and fetus:

- Carbon monoxide in tobacco smoke crosses the placenta and reduces hemoglobin's ability to carry oxygen.
- Nicotine causes generalized vasoconstriction, decreasing uterine perfusion.
- Women who smoke may have a poorer diet, and cigarette smoking can interfere with the assimilation of essential vitamins and minerals such as calcium, vitamin B_{12}, and vitamin C.
- Pregnant women who smoke have an increased risk of miscarriage, stillbirth, placenta previa, placental abruption, premature rupture of membranes, and preterm labor and birth.

The fetus of a woman who smokes is more likely to have low birth weight from intrauterine growth restriction. The infant of a mother who smokes is more likely to have respiratory or ear infections, allergies, chronic lung conditions such as asthma, and is twice as likely to die from sudden infant death syndrome (SIDS).

If a woman stops smoking by week 16 of pregnancy, she has no greater risk for a low-birth-weight infant than women who have never smoked. Not smoking after the birth will contribute to a healthier infant and child.

Smoking cessation counseling should be offered to all women who smoke. Nurses and other health care providers can use the five As of the Public Health Service guidelines—ask, advise, assess, assist, and arrange:

- Ask all women if they use tobacco.
- Advise a woman who smokes to quit.
- Assess her willingness to quit.
- Assist her to modify her smoking behaviors.
- Arrange for follow-up care.

Health care providers must reinforce the women's smoking cessation efforts at every prenatal visit. Cessation of smoking at any time during the pregnancy has positive health benefits.

> Cessation of smoking at any time during the pregnancy has positive health benefits.

ALCOHOL

In the United States, **alcohol** is the most common **teratogen**. Approximately 23% of pregnant women report using alcohol in the first trimester, 9% in the second trimester, and 6% in the third trimester.

> **Teratogen:** Causing birth defects.

Maternal complications of alcohol use during pregnancy are an increased risk of miscarriage, stillbirth, placental abruption, and preterm labor. Large amounts of alcohol consumption can affect maternal nutrition. Intestinal absorption of calcium, amino acids, and vitamins, particularly thiamin, folate, and vitamin K, is diminished.

Birth defects related to prenatal exposure to alcohol can occur early in the first trimester, often before the woman knows she is pregnant. Alcohol passes readily across the placenta to the fetus and interferes with its growth and development. Microcephaly; intrauterine growth restriction; facial anomalies; abnormalities of the heart, eyes, kidneys, or skeleton system; and mental retardation may result.

Women who are binge drinkers or alcoholics are at increased risk of having an infant with **fetal alcohol syndrome (FAS),** diagnosed when the child manifests problems of growth restriction, facial anomalies, and central nervous system involvement.

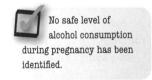

> No safe level of alcohol consumption during pregnancy has been identified.

No safe level of alcohol consumption during pregnancy has been identified. Pregnant women are advised not to drink any alcohol at all during pregnancy or while breastfeeding. The health care provider can identify at-risk drinking patterns with the use of a questionnaire such as **CAGE**. (See Table 57-1).

The social drinker given information about the effects of alcohol use is likely to quit. The woman who drinks to relieve depression or to elevate mood needs supportive counseling in addition to the education. The woman who is dependent on alcohol requires referral to an appropriate program for detoxification.

Table 57-1 CAGE Questionnaire to Identify Excessive Drinking

C	Have you ever felt you ought to **cut** down on your drinking?
A	Have people **annoyed** you by criticizing your drinking?
G	Have you ever felt bad or **guilty** about your drinking?
E	Have you ever had a drink first thing in the morning to steady your nerves or get rid of a hangover (**eye opener**)?

More than one positive response suggests the woman is at risk for alcohol abuse.

Adapted from Ewing, J. (1984). Detecting alcoholism: the CAGE questionnaire. *Journal of the American Medical Association, 252,* 1905.

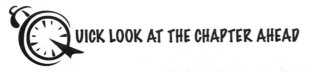

The unborn child of a pregnant woman who is a habitual user of illicit drugs may become passively addicted.

Marijuana, amphetamines, phencyclidine (PCP) and methylenedioxymethamphetamine (MDMA), commonly called "Ecstasy," and heroin have seriously negative effects on mother and infant, both immediate and long term, along with serious birth defects in the infant and later learning disabilities.

Methadone is commonly used in the treatment of heroin-addicted women by blocking withdrawal symptoms and cravings. But it has serious negative maternal and fetal effects, which in the newborn may be more severe than those associated with heroin.

The most significant problem for the drug-addicted infant is withdrawal. Therapeutic management includes dimming lights, decreasing noise, and swaddling.

The skin can be protected by mittens, sheepskin pads, and soft sheets.

Adequate nutrition and hydration can be promoted by small, frequent feedings and positioning to prevent regurgitation.

Medications to control withdrawal symptoms include phenobarbital, oral morphine sulfate solution, diazepam, and chlorpromazine.

58

Substance Abuse During Pregnancy: Part 2

TERMS

- ☐ neonatal abstinence syndrome
- ☐ marijuana
- ☐ amphetamines
- ☐ phencyclidine (PCP)
- ☐ methylenedioxy-methamphetamine (MDMA)
- ☐ cocaine
- ☐ heroin
- ☐ methadone

Almost 250,000 infants are born each year to women who use illicit drugs. Marijuana and cocaine are the most prevalent illicit drugs used during pregnancy. When the pregnant woman is a habitual user of illicit drugs, her unborn child may become passively addicted. Cocaine, heroin, and methadone use places the newborn at risk for complications after birth known as **neonatal abstinence syndrome**.

MATERNAL/FETAL EFFECTS OF ILLICIT DRUGS

Marijuana interferes with hormone production and can inhibit ovulation. Smoking marijuana increases carbon monoxide levels in maternal blood five times more than tobacco smoking, and decreases fetal oxygenation. Fetal exposure to marijuana has been associated with intrauterine growth restriction (IUGR), preterm birth, and learning disabilities in childhood.

Amphetamines are vasoconstrictive, decreasing blood flow to the maternal heart, brain, and uterus. Maternal effects include placental abruption, preterm labor, cardiac dysrhythmias, loss of appetite, and insomnia. IUGR and reduced fetal brain growth are associated with amphetamine use. After birth, the newborn may experience withdrawal.

Phencyclidine (PCP) and **methylenedioxymethamphetamine (MDMA)**, commonly called "Ecstasy," are drugs popular among adolescents and young adults. Both drugs produce euphoria.

Maternal effects of PCP and MDMA include elevated body temperature, decreased blood sodium, elevated blood pressure, and decreased levels of serotonin. Use of these drugs by mothers may be associated with neurological and behavioral problems in their children: IUGR, poor muscle control, and problems with long-term learning and memory.

> **Phencyclidine (PCP)** and **methylenedioxymethamphetamine (MDMA)**, commonly called "Ecstasy," are drugs popular among adolescents and young adults. Both drugs produce euphoria.

Cocaine use during pregnancy results in vasoconstriction, tachycardia, and hypertension. Placental vasoconstriction interferes with oxygenation to the fetus. Maternal complications include an increased risk of miscarriage, preterm labor, premature rupture of membranes, placental abruption, and stillbirth. Cardiovascular failure, intracerebral hemorrhage, respiratory failure, pulmonary edema, and seizures may also occur.

Fetal effects include IUGR; microcephaly; shorter body length; and congenital abnormalities of the heart, urinary tract, intestines, and central nervous system.

Newborns exposed to cocaine in utero may have lower Apgar scores and signs of withdrawal including exaggerated Moro reflex, tremors, prolonged crying, difficulty sleeping, sensitivity to environmental stimuli, poor response to comforting, and ineffective suck, leading to feeding problems.

Cocaine infants are at increased risk for SIDS. Long-term effects include learning disabilities.

Heroin use may inhibit ovulation, but decreasing heroin levels can then allow conception. Women who use heroin frequently report using more than one drug.

> Women who use heroin frequently report using more than one drug.

Maternal effects of heroin use include poor nutrition, iron deficiency anemia, increased risk of preterm labor, pregnancy-associated hypertension, breech presentation, placenta previa, placental abruption, premature rupture of membranes; and higher incidence of sexually transmitted, infections including HIV.

Fetal effects include IUGR, withdrawal symptoms, and increased risk of respiratory distress from meconium-stained amniotic fluid. Fetal lung maturity is accelerated because heroin stimulates production of surfactant.

Methadone is commonly used legally in the treatment of heroin-addicted women by blocking withdrawal symptoms and cravings. But maternal and fetal effects associated with methadone use include prematurity, rapid labor, placental abruption, IUGR, and fetal distress, and withdrawal symptoms in the newborn may be more severe than those associated with heroin.

NEONATAL ABSTINENCE SYNDROME

The most significant problem for the drug-addicted infant is withdrawal from heroin or methadone. Onset of symptoms occurs from 24 to 72 hours after birth, and can last up to 8 weeks. Manifestations occur in the neurological, metabolic, vasomotor, respiratory, and gastrointestinal systems. (See Table 58-1.) The severity of neonatal withdrawal symptoms is affected by the amount of heroin or methadone taken by

Table 58-1 Clinical Manifestations of Newborn Drug Withdrawal

Affected System	Clinical Manifestations
Central nervous system	High-pitched cry Short, restless sleep pattern Increased muscle tone with exaggerated reflexes Tremors or myoclonic jerks Agitation and irritability Skin excoriations on face, knees, elbows Convulsions
Metabolic/Vasomotor	Sweating Fever Frequent sneezing or yawning Mottling
Respiratory	Tachypnea Nasal flaring Nasal stuffiness
Gastrointestinal	Disorganized but vigorous suck Uncoordinated suck and swallow Frantic sucking of hands Exaggerated rooting reflex Drooling Regurgitation and projectile vomiting Diarrhea

the mother, the length of time she has been using drugs, and how soon before delivery the drugs were taken. An assessment tool called the Neonatal Abstinence Scoring System has been developed and is widely used in clinical practice.

> An assessment tool called the Neonatal Abstinence Scoring System has been developed and is widely used in clinical practice.

Therapeutic management of neonatal withdrawal includes reducing environmental stimuli that would trigger responses such as hyperactivity and irritability: dimming lights, decreasing noise, and swaddling. Swaddling restricts movement and prevents damage to the skin from excessive activity. The skin can be further protected from excoriation with mittens, sheepskin pads, and soft sheets.

Adequate nutrition and hydration can be promoted by small, frequent feedings and positioning on the right side or in semi-Fowlers after feeding to prevent regurgitation. Taking daily weights and monitoring of intake and output assess nutritional status.

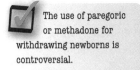
The use of paregoric or methadone for withdrawing newborns is controversial.

Medications used to control withdrawal symptoms include phenobarbital, oral morphine sulfate solution, diazepam, and chlorpromazine. The use of paregoric or methadone for withdrawing newborns is controversial.

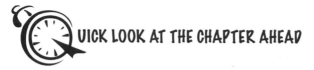

Women younger than 19 or older than 35 are at greater risk than those in between for maternal and fetal complications.

Adolescent women who become pregnant are incomplete in their physical and psychosocial development, and behave in ways detrimental to their health and the health of their babies.

There is a progression in pychosocial development throughout adolescence, from under age 15 to age 19. The younger adolescent female has difficulty dealing with the demands of pregnancy.

It is difficult for the adolescent woman to accomplish the developmental tasks of adolescence at the same time she is experiencing pregnancy and learning to assume the parenting role.

Adolescents over age 15 who receive early and consistent prenatal care are at no greater risk for problems during pregnancy than adult pregnant women.

Nursing care of the pregnant adolescent must be adapted to the developmental level of the young woman. After the birth, the early adolescent will need support and supervision as she cares for her infant. It is important to treat the middle adolescent as a young adult capable of participating in decision making. The late adolescent should be regarded as an equal partner in decision making.

Women of advanced maternal age have psychological and physical needs that are different from younger women. These women are more likely to have chronic health problems which place them at additional risk for obstetrical complications.

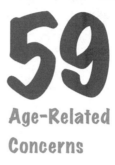

59

Age-Related Concerns

TERMS
- [ ] adolescent
- [ ] advanced maternal age
- [ ] medical-legal issues
- [ ] psychosocial development
- [ ] developmental tasks

However, the majority of women over 35 do have normal pregnancies, deliveries, and newborns.

Modifications of perinatal health care are necessary to meet the needs of women of advanced maternal age. Adjustments to the mothering role and the high energy demands of taking care of a newborn can be difficult for the older women.

Women at the extremes of childbearing years, younger than 19 or older than 35, are at more risk than those in between for maternal and fetal complications. These risks may be related to sociocultural and economic factors.

Almost 1 million **adolescent** women in the United States become pregnant each year and more than half of them give birth. Most of these pregnancies are unplanned, coming at a time when physical development and psychosocial development of the mothers are incomplete.

More than 500,000 live births occurred from women over age 35 in the year 2000. Women are postponing childbearing because of the trend toward later marriage, increased educational and career opportunities, more need for two-income families, and advances in reproductive technology. Women of **ad-vanced maternal age** have psychological and physical needs that are different from younger women.

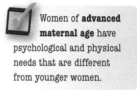
Women of **advanced maternal age** have psychological and physical needs that are different from younger women.

PREGNANCY BEFORE AGE 19

There are **medical-legal issues** related to teenagers that can affect their care. (See Table 59-1.) Adolescents may behave in ways that can affect their health negatively during pregnancy. Preconception concerns include

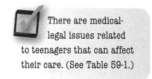
There are medical-legal issues related to teenagers that can affect their care. (See Table 59-1.)

- inadequate dietary intake with iron deficiency anemia
- increased use of tobacco, alcohol, and illicit drugs
- higher incidence of sexually transmitted infections
- vulnerability to intimate partner violence.

The adolescent may delay seeking prenatal care and be inconsistent with prenatal visits.

Because of concerns about weight gain, the adolescent may restrict caloric intake.

Physiological risks of adolescent pregnancy include preterm birth, delivery of low-birth-weight infant, pregnancy-induced hypertension, iron deficiency anemia, inadequate weight gain, and cephalopelvic disproportion.

Adolescents over age 15 who receive early and consistent prenatal care are at no greater risk for problems during pregnancy than adult pregnant women.

There is a progression in **pychosocial development** throughout adolescence. The

Adolescents over age 15 who receive early and consistent prenatal care are at no greater risk for problems during pregnancy than adult pregnant women.

Table 59-1 Medical-Legal Issues for Pregnant Teenagers

Issue	Description
Medical emancipation	Minors who are over age 13, are pregnant, are parents, live apart from their parents, or are financially independent may consent to certain medical treatments and procedures including contraception, diagnosis and treatment of STDs including HIV, prenatal care and delivery services, drug and alcohol treatment, and psychiatric care.
Legal emancipation	Teenagers less than 18, who are married, are pregnant, are parents, serve in the military, have financial independence, or do not live with their parents may be determined by law to have the legal rights of an adult.
Age of consent for sexual intercourse	The age at which a teenager may legally consent to sexual intercourse is determined by each state. The age varies from 14 to 18, with most states setting the age at 16.
Statutory sexual assault	Sexual intercourse between a minor and person who is 4 or more years older is considered a criminal offense as defined by state law.
Parental consent for abortion	In many states minors cannot receive pregnancy termination services without notification or consent of at least one parent.
Judicial bypass	The pregnant teenager may file a petition to a local judge for termination of pregnancy without notification or consent of her parents.
Adoption	In most states, adolescents can consent to relinquish their infants for adoption. However, in some states, the father of the baby must also give consent. Grandparents may have legal rights in some states.
Mandatory reporting of abuse	In most states mandatory reporting of intimate partner violence is not required of health care providers caring for women and teenagers. Conflict with mandatory reporting of child sexual abuse can occur if the adolescent is below the age of consent.

Adapted from Harner, H. M., Burgess, A. W., & Asher, J. B. (2001). Caring for pregnant teenagers: medicolegal issues for nurses. *Journal of Obstetric, Gynecologic, & Neonatal Nursing, 30*(2), 139–147.

early adolescent, under age 15, is a concrete thinker and has difficulty visualizing the future. She is dependent on her family for emotional and physical support, and perceives herself as being controlled by others. She has not yet developed an adult body image, so the physical changes of pregnancy can be threatening.

The middle adolescent, age 15 to 17, challenges authority, is strongly influenced by her peer group, and is capable of abstract thinking, but may have difficulty understanding the long-term implications of her actions. She is beginning to view herself as being in control of her future, but is not likely to be financially independent from her family.

The late adolescent, age 18 to 19, has a firm sense of self and can think abstractly. She begins to view control as coming from herself, increasing her ability to understand and accept the consequences of her behavior.

Developmental tasks to be achieved during adolescence are

- developing an adult identity and body image
- gaining autonomy and independence
- developing emotional intimacy in relationships
- gaining a sense of achievement with plans for the future.

It is difficult for the adolescent woman to accomplish the developmental tasks of adolescence at the same time she is experiencing pregnancy and learning to assume a parenting role. If her education is disrupted, the adolescent mother and her infant are more likely to live in poverty and to require public assistance.

Nursing care of the pregnant adolescent must be adapted to the developmental level of the young woman. A trusting nurse-client relationship is the foundation for effective intervention. When dealing with the early adolescent who is dependent on her family, evaluate the strength of family support. Include significant family members in any teaching and planning. Address questions, issues, and concerns in simple language, using audiovisuals and illustrations whenever possible to match the concrete thinking of the early adolescent.

Nursing care of the pregnant adolescent must be adapted to the developmental level of the young woman. A trusting nurse-client relationship is the foundation for effective intervention. When dealing with the early adolescent who is dependent on her family, evaluate the strength of family support. Include significant family members in any teaching and planning. Address questions, issues, and concerns in simple language, using audiovisuals and illustrations whenever possible to match the concrete thinking of the early adolescent.

Because the early adolescent may not be able to accept the reality of the unborn child, interventions such as listening to the fetal heart rate and having an ultrasound picture are important to promote mother-fetus bonding. After the birth, the early adolescent will need support and supervision as she cares for her infant.

The middle adolescent is able to understand more detailed information and may receive anticipatory guidance well. When possible, the father of the baby is encouraged to take part in perinatal experiences. It is important to treat the middle adolescent as a young adult capable of participating in decision making. Transition to the parenting role can be facilitated by teaching infant-care skills and encouraging her to assume as much responsibility for infant care as possible.

The late adolescent is an equal partner with health care providers in decision making. Nursing care for this age group is similar to the care of adult pregnant women.

PREGNANCY OVER AGE 35

Reproductive concerns for women over age 35 include decreased fertility, increased risk of genetic abnormalities, higher rates of multiple gestation, and greater incidence of pregnancy loss from miscarriage, ectopic pregnancy, and stillbirth. These women are more likely to have chronic health problems such as hypertension, diabetes, obesity, uterine fibroids, stress, or depression.

These health conditions place pregnant women at additional risk for the development of obstetrical complications such as gestational diabetes, pregnancy-induced hypertension, preterm labor, intrauterine growth restriction, placental abruption, abnormal fetal presentations, and macrosomia. In labor, the older woman is more likely to have labor induction, a non-reassuring fetal heart rate pattern, or cesarean delivery.

Although the risks are greater, the majority of women over 35 do have normal pregnancies, deliveries, and newborns.

Older women who have postponed childbearing tend to make the experience more positive. Because they tend to be better educated, they seek early prenatal care, have a higher concern for the health

> Although the risks are greater, the majority of women over 35 do have normal pregnancies, deliveries, and newborns.

of themselves and their baby, and express a greater readiness for child-bearing. The mature woman tends to be more collaborative, more asser-tive, and display positive health behaviors.

Some stressors for pregnant women of advanced maternal age may include caring for elderly parents simultaneously, lack of peer support system, social isolation postpartum, and concerns about balancing ca-reer and motherhood.

Modifications of perinatal health care are necessary to meet the needs of women of advanced maternal age. Preconceptual health care is more likely to include drugs or procedures to facilitate conception. Ge-netic testing for chromosomal abnormalities is more likely to be offered, and options for pregnancy outcomes discussed.

The older pregnant woman usually has increased psychological vul-nerability and higher anxiety about the dangers to herself and the fetus. Accurate information about risks, and support for behaviors promoting health may help reduce anxiety. Careful assessments by health care pro-viders and education of women about the signs and symptoms of po-tential problems lead to early detection and treatment of complications.

Adjustments to the mothering role and the high energy demands of taking care of a newborn can be difficult for older women. Nurses in the postpartum area can help older mothers by acknowledging that changes in lifestyle will occur, encourag-ing them to express their feelings, teaching infant-care skills, offering specific sugges-tions for obtaining adequate nutrition and rest, and recommending acceptance of help from partner, family, and friends.

> Nurses in the postpartum area can help older mothers by acknowledging that changes in lifestyle will occur, encouraging them to express their feelings, teaching infant-care skills, offering specific suggestions for obtaining adequate nutrition and rest, and recommending acceptance of help from part-ner, family, and friends.

PART XI • QUESTIONS

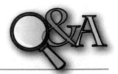

1. A nurse is reviewing prenatal information on several obstetrical clients. Which woman is most at risk for the development of postpartum depression?
   a. Gravida 1, Para 0, history of depression.
   b. Gravida 1, Para 0, unplanned pregnancy.
   c. Gravida 2, Para 1, recent relocation for husband's new employment.
   d. Gravida 3, Para 2, husband and wife both employed.

2. A new mother calls the pediatrician's office to ask about the safety of continuing to breastfeed while taking antidepressant medication for postpartum depression. What would be the response by the nurse?

   _____

   _____

   _____

3. Which pregnant women should be screened for intimate partner violence?
   a. All women who come for prenatal care.
   b. Hispanic, African American, or Native American women.
   c. Teenagers who have an unplanned pregnancy.
   d. Women who have a history of previous abuse.

4. What is the best nursing action to ensure the safety of a pregnant woman who has reported intimate partner violence (IPV)?
   a. Accurately describe injuries using a body map.
   b. Discuss a safety plan when alone with the woman.
   c. Insist that woman leave her partner.
   d. Provide a pamphlet entitled "Reporting Abuse."

5. List the four items in the CAGE questionnaire to identify excessive drinking.

   _____   _____

   _____   _____

6. A woman in week 32 of pregnancy asks the nurse if it is OK to have a glass of wine with dinner. What is the best response by the nurse?
   a. "Alcohol crosses the placenta and causes birth defects."
   b. "An occasional glass of wine will not harm the baby. It would be OK to drink wine with dinner."
   c. "Drinking alcohol during pregnancy will cause your baby to have fetal alcohol syndrome."
   d. "There is no safe level of alcohol consumption during pregnancy. You should not drink any alcohol while you are pregnant."

7. Maternal and fetal complications from the use of cocaine during pregnancy are the result of which physiologic response?
   a. Diminished hormone production.
   b. Elevated carbon monoxide levels.
   c. Generalized vasconstriction.
   d. Interference with assimilation of essential nutrients.

8. A nurse assesses a term newborn 52 hours after birth. Assessment data includes a high-pitched cry, tremors, frantic sucking of hands, and nasal stuffiness. What would be the priority nursing action?
   a. Assess the infant for signs of respiratory distress syndrome.
   b. Do further assessments for neonatal abstinence syndrome.
   c. Encourage the mother to feed the infant.
   d. Measure blood sugar level of the newborn.

9. A 14-year-old primigravida attends an adolescent prenatal clinic. For what obstetrical complication would this client be most at risk?
   a. Gestational diabetes.
   b. Macrosomia.
   c. Placenta previa.
   d. Pregnancy-induced hypertension.

10. Which health care intervention has the greatest impact on minimizing complications of pregnancy for adolescents or women of advanced maternal age?
    a. Adequate dietary intake with appropriate weight gain.
    b. Early and adequate prenatal care.
    c. Education about transition to the parenting role.
    d. Genetic testing for chromosomal abnormalities.

PART XI • ANSWERS AND RATIONALES

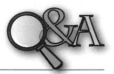

1. **The answer is a.** A significant predictor of postpartum depression (PPD) is a history of depression or bipolar illness. Although options b and c include other predictors of PPD, they are less significant risk factors. Option d does not include any risk factors for PPD.

2. **The answer should indicate although antidepressant medication is excreted in breastmilk, there is no indication that the infant's development is affected. Therefore, it is safe to continue to breastfeed.**

3. **The answer is a.** Every woman who receives prenatal care should be screened for IPV at the first visit, at least once each trimester, and at the postpartum checkup. The other options list women who are at risk for IPV, but these women should not be the only women screened.

4. **The answer is b.** All discussions about intimate partner violence should be done in an environment when the woman is alone with the nurse to provide confidentiality and to prevent the partner from knowing what the woman has reported. Option a is important documentation that should be done, but does not contribute to the woman's safety. Option c is incorrect because the decision to leave the abuser must be made by the woman. Option d is incorrect because any literature given must not be identifiable as an abuse resource.

5. **The answer should include the items cut, annoyed, guilty, and eye opener from the CAGE Questionnaire to Identify Excessive Drinking.**
   C   Have you ever felt you ought to **cut** down on your drinking?
   A   Have people **annoyed** you by criticizing your drinking?
   G   have you ever felt bad or **guilty** about your drinking?
   E   Have you ever had a drink first thing in the morning to steady your nerves or get rid of a hangover (**eye opener**)?

6. **The answer is d.** No safe level of alcohol consumption during pregnancy has been identified. Therefore, pregnant women are advised not to drink any alcohol during pregnancy or while breast-feeding. Option a is not the best choice because birth defects

related to prenatal exposure to alcohol usually occur early in the first trimester. Also, this response does not address the woman's question. Option b is an inappropriate choice because the nurse should not advise the consumption of any alcohol during pregnancy. Option c is not the best choice because fetal alcohol syndrome usually results from excessive consumption of alcohol in binge drinking or alcoholism.

7. **The answer is c.** Cocaine use during pregnancy causes vasoconstriction, leading to maternal and fetal complications such as preterm labor, placental abruption, cardiovascular failure, intrauterine growth restriction, and stillbirth. Option a is incorrect because marijuana and heroin may be associated with diminished hormone production leading to infertility. Option b is incorrect because smoking tobacco and marijuana increases carbon monoxide levels in maternal blood. Option d is incorrect because use of tobacco or alcohol interferes with intestinal absorption of essential vitamins and minerals.

8. **The answer is b.** The assessment data described are clinical manifestations of newborn withdrawal. Therefore the infant should be assessed further for neonatal abstinence syndrome. Option a is incorrect because the data do not suggest respiratory distress syndrome. Option c is not the most appropriate choice because hunger behavior may include sucking of the hands, but frantic sucking together with the other signs is associated with newborn withdrawal. Option d is incorrect because signs of hypoglycemia usually occur within the first 12 to 24 hours after birth. Tremors at 52 hours after birth are indicative of newborn withdrawal.

9. **The answer is d.** The adolescent pregnant woman is at risk for pregnancy-induced hypertension, preterm birth, delivery of a low-birth-weight infant, iron deficiency anemia, and cephalopelvic disproportion. The other options are obstetrical complications that are more prevalent in women of advanced maternal age.

10. **The answer is b.** Early and consistent prenatal care leads to early detection and treatment of complications in both adolescents and women of advanced maternal age. The other options listed are important interventions; however, adequate prenatal care is the single most important intervention for a positive pregnancy outcome.

XII

Selected Complications in the Newborn

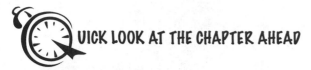

A premature infant is one born before 37 weeks of gestation. The organ systems of the preterm infant are immature, which influences the transition to extrauterine life and the ability to maintain adequate bodily functions.

Immediate complications of prematurity:

- Respiratory distress syndrome (RDS) from insufficient surfactant production in immature lungs.

- Apnea of prematurity (AOP) when breathing stops for longer than 20 seconds.

- Patent ductus arteriosus (PDA) when the ductus arteriosus does not close because of a diminished response to vasoconstrictive stimuli.

- Hypoglycemia because available glycogen stores in the liver are rapidly used up for maintenance of respiratory effort and thermoregulation.

- Intraventricular hemorrhage (IVH) in the fragile blood vessels in the brain.

- Necrotizing enterocolitis (NEC), a breakdown in the intestinal mucosal wall, leading to infection.

- Anemia from a lack of iron stores in the liver, decreased ability to produce red blood cells, accumulation of blood in cephalohematoma or bruises, and blood loss from obstetrical complications and frequent laboratory studies.

60
Prematurity: Overview

- Physiologic jaundice because the immature liver cannot conjugate bilirubin.

- Infections such as pneumonia, sepsis, and meningitis.

Long-term complications of prematurity:

- Bronchopulmonary dysplasia (BPD), associated with lung damage after prolonged use of therapies to treat RDS.

- Retinopathy of prematurity (ROP) from bleeding and scarring in the retina of the eye.

- Neurological deficits because of hypoxia and ischemia in the brain.

- Hearing loss ranging from moderate to profound in 1 to 4% of preterm infants.

 Because long-term complications affect the growth, development, and health status of children born prematurely, all nurses must be aware of the needs of these infants.

TERMS
- ☐ **respiratory distress syndrome (RDS)**
- ☐ **apnea of prematurity (AOP)**
- ☐ **patent ductus arteriosus (PDA)**
- ☐ **hypoglycemia**
- ☐ **intraventricular hemorrhage (IVH)**
- ☐ **necrotizing enterocolitis (NEC)**
- ☐ **anemia**
- ☐ **physiologic jaundice**
- ☐ **infections**
- ☐ **bronchopulmonary dysplasia (BPD)**
- ☐ **retinopathy of prematurity (ROP)**
- ☐ **neurological deficits**
- ☐ **hearing loss**

Prematurity is a serious problem in the United States, and the number of premature births is increasing. A premature infant is one born before 37 weeks of gestation.

About 84% of these infants are born between 31 and 36 weeks of gestation, and are considered to be moderately preterm. About 16% of premature infants are born between 24 and 30 weeks of gestation and are categorized as extremely preterm.

EFFECTS OF PREMATURITY

Organ systems of the preterm infant are immature, which influences the transition to extrauterine life and the ability to maintain adequate bodily functions. (See Table 60-1.) The ability of a preterm infant to adapt to life outside the uterus can be predicted by gestational age and birth weight.

The severity of clinical problems is associated with the degree of organ immaturity; organ maturity increases with gestational age.

IMMEDIATE COMPLICATIONS OF PREMATURITY

- **Respiratory distress syndrome (RDS)** is the result of insufficient surfactant production in immature lungs. Lung expansion cannot be maintained, producing widespread atelectasis. Inadequate pulmonary perfusion produces hypoxemia and acidosis. Prolonged hypoxia can effect oxygenation of other organ systems such as the brain, kidneys, and intestines.

- **Apnea of prematurity (AOP)** is a common problem in the first week of life and will usually resolve when the premature infant is 37 weeks post conception. AOP occurs when breathing stops for longer than 20 seconds or there are breathing pauses associated with cyanosis, bradycardia, pallor, or hypotonia.

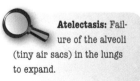
Atelectasis: Failure of the alveoli (tiny air sacs) in the lungs to expand.

- **Patent ductus arteriosus (PDA)** results when the ductus arteriosus does not close because of a diminished response to vasoconstrictive stimuli. The shunting of blood back to the lungs can lead to hypoxia, acidosis, heart failure, and pulmonary edema.

Table 60-1 Physiological Alterations in the Preterm Infant

System	Alterations
Respiratory	The respiratory system is the last to mature. There is inadequate surfactant production leading to decreased lung compliance, higher requirements for inspiratory pressure, and decreased gas exchange in collapsed alveoli. Also, the respiratory control center in the brainstem is immature.
Cardiovascular	The transition at birth from fetal to neonatal circulation may be delayed. Decreased constriction of pulmonary arterioles in response to decreased oxygen levels occurs because vascular musculature is underdeveloped. There is lowered pulmonary vascular resistance. Also, the ductus arteriosis may remain open and blood is shunted back to the lungs.
Thermoregulation	The ability to produce body heat is diminished because of decreased glycogen stores in the liver, less amounts of brown fat, and decreased muscle mass for voluntary muscular activity. Heat loss is increased because there is a high ratio of body surface to body weight, decreased amounts of subcutaneous fat for insulation, thinner and more permeable skin, and increased surface area from the nonflexed posture.
Gastrointestinal	The immature GI system has limited ability to convert certain essential amino acids, absorb saturated fats, and digest lactose. Caloric and fluid needs may be difficult to meet because of small stomach capacity and fatigue from sucking. The gag, sucking, and swallowing reflexes are poorly developed, leading to risk of aspiration.
Renal	The glomerular filtration rate is decreased because of decreased renal blood flow. Kidneys have limited ability to concentrate urine or to excrete excess amounts. There is predisposition to metabolic acidosis because of reduced ability to balance pH. The immature kidneys have difficulty excreting drugs.
Hepatic/Hematologic	Glycogen stores are diminished, increasing the risk for hypoglycemia. Decreased iron stores can lead to anemia. Conjugation of bilirubin is impaired, leading to hyperbilirubinemia.
Immune	There is increased risk for infection because few antibodies may be present for the passive immunity acquired in the third trimester. Skin integrity may be altered because the skin is fragile and invasive procedures are common.
Neurologic	Rapid brain growth occurs in the third trimester. The capillary walls in the brain are thin and fragile and hypoxia may lead to intraventricular hemorrhage. Diminished muscle tone associated with prematurity can influence the strength of reflexes. There is more disorganization in sleep/wake cycles and decreased ability to interact with the environment.

- **Hypoglycemia** can occur because available glycogen stores in the liver are rapidly used for maintenance of respiratory effort and thermoregulation.
- **Intraventricular hemorrhage (IVH)** occurs because the blood vessels in the brain are fragile and vulnerable to hypoxia from birth trauma, birth asphyxia, or respiratory distress. This is common in the very low-birth-weight infant, and many of these hemorrhages are asymptomatic. Severe bleeding can lead to hydrocephalus, hearing loss, blindness, cerebral palsy, or learning and behavioral problems.
- **Necrotizing enterocolitis (NEC)** is a breakdown in the intestinal mucosal wall, leading to infection. Although the cause is unknown, factors associated with NEC include ischemia of the bowel and oral feedings.
- **Anemia** results from a lack of iron stores in the liver, decreased ability to produce red blood cells, accumulation of blood in cephalohematoma or bruises, blood loss from obstetrical complications such as placenta previa or abruption, and blood loss from frequent laboratory studies.
- **Physiologic jaundice** is common because the immature liver cannot conjugate bilirubin. Bilirubin levels tend to rise more quickly and reach a higher level than in the term infant.
- **Infections** such as pneumonia, sepsis, and meningitis are likely to occur because the immune system is immature. Localized infection can easily become systemic.

LONG-TERM COMPLICATIONS OF PREMATURITY

- **Bronchopulmonary dysplasia (BPD)** is associated with lung damage after prolonged use of therapies to treat RDS: exposure to high oxygen concentrations, positive pressure ventilation, and endotracheal intubation. It is common in extremely premature infants.

  The scarring from this chronic lung condition may result in increased serum carbon dioxide levels, decreased serum oxygen levels, and the inability to wean from mechanical ventilation. Children with BPD have an increased incidence of respiratory infections, slower growth rates, and may develop chronic lung disease with symptoms similar to asthma.

- **Retinopathy of prematurity (ROP)** results from bleeding and scarring in the retina of the eye and may permanently impair vision. ROP is common in extremely premature infants. Most cases resolve spontaneously; laser therapy and cryotherapy may be needed to preserve vision in severe cases.

> Children with BPD have an increased incidence of respiratory infections, slower growth rates, and may develop chronic lung disease with symptoms similar to asthma.

- **Neurological deficits** may occur because of hypoxia and ischemia in the brain. Major long-term sequelae include mental retardation, seizures, cerebral palsy, and learning disabilities. Recent studies have shown that approximately 80% of infants born before 26 weeks of gestation have severe to moderate mental impairment.

> Recent studies have shown that approximately 80% of infants born before 26 weeks of gestation have severe to moderate mental impairment.

- **Hearing loss** ranging from moderate to profound occurs in 1 to 4% of preterm infants.

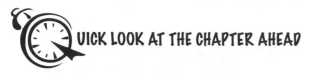

Accurate assessment of the preterm infant's gestational age, identification of specific newborn and family needs, and appropriate interventions are important.

The gestational age of a preterm infant can be estimated by scoring observations of neurological and physical maturity.

Maintenance of respiratory function is the primary need of the preterm infant.

Thermoregulation is another important need and directly affects respiratory function.

Management of hydration and nutrition through parenteral fluids, gavage feedings, bottle feeding, or breastfeeding is critical.

Breastmilk is the ideal food for the preterm infant because there is a more rapid rate of growth, it is more easily digested, and the anti-infective properties cannot be duplicated in formulas.

Preterm infants who are breastfed maintain more stable oxygen saturation levels, have fewer incidences of bradycardia, have more stable body temperatures, and have better coordination of breathing, sucking, and swallowing.

The preterm infant has special needs related to degree of prematurity. The physiologic alterations in these infants and the family responses to the birth of a high-risk newborn determine the priorities for nursing care. Accurate assessment of gestational age, identification of specific needs of the newborn and family, and provision of appropriate interventions are important to achieving the best possible outcome.

61

Nursing Care of the Preterm Infant: Part 1

TERMS
- [ ] **assessment of gestational age**
- [ ] **maintenance of respiratory function**
- [ ] **thermoregulation**
- [ ] **kangaroo care**
- [ ] **hydration and nutrition**
- [ ] **gavage feedings**
- [ ] **nonnutritive feedings**

The gestational age of a preterm infant can be estimated by scoring observations of neurological and physical maturity. (See Figure 61-1.)

Neuromuscular Maturity

	−1	0	1	2	3	4	5
Posture							
Square window (wrist)	<90°	90°	60°	45°	30°	0°	
Arm recoil		180°	140–180°	110–140°	90–110°	< 90°	
Popliteal angle	180°	160°	140°	120°	100°	90°	< 90°
Scarf sign							
Heel to ear							

Gestation by Dates _____ wks

_____ am

Birth Date _____ Hour_____pm

APGAR _____ 1 min_____ 5 min

Maturity Rating

score	weeks
−10	20
−5	22
0	24
5	26
10	28
15	30
20	32
25	34
30	36
35	38
40	40
45	42
50	44

Physical Maturity

Skin	sticky friable transparent	gelatinous red, translucent	smooth pink, visible veins	superficial peeling &/or rash, few veins	cracking pale areas rare veins	parchment deep cracking no vessels	leathery cracked wrinkled
Lenugo	none	sparse	abundant	thinning	bald areas	mostly bald	
Plantar Surface	heel–toe 40–50 mm: −1 < 40 mm: −2	> 50 mm no crease	faint red marks	anterior transverse crease only	creases ant. 2/3	creases over entire sole	
Breast	imperceptible	barely perceptible	flat areola no bud	stipped areola 1–2 mm bud	raised areola 3–4 mm bud	full areola 5–10 mm bud	
Eye/Ear	lids fused loosely: −1 tightly: −2	lids open pinna flat stays folded	sl. curved pinna; soft; slow recoil	well-curved pinna; soft but ready recoil	formed & firm instant recoil	thick cartilage ear stiff	
Genitals, male	scrotum flat, smooth	scrotum empty faint rugae	testes in upper canal rare rugae	testes descending few rugae	testes down good rugae	testes pendulous deep rugae	
Genitals, female	clitoris prominent labia flat	prominant clitoris small labia minora	prominent clitoris enlarging minora	major & minora equally prominent	majora large minora small	majora cover clitoris & minora	

Scoring Section

	1st Exam = X	2nd Exam = 0
Estimating gest. age by maturity rating	_____Weeks	_____Weeks
Time of exam	Date_____ am Hour____pm	Date_____ am Hour____pm
Age at exam	_____Hours	_____Hour
Signature of examiner	_____ M.D./R.N.	_____ M.D./R.N.

Figure 61-1 Estimation of gestational age by maturity rating.

Scoring system: Ballard, J.L., Khoury, J.C., Wedig, K., Wang, L., Eilers-Walsman, B.L., Lipp, R. (1991). New Ballard Score, expanded to include extremely premature infants. *Journal of Pediatrics, 119,* 417–423.

RESPIRATORY FUNCTION

Maintenance of respiratory function is *the* primary need of the preterm infant. Initiation and maintenance of respiration may require intubation, oxygen therapy, mechanical ventilatory assistance with positive airway pressure, or the administration of surfactant.

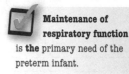

Maintenance of respiratory function is **the** primary need of the preterm infant.

The infant is placed in prone position when possible for improved chest expansion. If the supine position is used, care must be taken not to hyperextend the neck because this decreases tracheal diameter.

The infant is suctioned when necessary to remove secretions. It is important to maintain a stable body temperature to conserve the use of oxygen. Blood gases are closely monitored to determine the oxygenation status of the infant.

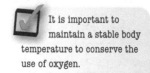

It is important to maintain a stable body temperature to conserve the use of oxygen.

Assessment for signs of respiratory distress such as nasal flaring, retraction, grunting, tachypnea, cyanosis, or low oxygenation saturation levels is ongoing. Continuous electronic respiratory and cardiac monitoring is used.

THERMOREGULATION

Thermoregulation is another important need of the premature infant and directly affects respiratory function. See Chapter 28 for a discussion of thermoregulation in the newborn. The preterm infant is at high risk for not being able to maintain adequate body temperature, and requires additional assistance.

It is essential to have a neutral thermal environment in which the infant can maintain a stable axillary temperature within the range of 36.5 to 37.5°C (97.7–99.5°F). This can be accomplished by the use of radiant warming panels or incubators.

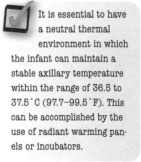

It is essential to have a neutral thermal environment in which the infant can maintain a stable axillary temperature within the range of 36.5 to 37.5°C (97.7–99.5°F). This can be accomplished by the use of radiant warming panels or incubators.

Other techniques to prevent heat loss in the preterm infant include use of plastic wrap over the infant under a radiant warmer to reduce drafts and conserve body fluids, warming the blankets or other equipment prior to use, and warming the oxygen before administration.

Skin-to-skin contact between a parent and the infant, known as **kangaroo care**, can assist the infant to maintain thermal stability.

Monitoring body temperature is important to detect hyperthermia as well as hypothermia; either condition is detrimental.

Serum glucose values are determined because changes in body temperature can cause hypoglycemia.

HYDRATION AND NUTRITION

Management of **hydration and nutrition** is critical for the preterm infant, and can be met in four ways: parenteral fluids, gavage feedings, bottle-feeding of formula or pumped breastmilk, or breastfeeding. Recent changes in the management of the nutritional needs of the preterm infant include minimal enteral feeding of small amounts of breastmilk to enhance intestinal maturation. Although nutritional needs are not met by enteral feeding alone, some nutrients and anti-infective components are provided in breastmilk.

Special parenteral fluids have been developed based on the needs of the preterm infant.

> **Gavage feedings:** Feeding through a tube placed in the mouth or nose to the stomach.

> Recent changes in the management of the nutritional needs of the preterm infant include minimal enteral feeding of small amounts of breastmilk to enhance intestinal maturation. Although nutritional needs are not met by enteral feeding alone, some nutrients and anti-infective components are provided in breastmilk.

Fluid Volume

Preterm infants are at high risk for fluid volume deficit because of high extracellular content, large body surface area, immature kidneys, and increased insensible water loss from phototherapy or a radiant warmer. Close monitoring of fluid status by daily weights, accurate measurement of intake and output, specific gravity of urine, and evaluation of serum electrolyte levels is important.

Caloric Requirements

Meeting the caloric requirements of the preterm infant can be a challenge. Caloric need per kilogram of body weight is higher than in the term infant.

> The stomach capacity of a preterm infant is limited; an overdistended stomach can lead to respiratory difficulty.

Caloric needs can be met by using commercially prepared parenteral solutions and formulas designed specifically to meet the needs of the preterm infant, or by breastmilk.

> It is very important to make sure that the energy expenditure to feed is not more than the amount of calories taken in.

The feeding method is determined by the gestational age, physical condition, and readiness to suck. A weight gain of one-half to 1 ounce per day after initial weight loss is evidence of adequate nutritional intake. **Nonnutritive sucking** through the use of a pacifier stimulates the suck reflex and improves sucking ability.

 Nonnutritive sucking through the use of a pacifier stimulates the suck reflex and improves sucking ability.

Breastmilk

Breastmilk is the ideal food for the preterm infant because it generates more rapid growth, it is easily digested, and its anti-infective properties cannot be duplicated in formulas. Preterm infants who are breastfed maintain more stable oxygen saturation levels, have fewer incidences of bradycardia, have more stable body temperatures, and have better coordination of breathing, sucking, and swallowing.

Before the infant can suck, the mother can pump her breasts, and the milk given by gavage feeding.

Mothers of preterm infants are encouraged to breastfeed when the infant demonstrates readiness:

Breastmilk is the ideal food for the preterm infant because it generates more rapid growth, it is easily digested, and its anti-infective properties cannot be duplicated in formulas. Preterm infants who are breastfed maintain more stable oxygen saturation levels, have fewer incidences of bradycardia, have more stable body temperatures, and have better coordination of breathing, sucking, and swallowing.

- a strong, vigorous suck
- coordination of sucking and swallowing
- presence of a gag reflex

- sucking on the gavage tube, hands, or a pacifier
- rooting
- being alert before the feeding
- sleeping after the feeding.

Guidance and support from nursing staff, lactation consultants, breastfeeding support groups, or more experienced mothers are helpful.

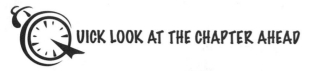

The preterm infant is best delivered in a tertiary care center. Postponing delivery, even a few days, increases the chance of survival and decreases health care costs.

A single course of corticosteroids given to the mother in preterm labor has been shown to significantly increase lung maturity and decrease the incidence of RDS. Also, surfactant replacement therapy given to the infant after birth is known to reduce mortality rates.

Because preterm infants have a higher risk for the development of infection, antenatal treatment of maternal infections and measures to protect the skin integrity of the infant are a high priority. Also, breastmilk provides antibodies against infection.

To minimize the risk for the development of retinopathy of prematurity (ROP), no higher concentrations of oxygen are administered than necessary to maintain adequate oxygen saturation levels. Decreasing environmental light and stimuli may also contribute to the prevention of ROP.

Prevention of events that cause fluctuations in cerebral blood flow can decrease the development of intraventricular hemorrhage (IVH).

Continuous electronic heart and respiratory monitoring detects periods of apnea and bradycardia. Gentle tactile stimulation, suctioning and oxygen, or a resuscitation bag and mask are used as required.

62

Nursing Care of the Preterm Infant: Part 2

If an infant develops necrotizing enterocolitis (NEC), oral feedings are stopped, a nasogastric tube is inserted to reduce gastric distension, and antibiotics are administered.

Nurses and other health care providers need to be aware of potential painful stimuli and provide pharmacological and non-pharmacological pain management.

Preterm infants are more susceptible to the stresses of the NICU environment. Modifications to reduce stress and overstimulation should be followed.

Kangaroo care enhances neurophysiological development and parent-infant attachment. Family-centered care is provided by encouraging the parents to partner with health care providers in the care of their infant.

Hospital stays for preterm infants are shorter, resulting in the discharge of smaller and less mature infants. Discharge planning and preparation of the parents are essential. See Chapters 40 and 41 for discussion of preterm labor management.

The nurse often is the health care provider who notices subtle changes in the infant's condition and reports these observations to the attending physicians for early recognition and treatment of any complications. (See Table 62-1.)

TERMS

- ☐ **corticosteroids**
- ☐ **sepsis**
- ☐ **skin integrity**
- ☐ **retinopathy of prematurity (ROP)**
- ☐ **intraventricular hemorrhage (IVH)**
- ☐ **necrotizing enterocolitis (NEC)**
- ☐ **pain management**
- ☐ **kangaroo care**
- ☐ **family-centered care**

PREVENTION OF COMPLICATIONS

A single course of **corticosteroids** given to the mother in preterm labor has been shown to significantly increase lung maturity and decrease the incidence of RDS. The efficacy of multiple courses of treatment has not been determined.

 Corticosteroids given to the infant after delivery have been associated with an increased risk of cerebral palsy and neurological developmental delays.

Table 62-1 Nursing Assessments for Complications

Complication	Nursing Assessments
Respiratory distress syndrome	Respiratory rate above 60 breaths per minute, retractions, central cyanosis, nasal flaring, expiratory grunting, diminished air exchange, and decreased oxygen saturation levels.
Apnea of prematurity	Periods of apnea for more than 20 seconds with or without color changes or bradycardia.
Patent ductus arteriosis	Systolic cardiac murmur at upper left sternal border, decreased oxygen saturation level with or without color change, increased respiratory rate, increased peripheral pulses.
Intraventricular hemorrhage	Periods of apnea, bradycardia, drop in hematocrit, diminished sucking reflex, twitching, lethargy, decreased muscle tone, full anterior fontanel, separated cranial sutures, seizures.
Necrotizing enterocolitis	Feeding intolerance, increased gastric residue that may be bile-stained, abdominal distention, increased abdominal girth, decreased or absent bowel sounds, blood in the stool, temperature instability, periods of apnea, and bradycardia.
Sepsis	Increase or decrease in white blood cell count with a shift to the left, lethargy, periods of apnea, temperature instability, feeding intolerance, and color changes—cyanotic, ashen, or mottled.
Hypoglycemia	Jitteriness, tachycardia, increased respiratory effort, irritability, poor feeding, high-pitched or weak cry, lethargy, low blood sugar level.
Physiologic jaundice	Yellow color of skin and sclera, increased levels of serum bilirubin.
Anemia	Low hemoglobin and hematocrit levels, poor feeding, decreased oxygen saturation level, dyspnea, tachycardia, tachypnea, pallor, poor weight gain, systolic murmur, diminished activity.

Also, surfactant replacement therapy given to the infant after birth is known to reduce mortality rates; however, the best type of surfactant to use and the optimal time for the initial dose continue to be studied.

Infection

Because preterm infants have a higher risk for the development of infection, antenatal treatment of maternal infections is a high priority. For a discussion on maternal infections during pregnancy, see Chapter 50. To prevent the development of postnatal **sepsis**, good handwashing, adequate housekeeping, and proper handling of equipment and supplies are necessary.

Measures to protect **skin integrity** of the infant will reduce the risk of infection, such as minimal use of adhesives, prevention of loss of moisture from the skin, avoiding dehydration, and frequent assessing for signs of skin breakdown. Also, the use of breastmilk for nourishment will provide antibodies against infection.

Retinopathy of Prematurity

To minimize the risk for the development of **retinopathy of prematurity (ROP)**, the nurse administers no higher concentrations of oxygen than necessary to maintain adequate oxygen saturation levels. Decreasing environmental light and stimuli may also contribute to the prevention of ROP. The infant's eyes are assessed by an ophthalmologist periodically for signs of ROP.

Intraventricular Hemorrhage

Prevention of events that cause fluctuations in cerebral blood flow can decrease the development of **intraventricular hemorrhage (IVH)**. Maintaining adequate oxygenation, preventing acidosis or electrolyte imbalances, limited and careful suctioning, elevation of the head of the bed, good body alignment, avoiding interventions that may cause crying, prevention of hypoglycemia, and decreasing external stimuli are all interventions to prevent IVH.

MANAGEMENT OF APNEA AND BRADYCARDIA

Continuous electronic heart and respiratory monitoring will detect periods of apnea and bradycardia. If gentle tactile stimulation is not sufficient to initiate breathing, the nose and oral pharynx are suctioned and oxygen administered. Then, if breathing does not begin, a resuscitation bag and mask are used.

Infants who have frequent apneic episodes may be given theophylline or caffeine to stimulate the central nervous system and maintain breathing. These infants are monitored for signs of toxicity and have serum drug levels measured regularly.

MANAGEMENT OF NECROTIZING ENTEROCOLITIS

If an infant develops **necrotizing enterocolitis (NEC)**, oral feedings are stopped, a nasogastric tube is inserted to reduce gastric distension, and antibiotics are administered. Nutritional and fluid needs are met parenterally. Surgery may be necessary to remove the necrosed portions of the intestine. Nursing care of necrotizing enterocolitis includes leaving the infant loosely diapered, positioning on back or side, good handwashing technique, and contact isolation.

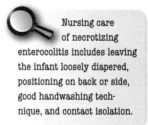
Nursing care of necrotizing enterocolitis includes leaving the infant loosely diapered, positioning on back or side, good handwashing technique, and contact isolation.

PAIN MANAGEMENT

Behavioral responses to pain in the newborn have been studied and assessment tools developed. The appropriateness of these tools to the preterm infant has not yet been determined. Nurses and other health care providers need to be aware of potential painful stimuli and provide pharmacological and non-pharmacological pain management. Strategies for pain management to reduce stress include non-nutritive sucking, use of sucrose on a pacifier, and environmental interventions such as lowering lights, reducing noise, providing soft music, and swaddling.

Nurses and other health care providers need to be aware of potential painful stimuli and provide pharmacological and non-pharmacological pain management.

DEVELOPMENTAL CARE

Maturation of body systems continues after birth in the preterm infant. Because preterm infants are born before the central nervous system is fully developed, they are more susceptible to the stresses of the NICU environment. Modifications to reduce stress and overstimulation include variations in environmental lighting, reduced noise levels, periods of uninterrupted sleep, nesting with rolled blankets or other supportive devices, swaddling, non-nutritive sucking, touch, positioning, and providing objects for the infant to grasp.

Kangaroo care enhances neurophysiological development and parent-infant attachment. The infant, dressed only in a diaper, is placed on the parent's bare chest for skin-to-skin contact. The parent drapes clothing or a blanket over the infant to maintain warmth. It is called "kangaroo" care because a marsupial-like pouch is formed by the draped clothing or blanket.

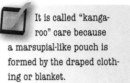
It is called "kangaroo" care because a marsupial-like pouch is formed by the draped clothing or blanket.

Neurophysiological behaviors of the infant are more organized as demonstrated by maintenance of body temperature, and more stable heart and respiratory rates with higher oxygen saturation levels.

Attachment is promoted in parents who participate in kangaroo care. They feel closer to their infants and are providing caregiving that no one else can do.

The benefits of kangaroo care have been demonstrated for up to 6 months; mothers are more sensitive to infant cues and infants score higher on developmental indices.

FAMILY-CENTERED CARE

The parents should be encouraged to partner with health care providers in the care of their infant. Early and frequent interactions with the infant, providing care to the infant when possible, and participation in decision making provide the parents with opportunities to assume the parenting role and develop confidence in their ability to parent their child. Ongoing support for the parents by nurses, health care providers, and parent support groups can help them cope with the stress, anxiety, or depression associated with the birth of a preterm infant.

Because of improvements in care and the availability of home care services, hospital stays for preterm infants are shorter, resulting in the discharge of smaller and less mature infants. Discharge planning and preparation of the parents are therefore essential. Criteria for discharge include maintenance of a stable body temperature in an open crib; ability of the infant to coordinate breathing, sucking, and swallowing; adequate amounts of intake with a sustained pattern of weight gain; and stable cardiorespiratory functioning.

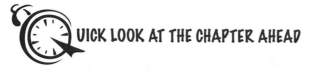
With current management strategies and good control of blood sugars, the effects of diabetes on the fetus and the mother can be minimized.

During times of maternal hyperglycemia, the fetus responds to high glucose levels with increased pancreatic beta cell production and increased insulin levels.

The infant of a diabetic mother (IDM) is typically large for gestational age, plump and full-faced, ruddy in color, with a large placenta and thick umbilical cord.

Careful assessment of the IDM is performed to detect complications and to plan appropriate interventions. The affected arm and shoulder of a fractured clavicle from shoulder dystocia may be immobilized by pinning the sleeve to the front of the shirt. Caution is used when bathing and dressing the infant. A fractured clavicle usually heals spontaneously without surgery or casting. Treatment of brachial plexus injury involves preventing contractures through range-of-motion exercises and maintaining correct alignment of the arm. Spontaneous recovery usually occurs in 3 to 6 months. Permanent damage may require surgery.

IDMs have an increased risk for RDS because of delayed maturity of the respiratory system. Management is similar to the management in the preterm infant.

63

Infant of Diabetic Mother

Hypoglycemia is the most common complication of IDMs. The risk for hypoglycemia is managed with frequent assessments of blood sugar levels and early feedings.

Hypocalcemia and hypomagnesemia may develop in IDMs. If laboratory results confirm low serum levels of calcium or magnesium, these electrolytes are administered intravenously.

Polycythemia can occur when hyperglycemia in the mother leads to increased levels of sugar and insulin in the fetus.

The incidence of congenital abnormalities is two to four times greater in IDMs, but can be decreased with good control of maternal blood sugars.

 When caring for the infant of the diabetic mother, the nurse's role is to recognize effects of diabetes on the newborn, assess for complications, and provide nursing interventions to manage symptoms.

TERMS

- [ ] maternal hyperglycemia
- [ ] infant of a diabetic mother (IDM)
- [ ] macrosomia
- [ ] shoulder dystocia
- [ ] respiratory distress syndrome (RDS)
- [ ] hypoglycemia
- [ ] hypocalcemia
- [ ] hypomagnesemia
- [ ] polycythemia
- [ ] congenital abnormalities

Before insulin was discovered, pregnancy in the diabetic woman was rare. If a pregnancy occurred, major complications to both mother and infant were common. With current management strategies and good control of blood sugars, the effects of diabetes on the mother and the fetus can be minimized.

FETAL AND NEONATAL EFFECTS

During times of **maternal hyperglycemia**, the fetus responds to high glucose levels with increased pancreatic beta cell production and increased insulin levels. This stimulates linear growth, increased weight of visceral organs, and an increase in adipose tissue.

The **infant of a diabetic mother (IDM)** is typically large for gestational age, plump and full-faced, ruddy in color, with a large placenta and thick umbilical cord. Even though the birth weight may be within the expected range for a term infant, the IDM may exhibit characteristics of prematurity because of gestational age.

Macrosomia in the IDM contributes to an increased likelihood of cesarean delivery, shoulder dystocia, birth trauma, and longer second stage of labor. See Chapter 46 for discussion of diabetes during pregnancy with fetal and neonatal risks.

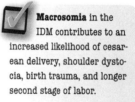

Macrosomia in the IDM contributes to an increased likelihood of cesarean delivery, shoulder dystocia, birth trauma, and longer second stage of labor.

COMMON COMPLICATIONS

Careful assessment of the IDM is performed to detect complications and to plan appropriate interventions. (See Table 63-1.) Individual health care agencies develop protocols for the frequency of assessments, especially for blood sugar levels.

The complications most often seen in IDMs include birth trauma, respiratory distress syndrome, hypoglycemia, hypocalcemia, hypomagnesemia, polycythemia, hyperbilirubinemia, and congenital malformations.

The complications most often seen in IDMs include birth trauma, respiratory distress syndrome, hypoglycemia, hypocalcemia, hypomagnesemia, polycythemia, hyperbilirubinemia, and congenital malformations.

Table 63-1   Nursing Assessment for Complications

Complication	Nursing Assessment
Fractured clavicle	Elicit Moro reflex to determine if there is decreased movement of affected arm. Palpate for crepitis of clavicle. Observe for swelling or hematoma at the fracture site. Assess for crying when clavicle or arm is moved.
Brachial plexus injury	Observe for lack of active motion in affected arm. Arm and shoulder are adducted and internally rotated with elbow extended and forearm pronated. Elicit Moro reflex; reflex is absent on affected side.
Respiratory distress syndrome	Observe for respiratory rate above 60 breaths per minute, retractions, central cyanosis, nasal flaring, expiratory grunting, diminished air exchange, and decreased oxygen saturation level.
Hypoglycemia	Observe for jitteriness, irritability, tachycardia, increased respiratory effort, poor feeding, lethargy, high-pitched or weak cry, and low blood sugar level.
Hypocalcemia	Observe for tremors, jitteriness, seizure activity, and low level of serum calcium.
Hypomagnesemia	Observe for tremors, jitteriness, seizure activity, and low level of serum magnesium.
Hyperbilirubinemia	Observe for yellow color of skin and sclera and increased level of serum bilirubin.
Congenital abnormalities	Perform careful head-to-toe assessment to detect congenital malformations.

Birth Trauma

Birth trauma from **shoulder dystocia** is associated with macrosomia in the IDM. The potential for fractured clavicle or brachial plexus injury increases with shoulder dystocia. A fractured clavicle is confirmed by X ray. The affected arm and shoulder may be immobilized by pinning the sleeve to the front of the shirt. Caution is used when bathing and dressing the infant. A fractured clavicle usually heals spontaneously without surgery or casting.

With brachial plexus injury, spontaneous recovery usually occurs within 3 to 6 months. Treatment involves preventing contractures through range-of-motion exercises and maintaining correct alignment of the arm. Permanent damage may require surgery.

Respiratory Distress Syndrome

IDMs have an increased risk for **respiratory distress syndrome** because of delayed maturity of the respiratory system, with decreased surfactant production. Management of respiratory distress syndrome (RDS) in the IDM is similar to its management in the preterm infant. (See Chapter 61.)

Hypoglycemia

Hypoglycemia is the most common complication of IDMs; from 25 to 40% of these infants experience low blood sugar in the first few hours of life. Because the infant continues to produce large amounts of insulin, the blood glucose is quickly depleted unless early feeding is initiated. Although protocols may vary, frequent monitoring of blood sugar levels in the first 12 to 24 hours of life normally is done. Within 24 hours after birth, insulin production usually stabilizes and the risk of hypoglycemia decreases.

The risk for hypoglycemia is managed with frequent assessments of blood sugar levels and early feedings. To prevent a drop in blood sugar, feedings are begun as soon as possible after birth. If there are signs of respiratory distress, intravenous or gavage feedings might be needed instead of breast or bottle feeding.

Hypocalcemia and Hypomagnesemia

Hypocalcemia and **hypomagnesemia** developing in IDMs is related to decreased parathyroid hormone production. Signs are similar to those of hypoglycemia, but usually occur later than 24 hours after birth. If symptoms persist in the presence of normal blood sugar levels, hypocalcemia is suspected. If laboratory results confirm low serum levels of calcium or magnesium, these electrolytes are administered intravenously.

Polycythemia

Polycythemia can occur when hyperglycemia in the mother leads to increased levels of sugar and insulin in the fetus. The resulting tissue hypoxia stimulates red blood cell production, increasing the hematocrit level. The potential for hyperbilirubinemia increases because there are more red blood cells to be broken down. If bruising occurs from a traumatic delivery, additional bilirubin must be conjugated and excreted. See Chapter 65 for a discussion of the management of jaundice.

Congenital Abnormalities

The incidence of **congenital abnormalities** is two to four times greater in IDMs. The most common malformations include cardiac, central nervous system, gastrointestinal, and musculoskeletal defects. With good control of maternal blood sugars, the incidence of congenital anomalies is decreased.

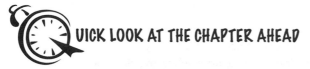

During pregnancy, a woman may be exposed to fetal red blood cells containing antigens different from her own. Her immune reaction is called isoimmunization.

When maternal antibodies against the antigens cross back into the fetal circulation, attach to, and break down the fetal erythrocytes, the fetus develops a hemolytic disease. One type is erythroblastosis fetalis, and a severe form of it is hydrops fetalis.

The most common type of hemolytic disease is ABO incompatibility or Rh incompatibility.

In ABO incompatibility, the mother has blood type O and the fetus has blood type A, B, or AB. Rarely is the disease severe, but there is no method of prevention.

In Rh incompatibility, the mother is Rh negative and the fetus is Rh positive. Negative consequences of Rh incompatibility can be prevented with the administration of Rh immunoglobulin (RhoGAM) to Rh-negative women during and after each pregnancy.

After delivery, the newborn is examined carefully for signs of erythroblastosis fetalis or hydrops fetalis and appropriate management instituted.

 Perinatal nurses need a thorough knowledge of the pathologic process of isoimmunization, methods of assessment and prevention, and management of the affected fetus or newborn.

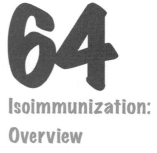

64

Isoimmunization: Overview

TERMS
- [ ] **pathologic jaundice**
- [ ] **isoimmunization**
- [ ] **erythroblastosis fetalis**
- [ ] **hydrops fetalis**
- [ ] **ABO incompatibility**
- [ ] **Rh incompatibility**
- [ ] **indirect Coombs test**
- [ ] **direct Coombs test**

Pathologic jaundice from hemolytic disease of the newborn was a major contributor to fetal or neonatal illness and death before the development of Rh immunoglobulin (RhoGAM). However, there is at least a 1% chance of isoimmunization occurring in women who have Rh negative blood type even with preventive measures.

PATHOPHYSIOLOGY

When a woman is exposed to red blood cells containing antigens different from her own, an immune reaction called **isoimmunization** can occur.

During pregnancy, a woman may be exposed to fetal red blood cells when the placental membrane is interrupted and fetal blood cells enter the maternal circulation. This introduction of fetal blood into the maternal circulatory system can happen with placental separation at the time of birth, during obstetrical procedures, or with hemorrhagic complications. A volume as small as 0.1 ml has been shown to cause isoimmunization. (See Table 64-1.)

> When a woman is exposed to red blood cells containing antigens different from her own, an immune reaction called **isoimmunization** can occur.

Hemolytic Diseases

Hemolytic disease occurs when maternal antibodies against antigens present on the fetal red blood cells cross back into the fetal circulation, attach to, and break down the fetal erythrocytes.

A condition known as **erythroblastosis fetalis,** or hemolytic disease of the newborn, develops with jaundice, anemia, and an increase in red blood cell production. The most common type of hemolytic disease of the newborn is produced by ABO incompatibility or Rh incompatibility.

Symptoms of a severe form of ertythroblastosis fetalis, called **hydrops fetalis,** include fetal edema with ascites, enlargement of the spleen and liver, and congestive heart failure. Polyhydramnios and thickening of the placenta may also be evident on ultrasound. If this disease causes multiple organ system failure, fetal or neonatal death can occur.

Table 64-1 Factors Contributing to Maternal-Fetal Blood Exchange

Delivery of the placenta
Non-symptomatic antepartal placental bleeds
Cesarean birth
Multiple gestation
Placenta previa
Placental abruption
Manual removal of the placenta
Intrauterine manipulation
Abortion
Ectopic pregnancy
Amniocentesis
Percutaneous umbilical blood sampling
Chorionic villus sampling
External cephalic version
Abdominal trauma
Trophoblastic disease

ABO Incompatibility

In **ABO incompatibility,** the mother has blood type O and the fetus has blood type A, B, or AB. In people with type O blood, antibodies against types A and B blood are developed naturally during childhood. These antibodies cross the placental barrier and break down fetal red blood cells. This blood incompatibility may result in neonatal jaundice, but rarely is the disease severe. There is no method of preventing this form of hemolytic disease.

Rh Incompatibility

Persons who have the D antigen on their red blood cells are designated as Rh positive; those without the D antigen are Rh negative. In **Rh incompatibility**, the mother is Rh negative and the fetus is Rh positive.

The typical picture is exposure to Rh-positive antigen with placental separation at the time of birth, production of antibodies postpartum, and development of hemolytic disease in an Rh-positive fetus during a subsequent pregnancy. This sequence of events can be prevented with the administration of Rh immunoglobulin (RhoGAM) to Rh-negative women during and after each pregnancy.

ASSESSMENT AND PREVENTION

Antepartal assessment of all pregnant women includes determination of Rh and ABO status on the first prenatal visit. If the woman is Rh negative, antibody titers with an **indirect Coombs test** are done to determine management.

If the indirect Coombs test is negative, usual management is repeating the antibody test at 28 weeks of gestation and administration of RhoGAM if antibody titers remain negative.

After delivery, if the newborn is Rh positive and the indirect Coombs test continues to be negative, postpartal administration of RhoGAM is appropriate.

> If the indirect Coombs test is positive during pregnancy, maternal antibodies have already developed and administration of RhoGAM is contraindicated.

In the case of a positive indirect Coombs test, serial maternal antibody titers are done every 2 to 4 weeks beginning at 18 weeks, then every 2 weeks during the third trimester. Increasing antibody titer levels indicates the need for further fetal assessment by percutaneous umbilical cord blood sampling for the presence of antibodies in the fetal blood, amniotic fluid analysis for the presence of bilirubin, and ultrasound for signs of hypdrops fetalis.

The presence of antibodies on fetal red blood cells is determined by the **direct Coombs test**. If fetal assessment indicates deterioration in the condition of the fetus, intrauterine fetal exchange transfusion or early delivery may be necessary. After delivery, the newborn is examined carefully for signs of erythroblastosis fetalis or hydrops fetalis and appropriate management instituted.

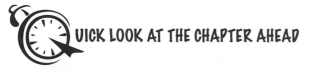

Jaundice appearing in the newborn during the first 24 hours of life is considered to be pathologic rather than physiologic.

The goal of therapy is to prevent the development of kernicterus, or bilirubin encephalopathy, the disposition of unconjugated bilirubin in the basal ganglia of the brain with permanent neurological damage. Unconjugated bilirubin cannot be excreted and builds up in the tissues.

Two treatments are used to decrease unconjugated serum bilirubin. Phototherapy, exposure to ultraviolet light, converts unconjugated bilirubin into products that can be excreted through feces and urine. Exchange transfusion involves alternating infusions of 5 to 20 ml of whole blood, then withdrawal of an equivalent amount of the infant's blood.

The progressive dilution of the infant's blood volume decreases the amount of bilirubin present, reduces the amount of antibodies, and provides undamaged red blood cells to carry oxygen.

The antibodies received from the mother are short-lived; therefore, when the transfused Rh negative red blood cells die, the Rh positive red blood cells produced by the infant will not be hemolyzed.

65

Isoimmunization: Management of the Newborn

TERMS
- [ ] jaundice—pathologic, physiologic
- [ ] kernicterus
- [ ] unconjugated bilirubin
- [ ] phototherapy
- [ ] fiberoptic blanket
- [ ] exchange transfusion

JAUNDICE

Observable **jaundice** occurs in newborns when the bilirubin level is 5 to 10 mg/dL. Progression of jaundice is cephalopedal: Jaundice begins in the face and head and moves downward. At serum bilirubin levels of approximately 10 mg/dL, the jaundice is at the umbilicus. If jaundice is present in the palms and soles, the serum level probably is greater than 15 mg/dL. When jaundice becomes apparent, total serum bilirubin level can be determined by transcutaneous bilirubinometry or by laboratory blood tests.

Jaundice appearing in the first 24 hours of life is considered to be **pathologic** rather than **physiologic**. See Chapter 30 for a discussion of changes in the hepatic system after birth, the conjugation of bilirubin, and the development of physiologic jaundice. The goal of therapy is to prevent the development of **kernicterus**, or bilirubin encephalopathy, the disposition of unconjugated bilirubin in the basal ganglia of the brain with permanent neurological damage.

> The goal of therapy is to prevent the development of **kernicterus**, or bilirubin encephalopathy, the disposition of unconjugated bilirubin in the basal ganglia of the brain with permanent neurological damage.

In term infants, kernicterus does not develop until bilirubin levels are above 20–25 mg/dL. In infants weighing less than 1000 grams, kernicterus can develop with bilirubin levels less than 10 mg/dL.

The clinical manifestations of kernicterus include lethargy, hypotonia, irritability, poor feeding, high-pitched cry, vomiting, and poor Moro reflex. Later signs include bulging anterior fontanel, fever, hypertonia, and seizures. Infants who survive may exhibit nerve deafness, cerebral palsy, and mental retardation.

Unconjugated bilirubin cannot be excreted and builds up in the tissues throughout the body. Initiation of treatment for hyperbilirubinemia is based on the gestational age and birth weight of the infant, the total serum bilirubin level, the rapidity of increases in serum bilirubin level, and age in number of hours since birth.

Two treatments are used to decrease unconjugated serum bilirubin: phototherapy and exchange transfusion.

PHOTOTHERAPY

Phototherapy, exposure to ultraviolet light, converts unconjugated bilirubin into products that can be excreted through feces and urine. The serum level of bilirubin at which phototherapy is initiated is a matter of clinical judgment by the physician, but it is often begun when bilirubin levels reach 12 to 15 mg/dL in the first 48 hours of life in a term newborn. In the preterm infant, phototherapy may be started at lower serum levels.

The infant, dressed only in a diaper, is placed under a radiant warmer or in an isolette with high-intensity lights for ultraviolet radiation. (See Figure 65-1.) The infant's eyes are covered, the mask positioned carefully to prevent nasal obstruction, and the infant carefully monitored for signs of dehydration. Nursing care includes monitoring infant and environmental temperatures and monitoring the intensity of the light reaching the infant's skin. The eye patches need to be removed when the parents are interacting with the infant.

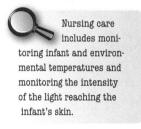

Nursing care includes monitoring infant and environmental temperatures and monitoring the intensity of the light reaching the infant's skin.

Another way to provide phototherapy is to wrap the infant, dressed only in a diaper, in a **fiber-optic blanket**. This blanket is then covered with a regular blanket. The fiber-optic blanket can be used for hospital or home care. Eye patches are not needed with this method of phototherapy,

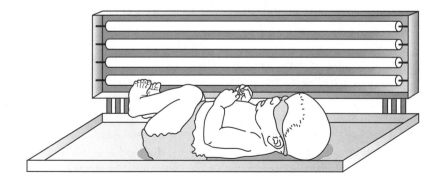

Figure 65-1 An infant under phototherapy.

and dehydration is not as likely to occur. Parents are usually less alarmed by this method of treatment because the infant is more accessible.

Some nursing considerations when an infant is receiving phototherapy include feeding the infant frequently to promote hydration and elimination, assessing skin irritation of the diaper area from loose stools, and assessing for signs of kernicterus.

> During phototherapy, cyanosis may be masked by the light; therefore, respiratory status should be assessed with the phototherapy lights turned off.

During phototherapy, cyanosis may be masked by the light; therefore, respiratory status should be assessed with the phototherapy lights turned off. A bronze discoloration of the skin or a maculopapular rash may be associated with phototherapy.

Parent-infant attachment is promoted by explanations of the therapy, allowing parents to express their anxieties, and encouraging parents to participate in the infant's care.

EXCHANGE TRANSFUSION

An **exchange transfusion** is done with Rh negative blood, usually through an umbilical venous catheter. The procedure involves alternating infusions of 5 to 20 ml of whole blood, then withdrawal of an equivalent amount of the infant's blood.

Indications for exchange transfusion are a positive direct Combs test, cord blood hemoglobin concentration below 12 g/100 ml, rapidly increasing serum bilirubin levels despite phototherapy, serum bilirubin levels of 17–22 mg/dL in a term infant, or 15 mg/dL in a premature infant.

 An infant with signs of hydrops fetalis or signs of cardiac failure should have an immediate exchange transfusion.

Complications of exchange transfusion include transfusion reaction, perforation of the blood vessel by the catheter, or infection.

The total procedure lasts 45 to 90 minutes, the total amount of blood exchanged is about twice the infant's blood volume, and the volume removed is about 85% of the infant's red blood cells.

Progressive dilution of the infant's blood volume decreases the amount of bilirubin present, reduces the amount of antibodies, and provides undamaged red blood cells to carry oxygen. The antibodies received from the mother are short-lived; therefore, when the transfused Rh negative red blood cells die, the Rh positive red blood cells produced by the infant will not be hemolyzed.

PART XII · QUESTIONS

1. Which therapy would the nurse use to reduce the incidence of respiratory distress syndrome (RDS) in a preterm infant?
   a. Administering corticosteroids to the mother prenatally.
   b. Giving corticosteroids to the preterm infant after birth.
   c. Limiting painful procedures that would stimulate crying.
   d. Maintaining adequate oxygen saturation levels.

2. List three reasons why a premature infant has difficulty maintaining a stable body temperature.

   _____

   _____

   _____

3. For which complication is the premature infant who develops respiratory distress syndrome at high risk?
   a. Anemia.
   b. Bronchopulmonary displasia.
   c. Hyperbilirubinemia.
   d. Patent ductus arteriosis.

4. When feeding a premature infant, what should the nurse remember?
   a. Gavage feedings should be done until 32 weeks gestation.
   b. Premature infant formula is the ideal food.
   c. Respiratory difficulty can occur with an overdistended stomach.
   d. Use of a pacifier will depress the infant's sucking ability.

5. The nurse assesses a premature infant and collects the following data: temperature 36.1°C (97.0°F), pulse 112 beats per minute, respirations 58 breaths per minute, and abdominal distention. What further nursing assessment would be most appropriate?

a. Auscultate for cardiac murmur.
b. Determine blood sugar level.
c. Palpate anterior fontanel.
d. Test stool for blood.

6. A father sits in a rocking chair in the NICU. His premature infant is placed on his bare chest and the father closes his shirt over the infant. What benefits to the infant can result from this intervention?

_____

_____

_____

7. A woman diagnosed with gestational diabetes delivers at 39 weeks of gestation. What nursing intervention for the newborn would be most important shortly after birth?
a. Assess for jaundice.
b. Elicit Moro reflex.
c. Evaluate for hypocalcemia.
d. Initiate early feedings.

8. A fractured clavicle is confirmed by X ray in a newborn infant. What nursing care would be most appropriate?
a. Maintain infant NPO in preparation for surgery.
b. Position affected arm above the infant's head.
c. Support the arm by pinning the sleeve to the shirt.
d. Teach range-of-motion exercises to the parents.

9. The nurse reviews the charts of several postpartum patients. Which patient is a candidate to receive Rh immunoglobulin (RhoGAM)?
a. Mother Rh positive, infant Rh negative, direct Coombs negative
b. Mother Rh negative, infant Rh positive, indirect Coombs positive
c. Mother Rh negative, infant Rh positive, direct Coombs negative
d. Mother Rh positive, infant Rh negative, indirect Coombs negative

10. What evidence on ultrasound indicates that a fetus with erythro-blastosis fetalis has progressed to hydrops fetalis?

_____

_____

_____

11. The nurse observes jaundice in a term newborn who is 16 hours old. Rank the following nursing actions in order of priority.

_____ Measure serum bilirubin level with transcutaneous bilirubinometry.

_____ Notify infant's primary care provider.

_____ Obtain equipment necessary for phototherapy.

_____ Review antepartal record for maternal blood type and Rh.

12. At the beginning of the shift, a nurse assumes care for an 2-day-old infant in an isolette receiving phototherapy. Assessment data include auxillary temperature 100.2°F (37.9°C), pulse 148 beats per minute, respirations 52 breaths per minute, 3 voidings, and 2 loose stools in the previous 8-hour shift. What further data is the most important to collect?

a. Current serum bilirubin level.

b. Infant's weight gain pattern.

c. Signs of kernicterus.

d. Temperature within the isolette.

PART XII • ANSWERS AND RATIONALES

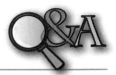

1. **The answer is a.** Corticosteroids given to the mother prenatally stimulate the production of surfactant in the fetal lungs. RDS results from inadequate surfactant production. Option b is incorrect because corticosteroids are not given to the infant after delivery because of the association with an increased risk of cerebral palsy. Option c is incorrect because crying is associated with an increased risk of intraventricular hemorrhage and does not stimulate surfactant production. Option d is incorrect because maintaining adequate oxygen saturation levels is a goal of therapy but it would not reduce the incidence of RDS.

2. **The correct answer should include any three of the following:**
    *   Decreased liver glycogen stores
    *   Less brown fat
    *   Decreased muscle mass
    *   High ratio of body surface to body weight
    *   Decreased subcutaneous fat
    *   Thin, more permeable skin
    *   Nonflexed posture with increased surface area.

3. **The answer is b.** Bronchopulmonary dysplasia is associated with lung damage after prolonged use of therapies to treat RDS. The other options are not complications of RDS.

4. **The answer is c.** An overdistended stomach can press on the diaphragm and lead to respiratory difficulty. Option a is incorrect because gavage feedings should be given until behaviors indicating readiness for nipple feeding are demonstrated. Although gestational age is considered, this is evaluated individually for each infant. Option b is incorrect because breastmilk is the ideal food for the preterm infant. Specialized premature infant formulas would be used if the mother is unable or unwilling to breastfeed. Option d is incorrect because non-nutritive sucking with a pacifier provides stimulation of the suck reflex and improves the sucking ability.

5. **The answer is d.** The assessment data given, especially abdominal distension, are suggestive of necrotizing enterocolitis (NEC). Testing the stool for blood is an appropriate nursing assessment. The other options are incorrect because they are not assessments associated with NEC: Option a is an assessment for patent ductus arteriosis, option b is an assessment for hypoglycemia, and option c is an assessment for intraventricular hemorrhage.

6. **The answer should include the statement that neurophysiological behaviors of the infant are more organized. There is better maintenance of body temperature, more stable heart and respiratory rates, and higher oxygen saturation levels.**

7. **The answer is d.** Infants of diabetic mothers are at high risk to develop hypoglycemia in the first few hours of life. Early feedings provide glucose to prevent a drop in blood sugar. Option a is incorrect because jaundice usually will not develop for 2 to 3 days after birth. Option b is not the best choice because the Moro reflex is a component of physical assessment of all newborns. Option c is incorrect because symptoms of hypocalcemia are not usually evident until more than 24 hours after birth.

8. **The answer is c.** Pinning the sleeve to the front of the shirt would immobilize the clavicle area to prevent pain and promote healing. Option a is incorrect because fractured clavicles usually heal without surgery. Option b is incorrect because positioning the arm above the head would be painful for the infant and would not promote proper alignment of the clavicle for healing. Option d is incorrect because immobilization promotes healing of the clavicle; range-of-motion exercises would be contraindicated.

9. **The answer is c.** For a woman to receive Rh immunoglobulin (RhoGAM) in the postpartum period, she must be Rh negative, her infant must be Rh positive, and the direct Coombs test must be negative, indicating no antibody production. In options a and d, the mother is Rh positive, so isoimmunization will not occur. In option b, the positive indirect Coombs indicates antibody production by the mother, and RhoGAM is contraindicated.

10. **The answer should include at least three of the following: fetal edema with ascites, enlargement of the spleen and liver, congestive heart failure, polyhydramnios, and thickening of the placenta.**

11. **The correct ranking is 1, 3, 4, 2.**

    <u> 1 </u>   Measure serum bilirubin level with transcutaneous bilirubinometry.

    <u> 3 </u>   Notify infant's primary care provider.

    <u> 4 </u>   Obtain equipment necessary for phototherapy.

    <u> 2 </u>   Review antepartal record for maternal blood type and Rh.

    The nurse should gather further assessment data of serujm bilirubin level and maternal blood type and RH before contacting the primary health care provider. Phototherapy equipment should be available in case phototherapy is ordered.

12. **The answer is d.** Data given in the question include an elevated auxillary temperature. Temperature elevations in the infant can occur if the environmental temperature is too high or as a result of dehydration. The data given do not indicate excessive output leading to dehydration. Therefore, the environmental temperature within the isolette needs to be assessed and regulated if too high. The other options are not of highest priority for the data given.

References
and Index

REFERENCES

General References

Gilbert, E. S., & Harmon, J. S. (2003). *Manual of high risk pregnancy and delivery* (3rd ed.). St. Louis: Mosby.

Heppard, M. C. S., & Garite, T. J. (2002). *Acute obstetrics: A practical guide* (3rd ed.). St. Louis: Mosby.

Hockenberry, M., Wilson, D., Winkelstein, M. L., & Kline, N. E. (2003). *Wong's nursing care of infants and children* (7th ed.). St Louis: Mosby.

Lowdermilk, D. L., & Perry, S. E. (2004). *Maternity and Women's Heath Care* (8th ed.). St. Louis: Mosby.

Mandeville, L. K., & Troiano, N. H. (1999). *AWHONN High-Risk and Critical Care Intrapartum Nursing* (2nd ed.). Philadelphia: Lippincott.

Martin, E. J. (2002). *Intrapartum management modules: a perinatal education program* (3rd ed.). Philadelphia: Lippincott Williams & Wilkins.

Mattson, S., & Smith, J. E. (Eds.) (2004). *AWHONN Core curriculum for maternal-newborn nursing* (3rd ed). St. Louis: Elsevier.

Olds, S. B., London, M. L., & Ladewig, P. W. (2004). *Clinical handbook: Maternal-newborn nursing & women's health care* (7th ed.). Upper Saddle River, NJ: Pearson Prentice Hall.

Olds, S. B., London, M. L., Ladewig, P. W., & Davidson, M. R. (2004). *Maternal-newborn nursing & women's health care* (7th ed.). Upper Saddle River, NJ: Pearson Prentice Hall.

Pillitteri, A. (2003). *Maternal and child health nursing: Care of the childbearing & childrearing family* (4th ed.). Philadelphia: Lipppincott Williams & Wilkins.

Simpson, K. R., & Creehan, P. A. (2001). *AWHONN perinatal nursing* (2nd ed.). Philadelphia: Lippincott.

Chapter 4

Hatcher, R. A., Zieman, M., Cwiak, C., Darney, P. D., Creinin, M. D., & Stosur, H. R. (2004). *A pocket guide to managing contraception.* Tiger, Georgia: Bridging the Gap Foundation. Can be retrieved from www.managingcontraception.com.

Chapter 5

Hatcher, R. A., Zieman, M., Cwiak, C., Darney, P. D., Creinin, M. D., & Stosur, H. R. (2004). *A pocket guide to managing contraception.* Tiger, Georgia: Bridging the Gap Foundation. Can be retrieved from www.managingcontraception.com.

Hutti, M. H. (2003). New and emerging contraceptive methods. *AWHONN Lifelines, 7* (1), 32–39.

Lindberg, C. E. (2003). Emergency contraception for prevention of adolescent pregnancy. *The American Journal of Maternal/Child Nursing, 28* (3), 199–204.

Woodson, S. (2003). Is emergency contraception going over-the-counter? *AWHONN Lifelines, 7* (6), 506–511.

Chapter 6

Bidwell, L. D. M., & Vander Mey, B. J. (2000). *Sociology of the family: investigating family issues.* Boston: Allyn & Bacon.

United States Census Bureau (2000). *Statistical abstract of the U. S.* Washington, D. C.: U. S. Dept. of Commerce.

Chapter 7

Hitchcock, J. E., Schubert, P. E., & Thomas, S. A. (1999). *Community health nursing: Caring in action.* Albany, NY: Delmar.

Stanhope, M. S., & Lancaster, J. (2000). *Community and public health nursing* (5th ed.). St. Louis: Mosby.

Chapter 8

D'Avanzo, C., & Geissler, E. M. (2003). *Pocket guide to cultural assessment* (3rd ed.). St. Louis: Mosby.

DeLuane, S. C., & Ladner, P. K. (2002). *Fundamentals of nursing: Standards and practice* (2nd ed.). Albany, NY: Delmar.

Mattson, S. (2000). Striving for cultural competence: Providing care for the changing face of the U. S. *AWHONN Lifelines. 4* (3), 48–52.

Mattson, S. (2000). Working toward cultural competence: Making the first steps through cultural assessment. *AWHONN Lifelines. 4* (4), 41–43.

Mattson, S. (2000). Providing culturally competent care: Strategies and approaches for perinatal clients. *AWHONN Lifelines. 4* (5), 37–39.

Ottani, P. A. (2002). Embracing global similarities: A framework for cross-cultural obstetric care. *Journal of Obstetric, Gynecologic, & Neonatal Nursing, 31*, 33–38.

Purnell, L. D., & Paulanka, B. J. (2003). *Transcultural health care: A culturally competent approach* (2nd ed.). Philadelphia: F. A. Davis.

Spector, R. E. (2004). *Cultural diversity in health & illness (*6th ed.). Upper Saddle River, NJ: Pearson Prentice Hall.

Chapter 9

Moore, K. L., & Persaud, T. V. N. (1998). *The developing human: Clinically oriented embryology* (6th ed.) Philadelphia: Saunders.

Thies, K. M., & Travers, J. F. (2001). *Growth and development through the life span.* Thorofare, NJ: Slack, Inc.

Chapter 11

Rubin, R. (1984). *Maternal identity and the maternal experience.* New York: Springer.

Chapter 14

American College of Obstetricians and Gynecologists (2002). *Nutrition during pregnancy.* Retrieved June 5, 2003, from http://www/medem.com/MedLB/article

March of Dimes Quick Reference: Fact Sheets (N. D.). *Peanuts, folic acid and peanut allergies.* Retrieved June 5, 2003, from http://www.marchofdimes.com/printableArticles/681_1819.asp

Purnell, L. D., & Paulanka, B. J. (2003). *Transcultural health care: A culturally competent approach* (2nd ed.). Philadelphia: F. A. Davis.

Chapter 18

Minato, J. F. (2000). Is it time to push? Examining rest in second-stage labor. *AWHONN Lifelines, 4* (6), 20–23.

Roberts, J. E. (2003). A new understanding of the second stage of labor: Implications for nursing care. *Journal of Obstetric, Gynecologic, & Neonatal Nursing, 32* (6), 794–801.

Chapter 20

Simpson, K. R., & Creehan, P. A. (2001). *AWHONN: Perinatal Nursing* (2nd ed.). Philadelphia: Lippincott.

Chapter 21

Hunter, L. P. (2002). Being with woman: A guiding concept for the care of laboring women. *Journal of Obstetric, Gynecologic, & Neonatal Nursing, 31* (6), 650–657.

Kennedy, H. P., & Shannon, M. T. (2004). Keeping birth normal: Research findings on midwifery care during childbirth. *Journal of Obstetric, Gynecologic, & Neonatal Nursing, 33* (5), 554–560.

Minato, J. F. (2000). Is it time to push? Examining rest in second-stage labor. *AWHONN Lifelines, 4* (6), 20–23.

Roberts, J. E. (2003). A new understanding of the second stage of labor: Implications for nursing care. *Journal of Obstetric, Gynecologic, & Neonatal Nursing, 32* (6), 794–801.

Simkin, P. (2002). Supportive care during labor: A guide for busy nurses. *Journal of Obstetric, Gynecologic, & Neonatal Nursing, 31* (6), 721–732.

Chapter 22

Alexander, J. M., Sharma, S. K., McIntire, D. D., & Leveno, K. J. (2002). Epidual analgesia lengthens the Friedman active phase of labor. *Obstetrics & Gynecology, 100*, 46–50.

Plunkett, B. A., Lin, A., Wong, C. A., Grobman, W. A., & Peaceman, A. M. (2003). Management of the second stage of labor in nulliparas with continuous epidural analgesia. *Obstetrics & Gynecology, 102*, 109–114.

Poole, J. H. (2003). Analgesia and anesthesia during labor and birth: Implications for mother and fetus. *Journal of Obstetric, Gynecologic, & Neonatal Nursing, 32* (6), 780–793.

Chapter 23

Gabbe, S. G., Niebyl, J. R., Simpson, J. L. (Eds.) (1996). *Obstetrics: Normal & Problem Pregnancies* (3rd ed.). New York: Churchill Livingstone.

Chapter 24

Purnell, L. D., & Paulanka, B. J. (2003). *Transcultural health care: A culturally competent approach* (2nd ed.). Philadelphia: F. A. Davis.

Spector, R. E. (2004). *Cultural diversity in health & illness (*6th ed.). Upper Saddle River, NJ: Pearson Prentice Hall.

Stolte, K. M. (1996). *Wellness: Nursing diagnosis for health promotion.* Philadelphia: Lippincott.

Chapter 38

Armstrong, D. S. (2004). Impact of prior perinatal loss on subsequent pregnancies. *Journal of Obstetric, Gynecologic, & Neonatal Nursing, 33* (6), 765–773.

Cote-Arsenault, D. (2003). The influence of perinatal loss on anxiety in multigravidas. *Journal of Obstetric, Gynecologic, & Neonatal Nursing, 32* (5), 623–629.

Chapter 39

Oates-Whitehead, R. M., Haas, D. M., & Carrier, J. A. K. (2003). Progesterone for preventing miscarriage (Cochrane Review) [Electronic Version]. *The Cochrane Library, 4, 2003.* Chichester, UK: John Wiley & Sons, Ltd.

Chapter 40

American College of Obstetrics and Gynecologists (2003). Progesterone recommended in certain high risk pregnancies to help prevent preterm birth. *ACOG News Release.* Retrieved from http:// www.acog. org/from_home/publications/press_releases/nr10-31

Bernhardt, J., & Dorman, K. (2004). Pre-term birth risk assessment tools: Exploring fetal fibronectin and cervical length for validating risk. *AWHONN Lifelines, 8* (1), 36–44.

Church-Balin, C., & Damus, K. (2003). Preventing prematurity. *AWHONN Lifelines, 7* (2), 97–101.

Goldenberg, R. L. (2002). The management of preterm labor. *Obstetrics & Gynecology, 100,* (5), 1020–1037.

Moore, M. L. (2003). Preterm labor and birth: What have we learned in the past two decades? *Journal of Obstetric, Gynecologic, & Neonatal Nursing, 32* (5), 638–349.

Moos, M. K. (2004). Understanding prematurity: Sorting fact from fiction. *AWHONN Lifelines, 8* (1), 32–37.

Chapter 41

Goldenberg, R. L. (2002). The management of preterm labor. *Obstetrics & Gynecology, 100* (5), 1020–1037.

Maloni, J. A. (2002). Astronauts & pregnancy bedrest. *AWHONN Lifelines, 6* (4), 318–323.

Maloni, J. A., Brezinski-Tomasi, J. E., & Johnson, L. A. (2001). Antepartum bedrest: Effect upon the family. *Journal of Obstetrics, Gynecologic, & Neonatal Nursing, 30* (2), 165–173.

Maloni, J. A., & Park, S. (2005). Postpartum symptoms after antepartum bedrest. *Journal of Obstetrics, Gynecologic, & Neonatal Nursing, 34* (2), 163–171.

Moos, M. K. (2004). Understanding prematurity: Sorting fact from fiction. *AWHONN Lifelines, 8* (1), 32–37.

Sprague, A. E. (2004). The evolution of bedrest as a clinical intervention. *Journal of Obstetrics, Gynecologic, & Neonatal Nursing, 33* (5), 542–549.

Chapter 43

Levine, R. J., Karumanchi, S. A., et al. (2004). Circulating angiogenic factors and the risk of preeclampsia. *The New England Journal of Medicine, 350* (7), 672–683

Peters, R. M., & Flack, J. M. (2004). Hypertensive disorders of pregnancy. *Journal of Obstetric, Gynecologic, & Neonatal Nursing, 33* (2), 209–220.

Sibai, B. M. (2003). Diagnosis and management of gestational hypertension and preeclampsia. *Obstetrics & Gynecology, 102* (1), 181–192.

Chapter 44

Nick, J. M. (2004). Deep tendon reflexes, magnesium, and calcium: Assessments and implications. *Journal of Obstetric, Gynecologic, & Neonatal Nursing, 33* (2), 221–230.

Peters, R. M., & Flack, J. M. (2004). Hypertensive disorders of pregnancy. *Journal of Obstetric, Gynecologic, & Neonatal Nursing, 33* (2), 209–220.

Sibai, B. M. (2003). Diagnosis and management of gestational hypertension and preeclampsia. *Obstetrics & Gynecology, 102* (1), 181–192.

Chapter 45

Mercer, B. (2003). Preterm premature rupture of the membranes. *Obstetrics & Gynecology, 101* (1), 178–193.

Chapter 46

Gabbe, S. G., & Graves, C. R. (2003). Management of diabetes mellitus complicating pregnancy. *Obstetrics & Gynecology, 102* (4), 857–868.

Kim, C., Newton, K. M., & Knopp, R. H. (2002). Gestational diabetes and the incidence of Type 2 diabetes. *Diabetes Care, 25,* 1862–1868.

MacNeill, S., Dodds, L., Hamilton, D. C., Armson, B. A., & VandenHof, M. (2001). Rates and risk factors for recurrence of gestational diabetes. *Diabetes Care, 24,* 659–662.

Chapter 47

Diabetes and Pregnancy. American Diabetes Association. Retrieved from http://www.diabetes.org/gestational-diabetes/pregancy. jsp

Langer, O., Conway, D. L., Berkus, M. D., Xenakis, E. M. J., Gonzales, O. (2000). A comparison of glyburide and insulin in women with gestational diabetes mellitus. *New England Journal of Medicine, 343,* 1134–1138.

Take charge of your diabetes. National Center for Chronic Disease Prevention and Health Promotion. Retrieved from http://www.cdc. gov/diabetes/pubs/tcyd/pregnant. htm

Chapter 48

Centers for Disease Control & Prevention. Severe Acute Respiratory Syndrome (SARS). Retrieved from www.cdc.gov/ncidod/sars/

Centers for Disease Control & Prevention. Targeted tuberculin testing and treatment of latent tuberculosis infection. Retrieved from www.cdc.gov/epo/mmwr/preview/mmwrhtml/rr4906a1.htm

Centers for Disease Control & Prevention. Treatment of tuberculosis. Retrieved from www.cdc.gov/mmwr/preview/mmwrhtml/rr5211a1.htm

Dombrowski, M. P., Schatz, M., Wise, R., Momirova, V., Landon, M., Mabie, W., et al. (2004). Asthma during pregnancy. *Obstetrics & Gynecology, 103,* 5–12.

Gilljam, M., Antoniou, M., Shin, S., Dupuis, A., Corey, M., & Tullis, D. E. (2000). Pregnancy in cystic fibrosis. Fetal and maternal outcome. *Chest, 118* (1), 85–90.

Goss, C. H., Rubenfeld, G. D., Otto, K., & Aitken, M. L. (2003). The effect of pregnancy on survival in women with cystic fibrosis. *Chest, 124,* 1460–1468.

Schneider, E., Duncan, D., Reiken, M., Perry, R., Messick, J., Sheedy, C., et al. (2004). SARS in pregnancy. *AWHONN Lifelines, 8* (2), 122–128.

Shek, C. C., Ng, P. C., Fung, G. P. G., Cheng, F. W. T., Chan, P. K. S., Peiris, M. J. S. et al. (2003). Infants born to mothers with severe acute respiratory syndrome. *Pediatrics, 112* (4), e254.

Chapter 49

Claster, S., & Vichinsky, E. P. (2003). Managing sickle cell disease. *British Medical Journal, 327,* 1151–1155.

Elkayam, U., & Gleicher, N. (1998). *Cardiac problems in pregnancy: diagnosis and management of maternal and fetal heart disease* (3rd ed.). New York: Wiley-Liss.

Chapter 50

Minkoff, H. (2003). Human immunodeficiency virus infection in pregnancy. *Obstetrics & Gynecology, 101,* 797–810.

Schrag, S., Gorwitz, R., Fultz-Butts, K., & Schuchat,A. (2002). Prevention of perinatal group B streptococcal disease: Revised guidelines from CDC. Retrieved from www.cdc.gov/mmwr/preview/mmwrhtml/rr5111a1.htm

Chapter 51

Heffner, L. J., Elkin, E., & Fretts, R. C. (2003). Impact of labor induction, gestation age, and maternal age on Cesarean delivery rates. *Obstetrics & Gynecology, 102,* 287–293.

Pozaic, S. (1999). Induction and augmentation of labor. In Mandeville, L. K., & Troiano, N. H. (Eds.), *AWHONN High Risk & Critical Care Intrapartum Nursing* (2nd ed.) (pp. 139–158). Philadelphia: Lippincott.

Simpson, K. R., & Atterbury, J. (2003). Trends and issues in labor induction in the United States: Implications for clinical practice. *Journal of Obstetric, Gynecologic, and Neonatal Nursing, 32* (6), 767–779.

Chapter 52

Cockey, C. D. (2003). Pros and cons of elective Cesarean. *AWHONN Lifelines, 7* (6), 500–501.

Dauphinee, J. D. (2004) VBAC: Safety for the patient and the nurse. *Journal of Obstetric, Gynecologic, & Neonatal Nursing, 33* (1), 105–115.

Chapter 54

Curran, C. A. (2003). Intrapartum emergencies. *Journal of Obstetric, Gynecologic, & Neonatal Nursing, 32* (6), 802–813.

Hall, S. P. (1997). The nurses's role in the identification of risks and treatment of shoulder dystocia. *Journal of Obstetric, Gynecologic, & Neonatal Nursing, 26* (1), 25–32.

Chapter 55

American Psychiatric Association (1994). *The diagnostic and statistical manual of mental disorders* (4th ed.). Washington, D. C.: American Psychiatric Association.

Beck, C. T. (2002). Revision of the postpartum depression predictors inventory. *Journal of Obstetric, Gynecologic, & Neonatal Nursing, 31* (4), 394–402.

Beck, C. T. (2002). Theoretical perspectives of postpartum depression and their treatment implications. *The American Journal of Maternal/Child Nursing, 27* (5), 282–287.

Bozoky, I., & Corwin, E. J. (2002). Fatigue as a predictor of postpartum depression. *Journal of Obstetric, Gynecologic, & Neonatal Nursing, 31* (4), 436–443.

Carolan, M. (2003). The graying of the obstetric population: Implications for the older mother. *Journal of Obstetric, Gynecologic, & Neonatal Nursing, 32* (1), 19–27.

Goodman, J. H. (2004). Postpartum depression beyond the early postpartum period. *Journal of Obstetric, Gynecologic, & Neonatal Nursing, 33* (4), 410–420.

Maley, B. (2002). Creating a postpartum depression support group. *AWHONN Lifelines, 6* (1), 62–65.

Sichel, D., & Driscoll, J. W. (1999). *Women's moods: What every woman must know about hormones, the brain, and emotional health.* New York: Quill.

Wisner, K. L., Parry, B. L., & Piontek, C. M. (2002). Postpartum depression. *The New England Journal of Medicine, 347* (3), 194–199.

Wroblewski, M., & Tallon, D. (2004). Implementing a comprehensive postpartum depression support program. *AWHONN Lifelines, 8* (3), 248–252.

Chapter 56

American College of Obstetricians and Gynecologists (2004). ACOG Violence Against Women Page Fact Sheet: Interpersonal violence against women throughout the lifespan. Retrieved from http://www.acog.org

Bohn, D. K., Tebben, J. G., & Campbell, J. C. (2004). Influences of income, education, age, and ethnicity on physical abuse before and during pregnancy. *Journal of Obstetric, Gynecologic, & Neonatal Nursing, 33* (5), 561–571.

Campbell, J. C. (2004). Danger assessment. Retrieved from http://www.son. jhmi.edu/research/homicide/da-z.htm

Cockey, C. D. (2003). Screening for violence in pregnancy. *AWHONN Lifelines, 7* (6), 495–497.

Dienemann, J., Campbell, J., Wiederhorn, N., Laughon, K., & Jordan, E. (2003). A critical pathway for intimate partner violence across the continuum of care. *Journal of Obstetric, Gynecologic, & Neonatal Nursing, 32* (5), 594–603.

Furniss, K. (1997). Battered women: How nurses can help. *AWHONN Lifelines, 1* (4), 12–14.

Harner, H. M. (2004). Domestic violence and trauma care in teenage pregnancy: Does paternal age make a difference? *Journal of Obstetric, Gynecologic, & Neonatal Nursing, 33* (3), 312–319.

Holtz, H., & Furniss, K. K. (1993). The health care provider's role in domestic violence. *Trends in Health Care Law and Ethics, 8* (2), 47.

Lipsky, S., Holt, V. L., Easterling, T. R., & Critchlow, C. W. (2003). Impact of police-reported intimate partner violence during pregnancy on birth outcomes. *Obstetrics & Gynecology, 102*, 557–564.

Parker, B., McFarlane, J., & Soeken, K., et. al. (1993). Physical and emotional abuse in pregnant: A comparison of adult and teenage women. *Nursing Research, 42* (3), 173–178.

Renker, P. R. (2003). Keeping safe: Teenager's strategies for dealing with perinatal violence. *Journal of Obstetric, Gynecologic, & Neonatal Nursing, 32* (1), 58–67.

Schoening, A. M., Greenwood, J. L., McNichols, J. A., Heermann, J. A., & Agrawal, S. (2004). Effect of an intimate partner violence educational program on the attitudes of nurses. *Journal of Obstetric, Gynecologic, & Neonatal Nursing, 33* (5), 572–579.

Chapter 57

Albrecht, S. A. (2004). Achieving 'SUCCESS': Nursing care for pregnant women who smoke. *AWHONN Lifelines, 8* (3), 190–191.

Maloni, J. A. (2001). Preventing low birth weight: How smoking cessation counseling can help. *AWHONN Lifelines, 5* (1), 32–35.

March of Dimes (2004). Drinking alcohol during pregnancy. Retrieved from http://www.marchofdimes.com/printableArticles/681_1170.asp?pri

Mersy, D. J. (2003). Recognition of alcohol and substance abuse. *American Family Physician, 67*, 1529–1532, 1535–1536.

Morse, B., Gehshan, S., Hutchins, E. (1997). *Screening for substance abuse during pregnancy: Improving care, improving health.* Arlington, VA: National Center for Education in Maternal and Child Health.

Murray, E., & Wewers, M. E. (2004). Nurses can play a significant role in reducing tobacco use in the US. *AWHONN Lifelines, 8* (3), 200–206.

National Institute on Drug Abuse (2003). Pregnancy and drug use trends. Retrieved from http://www.nida.nih.gov/Infofax/pregnancytrends.html

Chapter 58

Dashe, J. S., Sheffield, J. S., Olscher, D. A., Todd, S. J., Jackson, G. L., & Wendel, G. D. (2002). Relationship between maternal methadone dosage and neonatal withdrawal. *Obstetrics & Gynecology, 100*, 1244–1249.

Kuschel, C. A., Austerberry, L., Cornwell, M., Couch, R., & Rowley, R. S. H. (2004). Can methadone concentrations predict the severity of withdrawal in infants at risk of neonatal abstinence syndrome? *Archives of Disease in Childhood: Fetal and Neonatal Edition, 89*, F390–F393.

Morse, B., Gehshan, S., Hutchins, E. (1997). *Screening for substance abuse during pregnancy: Improving care, improving health.* Arlington, VA: National Center for Education in Maternal and Child Health.

National Institute on Drug Abuse (2003). Pregnancy and drug use trends. Retrieved from http://www.nida.nih.gov/Infofax/pregnancytrends.html

Chapter 59

Alan Guttmacher Institute (2005). State policies in brief. Retrieved from http://www.agi-usa.org/

Bowers, N. A., & Gromada, K. K. (2004). Pregnancy after age 35. *AWHONN Lifelines, 8* (2), 99–100.

Callaghan, W. M., & Berg, C. J. (2003). Pregnancy-related mortality among women aged 35 years and older, United States, 1991–1997. *Obstetrics & Gynecology, 102*, 1015–1021.

Carolan, M. (2003). The graying of the obstetric population: Implications for the older mother. *Journal of Obstetric, Gynecologic, & Neonatal Nursing, 32* (1), 19–27.

DeLisser, R., & Trimmer, T. (2001). Teen talk: an intervention for pregnant and parenting adolescent. *AWHONN Lifelines, 5* (4), 36–41.

Drake, P. (1996). Addressing developmental needs of pregnant adolescent. *Journal of Obstetric, Gynecologic, & Neonatal Nursing, 25* (6), 518–524.

Harner, H. M., Burgess, A. W., & Asher, J. B. (2001). Caring for pregnant teenagers: Medicolegal issues for nurses. *Journal of Obstetric, Gynecologic, & Neonatal Nursing. 30* (2), 139–147.

Jacobsson, B., Ladfors, L., & Milsom, I. (2004). Advanced maternal age and adverse perinatal outcome. *Obstetrics & Gynecology, 104,* 727–733.

Jolly, M. C., Sebire, N., Harris, J., Robinson, S., & Regan, L. (2000). Obstetric risks of pregnancy in women less than 18 years old. *Obstetrics & Gynecology, 96,* 962–966.

March of Dimes (2004). Quick reference and fact sheets: Teenage pregnancy. Retrieved from http://www.marchofdimes.com/professionals

March of Dimes (2002). Quick reference and fact sheets: Pregnancy after 35. Retrieved from http://www.marchofdimes.com/professionals

Montgomery, K. S. (2003). Health promotion for pregnant adolescent. *AWHONN Lifelines, 7* (5), 433–444.

Montgomery, K. S. (2003). Nursing care of pregnant adolescent. *Journal of Obstetric, Gynecologic, & Neonatal Nursing, 32* (2), 249–257.

Neumann, M., & Graf, C. (2003). Pregnancy after age 35: Are these women at high risk? *AWHONN Lifelines, 7* (5), 422–430.

Renker, P. R. (2002). "Keep a blank face. I need to tell you what has been happening to me." Teens' stories of abuse and violence before and during pregnancy. *The American Journal of Maternal /Child Nursing, 27,* (2), 109–116.

Salihu, H. M., Shumpert, M. N., Slay, M., Kirby, R. S., & Alexander, G. R. (2003). Childbearing beyond maternal age 50 and fetal outcomes in the United States. *Obstetrics & Gynecology, 102,* 1006–1014.

Viau, P. A., Padula, C. A., & Eddy, B. (2002). An exploration of health concerns & health-promotion behaviors in pregnant women over age 35. *The American Journal of Maternal/Child Nursing, 27* (6), 328–334.

Chapter 60

Behrman, R. E., & Kliegman, R. M. (2002). *Nelson essentials of pediatrics* (4th ed.). Philadelphia: W. B. Saunders.

March of Dimes (2005). Outlook is bleak for the smallest premature babies: 80 percent have impairment, study shows. Retrieved from http://www.modimes.org/printableArticles/14458_14518.asp?printable=true

March of Dimes (2004). Preterm birth. Retrieved from http://www. modimes.org/printableArticles/14332_1157.asp?printable=true

Marino, B. S., Fine, K. S., & McMillan, J. A. (2004). *Blueprints: Pediatrics* (3rd ed.). Malden, MA: Blackwell Publishing.

Nemours Foundation (2002). Apnea of prematurity. Retrieved from http://www.kidshealth.org/parent/medical/lungs/aop. html

Chapter 61

Bakewell-Sachs, S., & Blackburn, S. (2003). State of the science: Achievements and challenges across the spectrum of care for preterm infants. *Journal of Obstetrical, Gynecologic, & Neonatal Nursing, 32* (5), 683–695.

Byers, J. F. (2003). Components of developmental care and the evidence for their use in the NICU. *The American Journal of Maternal/Child Nursing, 28* (3), 174–180.

Meade Johnson Nutritionals. (1999). Newborn maturity rating & classification. Retrieved from http://www.meadjohnson. com/professional/pdf/LB146REV_11_99.pdf

Chapter 62

Bakewell-Sachs, S., & Blackburn, S. (2003). State of the science: Achievements and challenges across the spectrum of care for preterm infants. *Journal of Obstetrical, Gynecologic, & Neonatal Nursing, 32* (5), 683–695.

Byers, J. F. (2003). Components of developmental care and the evidence for their use in the NICU. *The American Journal of Maternal/Child Nursing, 28* (3), 174–180.

Feldman, R., Eidelman, A. I., Sirota, L., & Weller, A. (2002). Comparison of skin-to-skin (kangaroo) and traditional care: Parenting outcomes and preterm infant development. *Pediatrics, 110* (1), 16–26.

Preyde, M., & Artdal, F. (2003). Effectiveness of apparent "buddy" program for mothers of very preterm infants in a neonatal intensive care unit. *Canadian Medical Association Journal, 168* (8), 969–973.

Chapter 63

Kicklighter, S. D. (2001). Infant of diabetic mother. Retrieved from http://www.emedicine.com/ped/topic845.htm

Salim, R., Hasanein, J., Nachum, Z., & Shalev, E. (2004). Anthropometric parameters in infants of gestational diabetic women with strict glycemic control. *Obstetrics & Gynecology, 1004*, 1021–1024.

Stotland, N. E., Hopkins, L. M., & Caughey, A. B. (2004). Gestational weight gain, macrosomia, and risk of cesarean birth in nondiabetic nulliparas. *Obstetrics & Gynecology, 1004*, 671–677.

Chapter 64

Behrman, R. E., & Kliegman, R. M. (2002). *Nelson Essentials of Pediatrics* (4th ed.). Philadelphia: Saunders.

Marino, B. S., Fine, K. S., & McMillan, J. A. (2004). *Blueprints Pediatrics* (3rd ed.). Malden, MA: Blackwell Publishing.

Moise, K. J. (2002). Management of rhesus alloimmunization in pregnancy. *Obstetrics & Gynecology, 100* (3), 600–611.

Neal, J. L. (2001). RhD isoimmunization and current management modalities. *Journal of Obstetric, Gynecologic, & Neonatal Nursing, 30* (6), 589–606.

Chapter 65

Behrman, R. E., & Kliegman, R. M. (2002). *Nelson Essentials of Pediatrics* (4th ed.). Philadelphia: Saunders.

Marino, B. S., Fine, K. S., & McMillan, J. A. (2004). *Blueprints Pediatrics* (3rd ed.). Malden, MA: Blackwell Publishing.

Moise, K. J. (2002). Management of rhesus alloimmunization in pregnancy. *Obstetrics & Gynecology, 100* (3), 600–611.

Neal, J. L. (2001). RhD isoimmunization and current management modalities. *Journal of Obstetric, Gynecologic, & Neonatal Nursing, 30* (6), 589–606.

Websites

March of Dimes: http://www.modimes.org/

Nursing Network on Violence Against Women International: http://www.nnvawi.org

http://www.not-2-late.com

Planned Parenthood: http://www.plannedparenthood.org/

Postpartum Support International. http://www.postpartum. net

INDEX